MAGNETIC RESONANCE IMAGING IN ORTHOPAEDICS AND RHEUMATOLOGY

EDITOR

David W. Stoller, M.D.

ASSOCIATE EDITORS

Harry K. Genant, M.D.

Clyde A. Helms, M.D.

Chris G. Goumas, M.D.

MAGNETIC

IN

AND

RESONANCE IMAGING
ORTHOPAEDICS
RHEUMATOLOGY

J. B. Lippincott Company   *Philadelphia*

London   Mexico City   New York   St. Louis   São Paulo   Sydney

Acquisitions Editor: Dean Manke
Sponsoring Editor: Delois Patterson
Indexer: Katherine Pitcoff
Compositor: The Clarinda Company
Printer/Binder: Halliday Lithograph

1 3 5 6 4 2

Library of Congress Cataloging-in-Publication Data

Magnetic resonance imaging in orthopaedics and
    rheumatology.

  Includes index.
   1. Orthopedia—Diagnosis.   2. Rheumatism—Diagnosis.
3. Magnetic resonance imaging.   I. Stoller, David W.
II. Title.   [DNLM: 1. Bone Diseases—diagnosis.
2. Joints—anatomy & histology.   3. Magnetic Resonance
Imaging.   4. Muscular Diseases—diagnosis.   5. Musculo-
skeletal System—anatomy & histology.   6. Musculoskeletal
System—pathology.   WE 141 M1953]
RD734.5.M33M34   1989   616.7'0757   88-13849
ISBN 0-397-59058-5

To my parents, Adele and Nat Stoller
For their love and support

Contributors List

John V. Crues III, M.D.
Director of MRI
Department of Radiology
Santa Barbara Cottage Hospital
Santa Barbara, California
Assistant Clinical Professor of
  Radiology
University of California at Los
  Angeles
School of Medicine
Los Angeles, California

Gregory W. Doyle, M.D.
Clinical Instructor
Department of Radiology
University of California at San
  Francisco
San Francisco, California

Harry K. Genant, M.D.
Professor of Radiology, Medicine,
  and Orthopaedic Surgery
Department of Radiology
University of California at San
  Francisco
San Francisco, California

Chris G. Goumas, M.D.
Chief Resident
Department of Radiology
University of California at San
  Francisco

Clyde A. Helms, M.D.
Associate Professor of Radiology
Department of Radiology
University of California at San
  Francisco
San Francisco, California

Philipp Lang, Cand. Med.
Visiting Scholar
University of California at San
  Francisco
San Francisco, California

Sheila G. Moore, M.D.
Assistant Professor of Radiology
Department of Radiology
Stanford University Medical Center
Stanford, California

Frank W. Morgan, M.D.
Department of Radiology
Santa Barbara Cottage Hospital
Santa Barbara, California

David W. Stoller, M.D.
Director, California Institute for
  Musculoskeletal Imaging
San Francisco, California
Assistant Clinical Professor of
  Radiology
University of California at San
  Francisco Medical Center
San Francisco, Caltfornia

Foreword

Magnetic resonance imaging (MRI) is probably the most important advance in diagnostic medicine since the discovery of x-rays at the end of the last century. Although the contributions of MRI to the study of disorders of the central nervous system (CNS) have initially captured most of the interest of the medical community and most of the available time on the small number of existing imagers, MRI of the musculoskeletal system has been rapidly gaining prominence and is challenging the supremacy of CNS MRI in the number of examinations performed.

The reasons for the use of MRI in the musculoskeletal system are even more compelling than in the examination of CNS. The musculoskeletal apparatus is a complicated system for stabilization of posture and locomotion and consists of multiple soft tissue structures: muscles, tendons, menisci, fat pads, bursae, fasciae, etc., in addition to bone marrow, cartilage, and cortical bone. To distinguish these from each other and see abnormalities in them has not been possible so far except by invasive methods such as surgery or arthroscopy.

The noninvasiveness of MRI and its ability to depict directly structures in all three orthogonal planes make the technique unique. Although generally no contrast media were needed, the recent introduction of and FDA approval of gadolinium DTPA has further added to the sensitivity of the method in detecting abnormalities. There is at present no better imaging approach for most of the afflictions of the spine and joints than MRI.

The compelling reasons for the musculoskeletal use of MRI have made this book needed and essential for the practice of musculoskeletal radiology and orthopedics. The primary author, Dr. Stoller, has shown great ability in attracting superb collaborators who have all adhered to an orderly, methodical, and highly detailed mode of presenting facts. The general format followed in the nine chapters starts with an outline and with the presentation of techniques and sequences used for the given anatomic region; then there are extensive and well-organized sections on anatomy with variants in all *three orthogonal planes, and pathology including trauma and inflammatory and neoplastic diseases. Every chapter concludes with a discussion of perspectives making the vision of the future exciting. The use of gadolinium DTPA, gradient echo, and STIR imaging is dealt with in many illustrations adding to the richness of depiction of pathology.*

A book with so much substance and so well illustrated is an amazing testimonial to the great and rapid advances of an imaging method that was totally new in 1981 and became clinically feasible only in 1983. The principal author and his collaborators have captured the important points of musculoskeletal MRI and have been able to convey their enthusiasm for the continuing advances of this spectacular technique in a detailed and complete textbook, that is not only instructive but also a joy to read.

Alexander R. Margulis, M.D.
Professor and Chairman
Department of Radiology
University of California at San Francisco

Foreword

All of us involved in the diagnosis and care of patients with pathology involving the musculoskeletal system are aware that MRI is one of the most—if not the most—important advance in musculoskeletal imaging to have arrived on the medical scene in the last 50 years. It has opened vistas of musculoskeletal diagnosis and approaches to treatment not dreamed of by orthopedists a few short years ago. Many of the "tried and true" radiologic procedures upon which we depended so heavily in the past have been rendered obsolete by MRI (and computed tomography). For example, MRI can diagnose intra-articular pathology of the knee more accurately than can arthrography and, frequently, more definitely than arthroscopy is able to without being invasive.

Dr. Stoller has ably addressed this comprehensive text not only to radiologists, but also to orthopedists. While most orthopedists of today frequently request MRI studies, they must in most cases blindly accept the radiologist's evaluation. This is because few (including myself until very recently) understand the technique and are unsophisticated in image interpretation. Dr. Stoller's text will go far in unraveling the mystery of MRI and demonstrating its clinical applications—today and for years to come.

At last, MRI enables us to visualize and identify not only the bony portions of the musculoskeletal system, but also bone marrow, blood and blood vessels, fat, cartilage, muscle, fascia and tendons, and ligaments—all without invasiveness. Many of the techniques described in this text were either originated or improved by Dr. Stoller and his co-authors. I am certain that this text will become essential for the library of not only the radiologist, but the orthopedist and any other specialist involved in the care of patients with diseases and disabilities of the musculoskeletal system.

William R. Murray, M.D.
Professor and Chairman
Department of Orthopaedic Surgery
University of California at San Francisco

Foreword

In 1901, the first Nobel prize in physics was awarded to Wilhelm Conrad Roentgen for his discovery of a short wave length form of energy, which he called the x-ray. The application of x-rays, which could pass through living tissues to record images on film, revolutionized medical diagnosis. Although the bones of the extremities were among the first structures to be so visualized, it is fair to state that most subsequent advances in x-ray technology resulted in improved diagnosis of conditions affecting visceral *as opposed to* parietal *structures. It was not by accident that the average radiologist is far more skilled in reading chest films and studies of the gastrointestinal or genitourinary tracts using contrast materials than at interpretation of skeletal abnormalities.*

Parietal structures such as red (hematopoietic) and yellow (fatty) bone marrow, skeletal muscle, tendons, joint structures such as articular capsules, ligaments, hyaline and fibrocartilages, and fat pads have largely remained a "black box," despite arthrography, discography, and other attempts to use injected contrast materials.

The decade of the 1980s has witnessed another revolution in medical diagnostic imaging, i.e., magnetic resonance. The hydrogen atoms in molecules characteristic of various parietal tissues behave differently when manipulated magnetically, thus effectively opening the black box. And, unlike x-ray technology, the use of magnetic fields to examine the physical state of hydrogen atoms produces neither tissue damage nor risk to the patient.

The chapters in this volume systematically examine the newly emerging diagnostic data. The authors have been at the cutting edge of this spectacular new technology since its inception. They provide more than 1,000 state-of-the-art high resolution images in just over 400 pages. The great sensitivity of magnetic resonance imaging has already produced some diagnostic dilemmas: for example, should prophylactic bone coring be performed in a femoral head showing the earliest changes of osteonecrosis? The answer certainly lies in longitudinal studies of the natural history of such changes.

Clearly all *radiologists and clinicians dealing with patients with musculoskeletal disorders* must *become familiar with this new knowledge, including its limitations. This volume is the most comprehensive treatment of magnetic resonance imaging of spinal, axial, and appendicular joints ever attempted and should become a classic reference work.*

Daniel J. McCarty, M.D.
Will and Cava Ross Professor and Chairman
Department of Medicine
Medical College of Wisconsin

Preface

Applications for magnetic resonance imaging (MRI) in the fields of orthopedics and rheumatology have shown exponential growth since its initial clinical introduction in 1983. With the development of advanced systems hardware, surface coil technology, and flexible software programs—including innovative fast scan pulse sequences—MRI has replaced computed tomography in many applications for the evaluation of disorders affecting the axial and appendicular skeleton. Developments in musculoskeletal MRI techniques and new clinical applications are advancing so rapidly, they presently outpace their discussions in the current clinical literature.

This book was written with the intent of providing a comprehensive knowledge base for specialists in radiology, orthopedics, and rheumatology who desire clinical expertise in imaging bone and joint disorders with MRI. Every effort was made to provide images of the highest quality, using advanced software applications, including fast scan techniques, STIR (short TI inversion recovery) sequences, and new surface coil designs.

The first chapter provides an excellent introduction, presenting the physics of MRI with special attention to musculoskeletal imaging. The second chapter discusses a wide spectrum of MR imaging applications in the pediatric patient, with a comprehensive introduction to the basic concepts of tumor imaging. The following chapters provide a regional approach to musculoskeletal imaging. Imaging of the ankle and foot; the knee; the hip; the shoulder; the hand, wrist, and elbow; the spine; and the temporomandibular joint are discussed. Disorders affecting all appendicular joints (such as trauma, arthritis, infection, and neoplasia) are covered within each anatomic region for both the appendicular and axial skeleton.

Magnetic Resonance Imaging in Orthopaedics and Rheumatology is a complete and current reference that addresses the growing need of radiologists, orthopedic surgeons, and rheumatologists to understand and incorporate new clinical applications of bone and joint imaging.

David W. Stoller, M.D.

Acknowledgments

In order to deliver a timely text with state-of-the-art image quality and technical updates, a number of individuals contributed their time—ignoring conventional constraints and burning the "midnight oil"—their knowledge, and their expertise.

I applaud and acknowledge the following individuals for their assistance:

Chris Goumas, M.D., resident in radiology, University of California, San Francisco, *for his time, effort, and enthusiasm in assisting in literature searches and manuscript and image preparation, generally performing the job of ten individuals. This project could not have been completed without his generosity and dedication as a special contributor.*

John V. Crues III, M.D., *for his efforts in writing Chapter 1, and for his expertise and case material for the chapters on the ankle, shoulder, and knee. John's generosity and character are much appreciated and admired.*

Bruce A. Porter, M.D., Director of First Hill Diagnostic Imaging Center, Seattle, Washington, *for providing all the STIR images using short TI inversion recovery techniques. Dr. Porter is a pioneer and leader within the field of body and marrow imaging, and his contribution to the success of this book is invaluable.*

Leonard Gordon, M.D., *for contributions to Chapter 7.*

Jerry H. Mink, M.D., *for his encouragement and support during my early experience with MRI and for his contribution of Figure 4-148.*

Sheila Moore, M.D., *for her contribution to Chapter 2.*

I would also like to acknowledge those who kindly contributed case material and illustrations:

Richard Turkanis, M.D.—rotator cuff tears and impingement.

Geremy McCreary, M.D., of the Medical Center Magnetic Imaging, Oakland, California—Figures 3-20, 3-26, and 7-12.

John Hunter, M.D.—Figure 5-39.

Neil Chavitz, M.D.—Figure 4-44.

Mel Senac, M.D.—juvenile rheumatoid arthritis of the knee.

Barbara Griffiths, M.D.—Figure 4-17.

Lynn Steinbach, M.D.—Figure 3-23 and case material from Letterman Army Medical Hospital.

Michael Schneider, M.D., of Los Robles Regional Medical Center—Figure 4-122.

Bob Princenthal of Humana Hospital West Hills—Figure 3-14.

Brenda G. Nichols, Ph.D., of Diasonics—Diasonics surface coils and imager, and assistance in providing clinical images using her shoulder coil design.

Ann Shimakawa, of General Electric—G.E. surface coils and imager.

I would like to thank the following individuals for their technical expertise and contributions:

Felix Wehrli, Ph.D., of General Electric—for his assistance in providing information on fast scan applications and cooperation in reviewing Chapter 1.

Richard Wada and the staff of the Educational Media Resources Photography Department of the University of California, San Francisco—they produced text images with unmatched professional quality and delivered them in record-breaking time.

Gamma Photographic Labs in San Francisco.

Luna Grafix, Inc.

The magnetic resonance imaging technicians at the University of California, San Francisco—Evelyn Proctor, Niles Bruce, Vesta March, Cathy McGarvey, Pauline Mattei, and Michael Collins.

Dean J. Manke, Vice President, Book and Looseleaf Publications at J. B. Lippincott, and Delois Patterson, Developmental Editor—their understanding and appreciation of the necessary quality helped bring this textbook to fruition.

Denice Nakano—many deadlines were met through her helpfulness in overseeing communications and dispatch of manuscript.

Special acknowledgment is given to Katherine Pitcoff, who served as my West Coast editor, tirelessly preparing manuscript for presentation to J. B. Lippincott.

David W. Stoller, M.D.

Contents

MAGNETIC RESONANCE IMAGING IN ORTHOPAEDICS AND RHEUMATOLOGY

John V. Crues III
Frank W. Morgan

Chapter 1 PHYSICAL AND TECHNICAL CONSIDERATIONS IN MAGNETIC RESONANCE IMAGING

OUTLINE

Since its development in the 1940s, nuclear magnetic resonance (NMR) has been used extensively to investigate the physical and chemical properties of matter. Damadian was among the first to suggest the use of NMR in medical diagnoses[1] and Lauterbur published the first NMR image in 1972.[2] The first use of clinical magnetic resonance (MR) imaging was in the early 1980s and has led to a revolution in medical imaging during this decade. In this chapter an overview of the technical aspects of MR imaging is presented. A more detailed discussion and list of references are presented by Crues and Shellock.[3]

BASIC CONCEPTS

The basic building block of the chemical elements is the atom. The atom is composed of a central nucleus of protons and neutrons with surrounding orbiting electrons. Nuclei that contain an odd number of protons or neutrons are actually small rotating magnets with very special magnetic properties. When placed in a large magnetic field, these nuclei (actually the magnetic moments of the nuclei) tend to align themselves in the direction of the magnetic field, just as a compass aligns with the magnetic field of the earth. In addition, spinning of these nuclei resembles the action of spinning tops; instead of aligning perfectly with the external magnetic field, the nuclei precess around the direction of the external magnetic field (Fig. 1-1). The frequency of this precession around the main magnetic field is given by the Larmor equation as:

$$\omega = \gamma \times B_0$$

In this equation ω is the precessional (Larmor) frequency, γ is the gyromagnetic ratio, and B_0 is the strength of the external magnetic field.

Although this equation holds for all magnetic nuclei placed in a magnetic field, different types of nuclei—that is, hydrogen nuclei versus phosphorus nuclei versus nitrogen nuclei, and so forth—possess unique gyromagnetic ratios. Because of the Larmor equation, nuclei with high gyromagnetic ratios precess at higher frequencies in a given magnetic field than do nuclei

with lower gyromagnetic ratios. Because hydrogen nuclei possess the largest gyromagnetic ratio known, and hydrogen is extremely abundant in the human body, most medical MR imaging is based on the hydrogen nucleus.

RESONANCE

In accordance with the rules of quantum mechanics, the hydrogen nucleus, which consists of a single proton, can exist in only two energy states in the presence of a magnetic field. The nucleus can either align itself in the direction of the main magnetic field (parallel) or in the direction opposite to the externally applied field (antiparallel, Fig. 1-2). The parallel state has lower energy than the antiparallel state and, if all else is equal, the nuclei will tend to align themselves with the main mag-

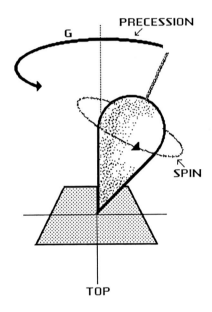

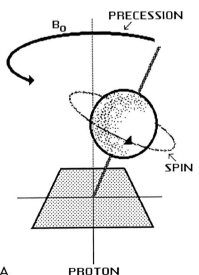

Figure 1-1

Nuclear motion in a magnetic field generated within an MR imager. **(A)** The hydrogen nucleus consists of a proton. The proton spins around its own intrinsic axis and, when placed in a magnetic field, precesses about the direction of the main magnetic field much like a top precesses about the direction of force exerted by a gravitational field. **(B)** Schematic diagram identifying location of radio frequency *(RF)* coils, gradient coils, and magnetic core in an MR imager.

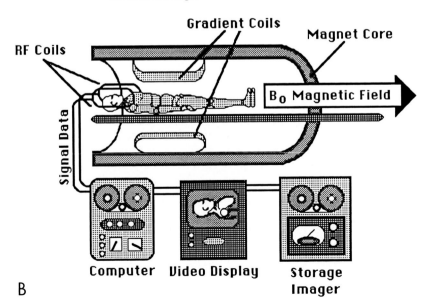

ANTIPARALLEL (SPIN DOWN)

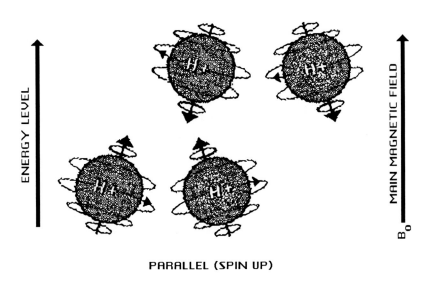

ENERGY LEVEL

MAIN MAGNETIC FIELD

B_0

PARALLEL (SPIN UP)

Figure 1-2
Nuclear alignment in a magnetic field. In the presence of an external magnetic field, hydrogen nuclei are constrained to align parallel or antiparallel to the external magnetic field. Just as a compass in equilibrium aligns itself with the magnetic field of the earth to be in the state of lowest energy, in equilibrium greater numbers of nuclei will be in the parallel than in the antiparallel orientation to minimize the overall energy of the nuclei.

netic field. If these nuclei are subjected to electromagnetic radiation of the proper frequency, the nuclei will be forced to make rapid transitions between the low and high energy states. This process is called *resonance* (Fig. 1-3).

The concept of nuclear magnetic resonance can be greatly simplified by using the concept of the *bulk mag-*

netization vector (M).[4] The bulk magnetization vector is the vector sum of the magnetic moments of all of the hydrogen nuclei in a sample of tissue. For a sample of tissue that is not placed in a large magnetic field, the nuclei are randomly oriented in space and therefore M is zero (Fig. 1-4A). Once the sample is placed in a large magnetic field, the nuclei tend to align themselves in the

BASELINE

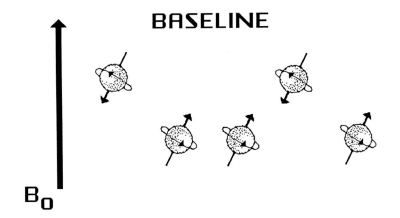

B_0

Figure 1-3
Nuclear magnetic resonance. In the baseline state in the presence of an externally applied magnetic field, more nuclei will be parallel than antiparallel. However, if the nuclei are exposed to an RF pulse of the proper energy (frequency), then nuclei will rapidly flip from parallel to antiparallel states. This condition is called resonance.

RESONANCE

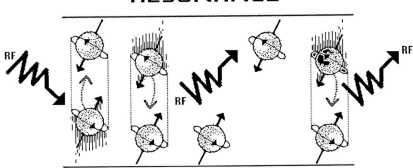

RF

RF

RF

Figure 1-4

The bulk magnetization vector. **(A)** The magnetic properties of a large collection of nuclei can be greatly simplified by use of the concept of the bulk magnetization vector. Nuclei that are not subject to an externally applied magnetic field are randomly oriented about one another. The vector sum of their magnetic moments cancel, and the net magnetization of the sample is zero. **(B)** In the presence of an external magnetic field, B_0, more nuclei will point in the direction of the magnetic field than in the direction opposite to the magnetic field. The vector sum is nonzero and points in the direction of the main magnetic field. This quantity is called the bulk magnetization vector.

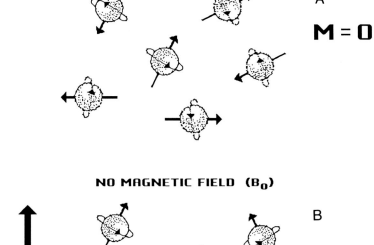

A

$M = 0$

NO MAGNETIC FIELD (B_0)

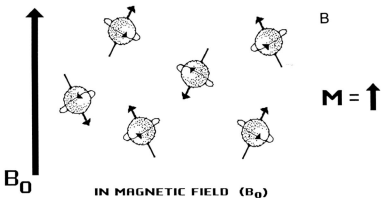

B

$M = \uparrow$

IN MAGNETIC FIELD (B_0)

Figure 1-5

The effect on the bulk magnetization vector of a 90° RF pulse. In the presence of an external magnetic field, nuclei tend to align themselves with the magnetic field, and the bulk magnetization vector points in the direction of the main magnetic field. However, after a 90° RF pulse, the number of parallel nuclei equals the number of antiparallel nuclei, and the Z component of the bulk magnetization vector becomes zero. The 90° pulse also forces the nuclei to precess in phase (see Fig. 1-6). The X–Y component of the bulk magnetization vector becomes nonzero. The resultant bulk magnetization vector points in the X–Y plane, a 90° rotation from the baseline position along the Z axis.

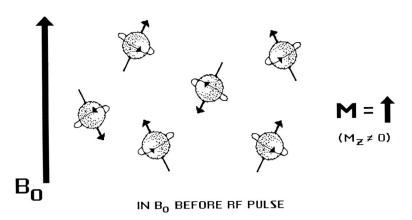

$M = \uparrow$

$(M_z \neq 0)$

IN B_0 BEFORE RF PULSE

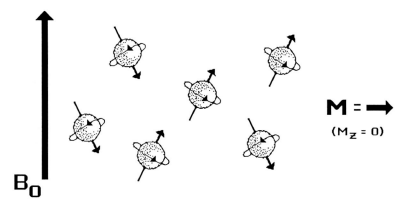

$M = \Rightarrow$

$(M_z = 0)$

IN B_0 AFTER 90° RF PULSE

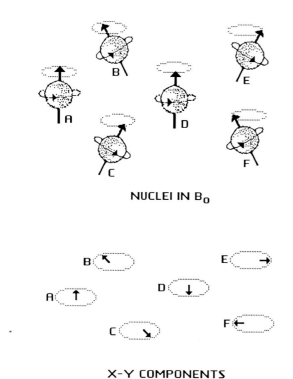

NUCLEI IN B$_0$

X–Y COMPONENTS

Figure 1-6

Nuclear precession. In an external magnetic field without exposure to an RF pulse, the nuclei precess randomly about one another. For each nucleus at one point in its "circle of precession" (as in *B*) another nucleus is directed oppositely within its "circle of precession" (as in *C*). The component of the nuclear moments in the direction perpendicular to the Z direction cancels and the X–Y component of the bulk magnetization vector is zero.

direction of the main magnetic field and the vector sum of all the nuclei will then be a large vector that points in the direction of the main magnetic field (Fig. 1-4B). Exposure to a radio frequency (RF) pulse of the proper frequency induces transitions between energy states, as described above. This tends to decrease the number of excess nuclei pointing in the direction of the main magnetic field, thus, decreasing the component of the bulk magnetization vector in the direction of the main magnetic field (Fig. 1-5).

Before the introduction of the RF pulse, the nuclei precess randomly (about one another) around the direction of the main magnetic field (Fig. 1-6). Therefore, the vector sum of the magnetic moments of the individual nuclei in a direction perpendicular to the main magnetic field *(X–Y component)* is zero. After the introduction of the RF pulse, the nuclei no longer precess randomly about one another because the RF pulse tends to cause nuclei to precess *in phase* with one another (Fig. 1-7). Since the nuclei are no longer randomly spaced around their "circles of precession," the vector sum of the magnetic moment of the nuclei is no longer zero in the X–Y plane. Thus, after introduction of an RF pulse, the *Z component* of M decreases and the vector is rotated away from the Z axis, as shown in Figure 1-8.

The degree of rotation of M from the Z axis *(nutation)* is determined by the strength and the duration of the RF pulse. These pulses are typically described in terms of the angle through which M is nutated. An RF pulse that rotates the vector 90° into the X–Y plane is therefore called a 90° pulse. An RF pulse of twice the duration, or the same duration and twice the magnitude, would invert the bulk magnetization vector, that is, rotate it 180° (Fig. 1-9).

Once the bulk magnetization vector has nutated into the X–Y plane, it rotates about the Z axis with a frequency given by the Larmor equation (Fig. 1-10). The importance of this is depicted in Figure 1-11. In Niagara Falls, electric energy is created by turning the energy of falling water into rotational mechanical energy via a turbine. The turbine rotates a magnet in the presence of surrounding electrical wires. The rotating magnet induces current in the surrounding wires at a frequency

Figure 1-7

The effect of a 90° RF pulse on nuclear phase. Before the 90° RF pulse, nuclei predominantly are in the parallel position and are randomly oriented around their "circles of precession." After the 90° RF pulse, equal numbers of nuclei are in the parallel and antiparallel orientations. The nuclei, however, are no longer oriented randomly around their "circles of precession," but precess pointing in the same direction. In this state the nuclei are said to be "in phase." The X–Y components no longer cancel one another, and the X–Y component of the bulk magnetization vector is no longer zero after the 90° pulse.

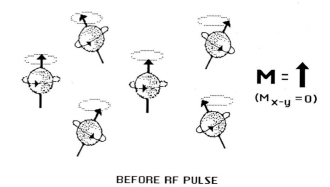

M = ↑
(M$_{x-y}$ = 0)

BEFORE RF PULSE

M = →
(M$_{x-y}$ ≠ 0)

AFTER RF PULSE

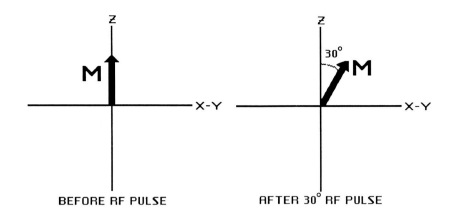

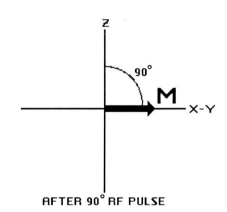

Figure 1-8

Nutation. RF pulses of increasing magnitude and duration at a frequency specified by the Larmor equation will cause the bulk magnetization vector to nutate away from the Z axis toward the X–Y plane. A small RF pulse may produce a 30° rotation, whereas a pulse of three times the magnitude or three times the duration will produce a 90° nutation.

Figure 1-9

The 90° and 180° RF pulses. The 90° pulse is the initial pulse in the standard spin echo sequence and a 180° pulse is used as a refocusing pulse in spin echo imaging. The 180° pulse is the initial pulse in the inversion recovery sequences that is followed by a 90° spin echo pulse for data acquisition.

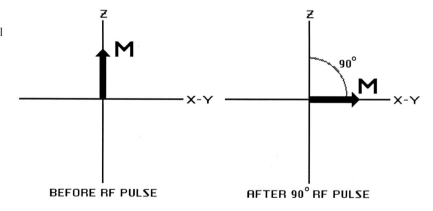

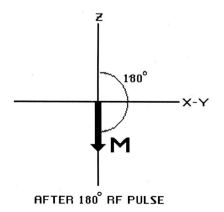

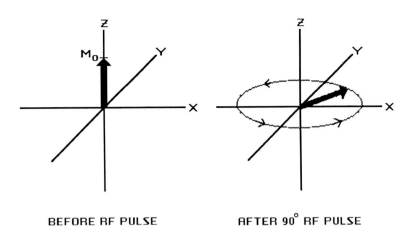

BEFORE RF PULSE   **AFTER 90° RF PULSE**

Figure 1-10

Rotation of the bulk magnetization vector. After nutation of the bulk magnetization vector into the X–Y plane following a 90° pulse, the bulk magnetization vector rotates around the Z axis at the Larmor frequency.

that is determined by its rotation rate. In a similar fashion, the rotating bulk magnetization vector induces electrical current in surrounding wires at a frequency determined by the Larmor frequency. This current is fed to a computer and is the signal used to construct images from NMR (see Fig. 1-1B).

T1 AND T2 RELAXATION

After termination of the RF pulse, M returns to the baseline state that is pointing in the Z direction (Fig. 1-12). Two processes occur that allow this to happen.

One process is called *T1 relaxation*. After the 90° pulse, the Z component of M is zero, which means that equal numbers of nuclei are parallel and antiparallel. T1 relaxation represents return to the equilibrium state, where a greater number of nuclei point parallel versus antiparallel to the Z direction. This is also called *longitudinal* or *spin-lattice relaxation*. In order for this to occur, excess nuclei in the antiparallel state must make the transition to the low-energy parallel state. According to quantum mechanical laws, this can only occur if induced by electromagnetic radiation at the Larmor frequency. In tissues, the RF used is derived from local atoms and molecules tumbling at the Larmor frequency.

Since large molecules tend to tumble slowly, that is, in the range of the Larmor frequency used by most resonance imagers, tissues containing large molecules, such as fat and protein, tend to have rapid T1 relaxation and therefore small values of T1 (the characteristic time required for M to return to near its equilibrium value along the Z axis; Fig. 1-13).[5]

T2 relaxation processes, on the other hand, are responsible for returning the X–Y component of the bulk magnetization vector, which is large after the 90° pulse, back to zero—its equilibrium value (Fig. 1-14). In other words, T2 processes, also called *spin-spin relaxation* or *transverse relaxation,* are responsible for causing the nuclei to precess out of phase with one another. If numerous nuclei precess in phase and are in precisely the same magnetic fields, they will precess in phase forever. However, if these nuclei experience slightly different magnetic fields, they will then precess at slightly different rotational rates. Nuclei in higher local magnetic fields will rotate more rapidly than nuclei in lower local magnetic fields, and these nuclei will soon lose phase with one another (Fig. 1-15). Substances with nuclei experiencing differing magnetic fields are associated with rapid dephasing and a rapid return of the X–Y component of bulk magnetization vector to zero. Such substances have a short T2, which is the characteristic time required for the X–Y component of the bulk magnetiza-

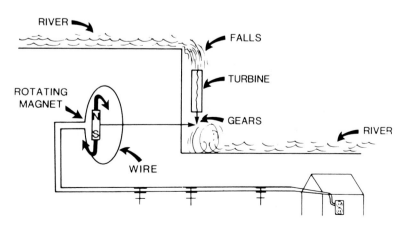

Figure 1-11

Electricity generation. Current is induced in wires by a rotating magnetic field. At an electricity generating plant the rotating magnetic field is produced by a rotating magnet. The energy required to rotate the magnet can be obtained from falling water, as at Niagara Falls, or from the burning of fossil fuels. In MR imaging, the rotating magnetic field is the bulk magnetization vector during resonance that induces current in the receiving coils that is then fed to the computer for image construction. (Crues JV III, Shellock FG: Technical considerations. In Mink JR, Reigher MA, Crues JV III (eds): Magnetic Resonance Imaging of the Knee, 5. New York, Raven Press, 1987)

tion vector to approximate zero after termination of the RF pulse (see Fig. 1-14). Since prominent magnetic field differences (gradients) occur in all matter at the atomic level, most solid substances possess short T2 values. However, fluids in which the nuclei are able to move randomly throughout space, tend to have long T2 values because the nuclei spend short periods of time in regions of low and high magnetic fields. Over the time course of an NMR pulse sequence, an average value results that tends to be very similar from nucleus to nucleus (Fig. 1-16). This process is called *motional narrowing* and is responsible for the long T2 of liquids within the body.

IMAGE PRODUCTION

Although by now it may be obvious that hydrogen nuclei within the human body can generate an electrical signal in a wire, how a small amount of current in a wire can be used to generate an image of the human body may not be quite so apparent. The most commonly used technique to make this transition is called the *two-dimensional Fourier transform technique*. The goal of MR imaging is to create a method by which the point of origin of an NMR signal can be determined so that a two-dimensional map can be constructed, in which the image intensity at a position on the map is determined by the strength of the NMR signal emanating from a specified location within the body.

In two-dimensional Fourier transform imaging, the spatial localization of signal in one direction (let's call it the X' direction) is determined by *frequency encoding*.

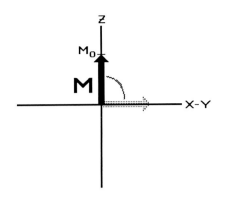

Figure 1-12

Relaxation. After termination of the 90° RF pulse, the bulk magnetization vector M returns to the baseline state, pointing in the Z direction.

Fullerton made a brilliant analogy between this technique and a harp.[6] If a harp and harpist are placed in one room, and a musician with perfect pitch is placed in an adjoining room, the musician could accurately tell the harpist which string was plucked (that is, how far the string is from the harpist's body) by the pitch of the sound emanating from the harp. In other words, the positions of the strings of the harp are encoded in the frequency of the sound they emit. Similarly, if a small magnetic field gradient is placed across the patient's body such that there is a slightly higher magnetic field on the patient's right side and a lower magnetic field on the patient's left side, signal returning from the patient's right side will be higher in frequency than signal emanating from the patient's left side. The computer can then use frequency differences to determine the location within the body from which the signal originates.

Unfortunately, frequency encoding can be used in

Figure 1-13

T1 relaxation. After termination of a 90° RF pulse, the Z component of the bulk magnetization vector returns to its baseline value logarithmically. T1 is the time required to return to approximately 63% of the baseline value.

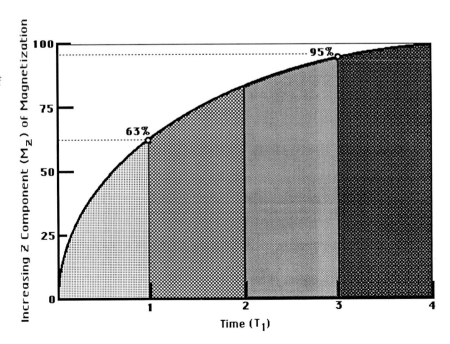

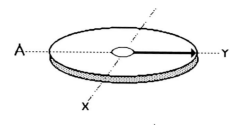

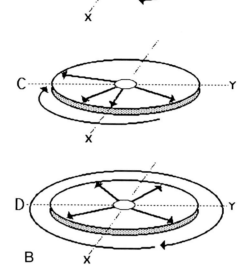

Figure 1-14

T2 relaxation. **(A)** After termination of the 90° excitation pulse, the X–Y component of M decreases exponentially with a time constant T2. **(B)** The exponential decay of the X–Y component of M is due to dephasing of nuclear spins from inhomogeneity of precession rates from variations in the strength of the magnetic field at the atomic level.

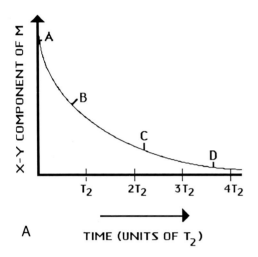

only one direction. In order to create a two-dimensional image of a slice through the body, spatial localization along two dimensions, that is, within an entire plane, must be specified. Spatial localization perpendicular to the X′ axis (call it the Y′ axis) is determined using *phase encoding*. Of all the technical aspects of two-dimensional Fourier transform imaging, phase encoding is probably the least intuitive. In order to achieve a more intuitive understanding of phase encoding, a simplified imaging model will be used to describe the encoding of information using phase relationships, rather than a more formal mathematical description of the technique.

A square wave function is a very simple function that is zero at all points except in the interval from zero to one in which its value is one (Fig. 1-17). This function accurately represents the signal intensity that would emanate from a slice from a square beaker of water placed within an MR imager (Fig. 1-18). A sine wave can be used to approximate this function, as shown schematically in Figure 1-19. A single sine wave, however, is a very rough approximation of the square wave that can be more closely reproduced if an additional sine wave (of three times the frequency of the first and one third its amplitude) is added to the original (Fig. 1-20). Note

that the higher frequency sine wave helps to sharpen the edges, which more closely resemble the sharp edges of a square wave. As higher frequency sine waves of the proper amplitude are added, the desired function can be more closely approximated. In general, the more frequency terms that are added to the equation, the more closely the square wave is reproduced.

The signal intensity from a square beaker of water can thus be closely approximated by a sequence of sine waves of the proper amplitudes and increasing frequencies. This is simply a physical analogue to the mathematical theorem of Fourier, which states that any well-behaved mathematical function can be reproduced by a series of sine and cosine functions. The advantage of Fourier's theorem is that it determines a way in which the proper amplitudes can be calculated for each sign and cosine frequency.

The problem in using a Fourier series to duplicate signal intensity in MR imaging is that a mechanism must be determined to calculate the coefficients that must be placed in front of each sine term in Fourier's series to properly duplicate the MR signal intensity. This problem is represented by the mathematical formula:

$$SI = A_0 + A_1 \sin Y' + A_2 \sin 2Y' \ldots.$$

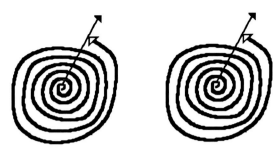

A. UNIFORM MAGNETIC FIELD

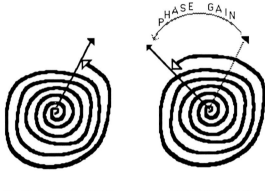

B. AVERAGE FIELD   HIGHER FIELD

Figure 1-15
Nuclear phase. **(A)** Nuclei in a perfectly uniform magnetic field will precess in phase indefinitely. **(B)** In a nonuniform magnetic field, nuclei in higher magnetic fields precess slightly faster and will "gain phase" relative to nuclei experiencing an average magnetic field.

This is a simplified Fourier series where SI is signal intensity, A's are the Fourier coefficients to be determined, and Y′ is the phase encoded direction.

In MR imaging, these coefficients can be directly measured. If an MR signal is obtained from these nuclei without the presence of a magnetic field gradient in the Y′ direction, then all of the nuclei will be in phase, (Fig. 1-21A), and the resulting signal will be proportional to the constant term in Fourier's series. If, however, a small magnetic field gradient is placed along the Y′ axis for a short period of time before the readout (frequency encoding) gradient, then the phase relationships of the nuclei along the Y′ direction will vary, (Fig. 1-21B). Note that if a line is drawn connecting the phase location of the nuclei, a low-frequency sine wave is depicted that is similar to the low-frequency sine used to approximate the step function in Figure 1-19. If a stronger phase encoding gradient is placed along the Y′ direction, the phase relationships between the nuclei along the Y′ direction more closely approximate the higher frequency components in the Fourier series of a step function (Fig. 1-21C).

The signal intensity that is returned from this strip of nuclei in the absence of a phase encoded gradient is proportional to A_0 in the Fourier series. The signal intensity that is returned after a small phase encoded gradient, such that the phase relationships are depicted as in Figure 1-21B, will be proportional to A_1 in the Fourier series. If larger and larger phase encoding gradients are placed on the sample, the returned signal intensity will be proportional to coefficients of higher and higher frequency components in the Fourier series. Therefore, the signal intensity versus position in the Y′ direction can be calculated using a Fourier series in which the amplitudes of the sine wave components are directly measured by the use of phase encoded gradients.

The Fourier coefficient for a given phase encoded gradient can be simultaneously measured for all slices along the X′ direction. Therefore, the signal intensity function in the Y′ direction can be calculated for every frequency (X′) interval simultaneously.

As described earlier for a standard step function (see Fig. 1-20), the spatial resolution along the Y′ dimension is determined by the highest number of frequency components used in calculating the signal intensity. Thus, the more phase encodings used, the better

Figure 1-16
Motional narrowing. **(A)** Strong magnetic field gradients exist at the atomic level. Nuclei fixed in space (solid) continuously experience a single magnetic field that is higher than average in some locations and lower in others. Nuclei in a high magnetic field precess rapidly, and those in a low magnetic field precess slowly, leading to rapid dephasing and a short T2. **(B)** Nuclei in fluids move through space during a pulse sequence and experience short intervals in high and low magnetic fields. These nuclei experience an overall average magnetic field that is uniform from nucleus to nucleus; dephasing occurs much more slowly than in solids. Typical fluids have long T2 relaxation times.

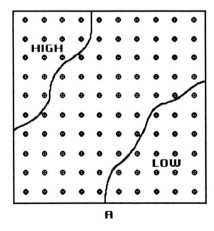

A

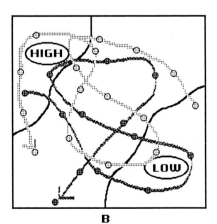

B

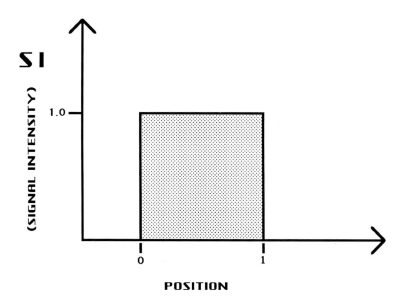

Figure 1-17

Square wave function. A square wave function is zero everywhere except between the interval from zero to one in which its value is one.

Figure 1-18

Signal intensity in a square beaker of water. In order to spatially localize the signal emanating from a square beaker of water, position along the X′ direction can be localized using frequency encoding as described in the text. Signal intensity along the Y′ direction, however, requires an additional spatial localizing technique called phase encoding. The signal intensity versus position along the phase encoded (Y′) axis for a square beaker of water is a simple square wave.

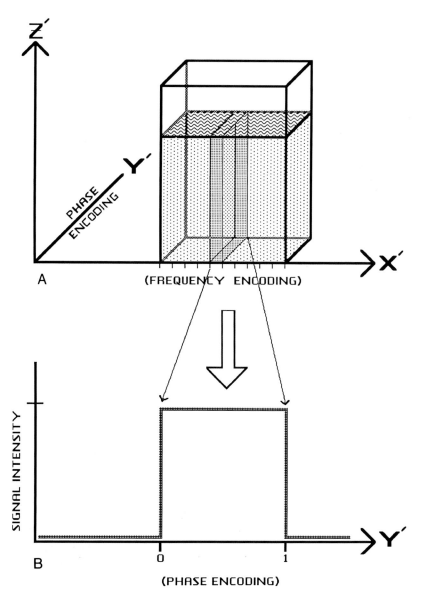

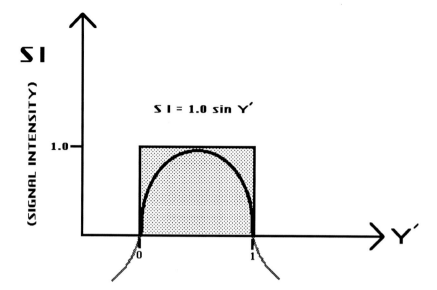

Figure 1-19

Low-frequency sine wave as an approximation to a square wave. This schematic diagram shows how a simple sine wave of the appropriate frequency can roughly approximate the square wave function.

Figure 1-20

Higher order approximations to a square wave. **(A)** A higher-frequency sine wave does not by itself provide an accurate approximation of a square wave. **(B)** The sum of the appropriately selected lower-frequency sine wave and a high-frequency sine wave, however, provides an improved approximation of a square wave than was obtained by either sine wave alone. In general, the greater the number of sine wave frequencies used to approximate a given function, the more accurate the approximation becomes.

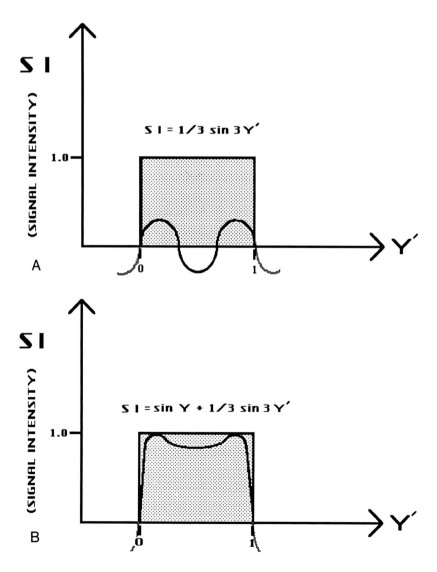

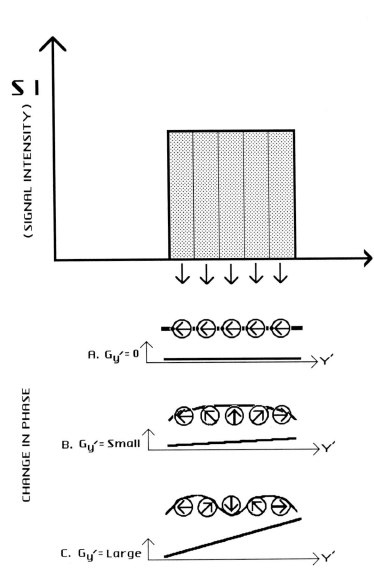

Figure 1-21

Calculation of Fourier coefficients by MR. *(A)* If no gradient is placed along the phase encoded axis, then the nuclei along this axis will be in phase at the time of signal sampling, and the resultant signal will be proportional to the A_0 Fourier coefficient. *(B)* If a small magnetic field gradient is placed along the phase encoded direction, then the nuclear phase along the Y′ direction will be slightly altered, and the resultant signal intensity will be proportional to the Fourier coefficient A_1. *(C)* Higher magnetic field gradients along the phase encoded direction will allow sampling of higher order Fourier coefficients.

the spatial resolution. Unfortunately, increasing the number of phase encodings increases the corresponding imaging time.

Although a simple rectangular beaker of water is used in this example, the technique can be used, similarly, for a more complicated sample, such as the human body, since a Fourier series can reproduce *any* well-behaved mathematical function, no matter how complicated it may be.

TISSUE CONTRAST

The basic principles discussed above can be used to obtain images with widely varying tissue contrast.[7] Five major chemical and physical properties of matter are predominantly responsible for imaging contrast among tissues. These five parameters are *hydrogen proton density, T1 relaxation time, T2 relaxation time, T2* relaxation time, and flow.*

Since the signal used to construct images with NMR emanates from the nucleus of hydrogen atoms (protons), if all else is equal, tissues with a higher density of protons per unit volume will emit greater signal and, consequently, will be brighter on subsequent images than tissue with a lower proton density. In most soft tissues within the body, the proton density differences are small, and therefore proton density is usually not a major source of contrast difference among tissues.

T1 relaxation is dependent on the presence of large macromolecules that vibrate near the Lamor frequency (see p. 2). Marked differences exist among tissues in the concentration of and interrelationship between macromolecules and hydrogen nuclei. Tissues with a strong interaction between hydrogen nuclei and the electromagnetic vibrations of macromolecules, such as the triglyceride appendages of fat molecules, exhibit short T1 relaxation times and are thus bright on a T1-weighted image. Other tissues, that have paramagnetic substances such as methemaglobin and gadolinium, also have short T1 relaxation times because the large magnetic field of the paramagnetic atoms enhances the interaction between macromolecules and water protons.[8] Fluids, such as urine and cerebrospinal fluid (CSF), contain few large macromolecules and possess very little interaction between macromolecules and the protons of water. Consequently, they have long T1 relaxation times. Pulse sequences that emphasize contrast between tissues based on T1 relaxation are called T1-weighted sequences (see below). Tissues with short T1 values are bright on T1-weighted MR images.

Contrast based on differences in T2 relaxation times has been instrumental in the acceptance of MR imaging over the past 10 years. Many abnormal processes, such as neoplasia and inflammation, produce increased free water within tissues. As discussed, because of motional narrowing (see p. 8), free water displays long T2 relaxation times, compared with normal tissue. T2-weighted pulse sequences (see the next page) emphasize the contrast difference between tissues based on T2 relaxation times, and tissues with long T2 relaxation times are bright. Thus, many common disease processes become conspicuous on T2-weighted images because of the high signal intensity, primarily due to increased free water.

Following an RF excitation pulse, the signal received decreases exponentially with the characteristic time called T2* (Fig. 1-22). This is called the *free induction delay* (FID). As we discussed under T2 relaxation, the etiology of the exponential loss in signal

Figure 1-22

The free induction decay. Free induction decay refers to the decay in signal intensity immediately after an excitation RF pulse. The envelope of the signal is determined by an exponential curve with a decay constant of T2*. The free induction decay is used as a signal for MR imaging when gradient echo images are performed. The free induction decay is, however, not used for image acquisition in standard spin echo and inversion recovery sequences. T2* decay is governed by all magnetic inhomogeneities at the atomic level, whereas, fixed magnetic inhomogeneities do not contribute to T2 decay. Thus, T2 decay is always more prolonged than T2* decay.

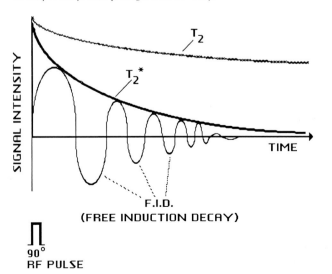

intensity is due to dephasing of the spins by local inhomogeneities in the magnetic field (see Fig. 1-14). However, T2* relaxation includes not only T2 relaxation due to inhomogeneities on a microscopic level from the physical–chemical nature of the sample, but also magnetic field inhomogeneities due to large fluctuations in the magnetic field from less than ideal primary magnets and other external magnetic field gradients. Thus, soft tissue contrast on T2*-weighted images is often poor because much of the contrast is secondary to changes that are independent of the physical–chemical properties of the tissues. T2* is usually markedly less than T2. Pulse sequences that measure T2* are discussed on p. 16.

The presence of flow can both increase and decrease the signal intensity on MR images. A complete description of the effects of flow on MR images is beyond the scope of this chapter, but many excellent reviews of this subject exist in the literature.[9]

PULSE SEQUENCES

In an attempt to fully exploit the numerous tissue parameters that can create contrast on MR images, multiple pulse sequences have been developed. The primary pulse sequences used in musculoskeletal imaging include spin echo, inversion recovery, and gradient echo techniques.

Virtually all MR imaging pulse sequences use some form of a *spin echo* in data acquisition. All spin echo techniques use at least one initial RF pulse called an *excitation pulse,* and either one or more additional *refocusing pulses* or a *gradient reversal* to generate a delayed signal pulse called a spin echo. In medical imaging it has become common practice to restrict the term spin echo pulse sequence to the subset of all spin echo techniques that utilizes a 90° RF excitation pulse followed by a 180° RF refocusing pulse to generate a spin echo as diagrammed in Figure 1-23. In addition to multiple technical reasons that favor the use of this type of spin echo pulse, this pulse also eliminates most of the signal loss due to external magnetic field inhomogeneities (T2* effects); yet does not affect signal intensity that is modified by the primary relaxation mechanisms of the tissues themselves, that is, T1 and T2 effects.

T1-Weighted Pulse Sequences

The mechanism by which a spin echo pulse sequence with a short recovery time (TR—the time between 90° excitation pulses) and a short echo time (TE—the time between a 90° excitation pulse and the spin echo) can be used to accentuate contrast differences between tissues with differing T1 values is illustrated in Figure 1-24. As the TR increases, however, the difference between signal intensities of tissues with differing T1 val-

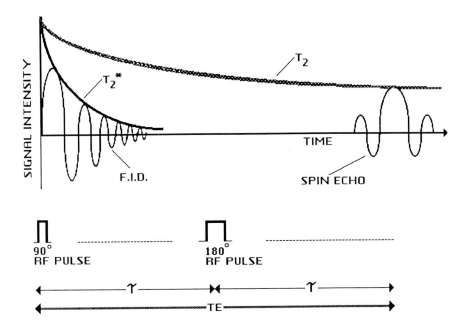

Figure 1-23
The spin echo pulse sequence. Standard spin echo pulse sequences consist of a 90° RF excitation pulse followed after τ msec by a 180° refocusing pulse. At 2 τ msec (TE) after the 90° excitation pulse, a spin echo is created. It is the spin echo that is recovered and utilized to calculate the image. The height of the spin echo is determined by T2 exponential decay.

ues is minimized, and the spin echo sequence becomes less efficient in distinguishing these tissues. Therefore, a spin echo sequence with a short TR and short TE is a good T1-weighted sequence. Typical pulsing parameters for a T1-weighted sequence is a TR between 200 and 600 msec and a TE of 15 to 30 msec.

Intermediate and T2-Weighted Pulse Sequences

On the other hand, spin echo pulse sequences with a long TE can efficiently distinguish tissues with differing T2 values, as illustrated in Figure 1-25. Long TR (minimal T1-weighting) and long TE spin echo pulse sequences are *T2-weighted* and are the most sensitive pulse sequences for disease processes associated with increased free water. Pulse sequences with a long TR

and short TE are *intermediately weighted*. Other terms commonly used for this pulse sequence include a *balance sequence*, a *density weighted sequence*, a *spin density weighted sequence,* and a *proton density weighted* image. This type of image generally has high signal-to-noise ratio (see p. 20) and is often best for delineating basic anatomy.

Typical pulsing parameters for an intermediate weighted sequence include a TR of 1500 to 2000 msec and a TE of 20 to 40 msec. T2-weighted sequences typically use a TR of 2000 msec and a TE of 60 to 80 msec.

Inversion Recovery Technique

The inversion recovery technique is another technique that is highly T1-weighted. The initial excitation pulse is a 180° excitation pulse that is followed by a standard

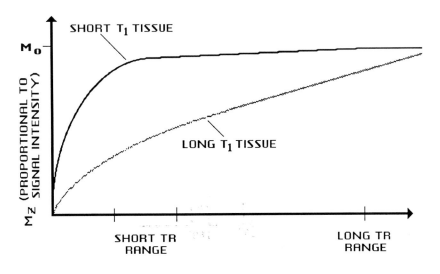

Figure 1-24
The T1-weighted spin echo sequence. If one evaluates the signal intensity obtained from tissues with differing T1 time constants, short TRs are associated with large differences in signal intensities from two tissues with differing TRs. After a long TR, all tissues, regardless of their T1 values recover most of their original Z component of bulk magnetization vector. However, only a short time after the initial 90° pulse, tissues with short T1s have recovered a significant amount of the original Z component of the bulk magnetization vector and they are bright, whereas tissues with long TRs are less bright, creating strong contrast between tissues with differing T1 values.

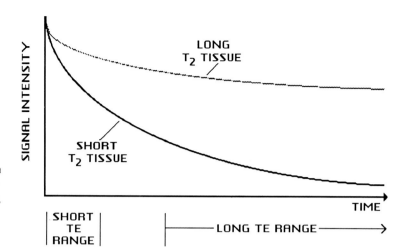

Figure 1-25

The T2-weighted spin echo pulse sequence. Spin echo pulse sequences with long TEs are efficient at distinguishing tissues with differing T2 values. In the short TE range, tissues with both long and short T2 values produce ample signal. However, as the TE is lengthened, tissues with short T2 values lose signal rapidly, whereas tissues with long T2 values maintain signal intensity, creating excellent contrast between tissues with differing T2 values.

spin echo pulse sequence at time "TI" after the initial 180° pulse, as shown in Figure 1-26. How this pulse sequence becomes a T1-weighted sequence is shown in Figure 1-27. To date, this particular pulse sequence has been sparingly used in the United States because the number of slices that can be obtained simultaneously has been limited and, until recently, no strong clear-cut advantages of the inversion recovery sequence over a T1-weighted spin echo sequence have been realized. However, because the strength of the signal that is returned from the spin echo sequence is proportional to the absolute magnitude of the Z component of the bulk magnetization vector at the instant of the 90° pulse, a TI can be determined for which fat, which has a short T1, will not emit a signal (see Fig. 1-27). This type of inversion recovery pulse sequence that has a short TI was initially used to eliminate the signal from subcutaneous fat that is responsible for motion artifacts in breathing. However, this technique—called *short TI inversion re-*

covery (STIR) technique—has recently been shown to be highly sensitive for diseases within the medullary space of bone because of its ability to suppress the signal from normal medullary fat and allow signal emanating from abnormal tissues to be better detected.

Gradient Recall Techniques

Over the last several years, gradient recall techniques have become increasingly popular, primarily because of their ability to increase the rate of data acquisition and decrease scan times.[10] A gradient recall sequence is depicted in Figure 1-28. The initial excitation pulse is an RF pulse that typically possesses a flip angle of less than 90°. If a 90° flip angle is used, the Z component of the bulk magnetization vector is zero after the excitation pulse (Fig. 1-29A). A period of time on the order of T1 is needed for the Z component of the bulk magnetization vector to recover and allow a second pulse se-

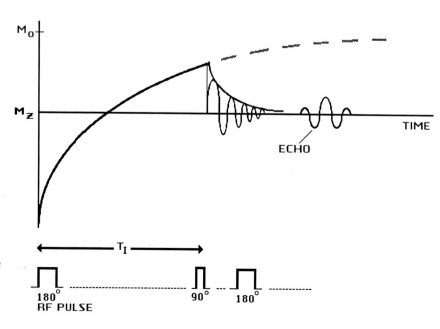

Figure 1-26

The inversion recovery pulse sequence. The inversion recovery pulse sequence is initiated by a 180° RF excitation pulse. After a time interval TI, a 90° pulse followed by a 180° refocusing pulse is used to create a standard spin echo that is sampled for image acquisition.

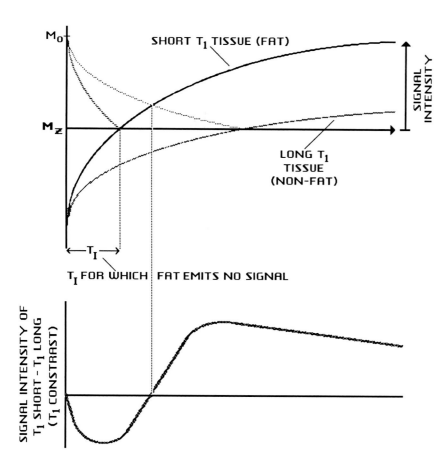

T_I FOR WHICH FAT EMITS NO SIGNAL

Figure 1-27

T1 contrast using inversion recovery pulse sequences. The strength of the signal intensity with standard inversion recovery pulse sequences is proportional to the absolute value of the Z component of the bulk magnetization vector at the time of signal sampling that is TI msec after the initial 180° excitation pulse. A short TI can be chosen so that tissues such as fat with short TR values will have a Z component of the bulk magnetization vector near zero at the time of tissue sampling. At this value, fat will emit no signal, whereas surrounding tissues with longer TRs will emit a signal. This can be used optimally to suppress unwanted fat signal when it overwhelms signal from abnormal surrounding tissue, as in bone marrow disease, or when it is responsible for unwanted motion artifacts.

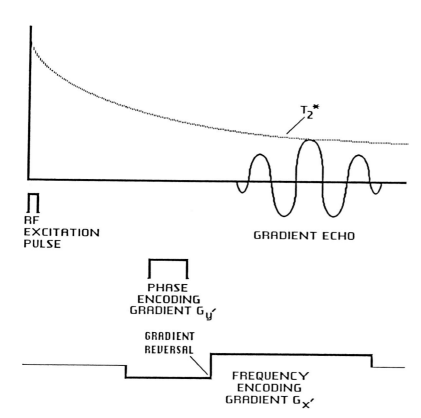

Figure 1-28

Gradient recall sequence. A highly schematic pulse sequence diagram of a theoretic gradient echo pulse sequence is shown. The sequence is initiated by an RF pulse that typically is less than 90°. It is followed by a dephasing gradient that is inverted which rephases the nuclei during data acquisition. This technique allows a phase encoded gradient as well as a frequency encoded gradient to be applied during sampling so that all necessary information to calculate a two-dimensional image using the two-dimensional Fourier transform method can be obtained during the course of a free induction decay.

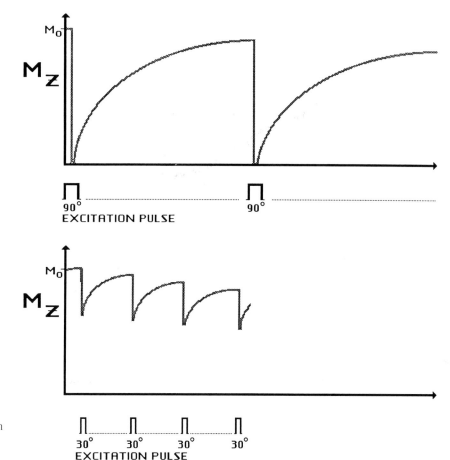

Figure 1-29

Small flip angle excitation pulses. After a standard 90° excitation pulse, the Z component of the bulk magnetization vector is zero. Time on the order of T1 is required for the Z component of bulk magnetization vector to recover, so that a second excitation pulse can generate sufficient signal. Smaller excitation pulses, such as a 30° pulse, do not decrease the Z component of bulk magnetization vector to zero, and additional excitation pulses can be used with TR values substantially less than T1.

quence to generate significant signal. If, however, the excitation pulse is less than 90°, the Z component of the bulk magnetization vector is not decreased to zero, and the subsequent excitation pulse can be separated from the first by a TR of significantly less than T1 (Fig. 1-29B). In addition, in order to maximize the resultant signal, the FID is used for data acquisition, instead of a standard spin echo with its associated long TE and signal dropoff.

In order to balance phase shifts from the readout (frequency encoding) gradient so that all phase shifts are only those specifically introduced by the phase encoding gradients, the initial readout gradient is negative, to cancel phase shifts introduced by the positive component of the frequency encoding gradient during acquisition of the signal.[11] Between the negative and positive gradient, a reversal occurs, consequently, the name *gradient reversal techniques* (see Fig. 1-28). Because of the use of partial flip angles, the TR values can be markedly shortened, to the range of 20 to 25 msec. Since image acquisition time is directly proportional to the value of TR, marked time savings over spin echo techniques can be realized. However, because the contrast parameters sampled by the gradient echo technique are

predominantly T2* effects (which, as discussed earlier, are not primarily determined by the physical–chemical properties of soft tissues), the high contrast between soft tissues obtained by spin echo technique is not routinely obtained with gradient echo images.

SURFACE COILS

The previous discussion has not detailed the actual hardware required to generate an MR image. Most of the hardware used in MR imaging is only of passing interest to the medical imager because the majority of the hardware is fixed from examination to examination and requires little operator intervention during a patient examination. This, however, is not true for *surface coils* that are critical in MR imaging of small parts, including joints (Fig. 1-30).

The most important fundamental determinant of image quality is the ratio between the signal emanated from a tissue versus the amount of noise received at the time of imaging. This ratio of signal divided by the noise is called the *signal-to-noise ratio (SNR)*. Many factors are important in the determination of SNR, including the

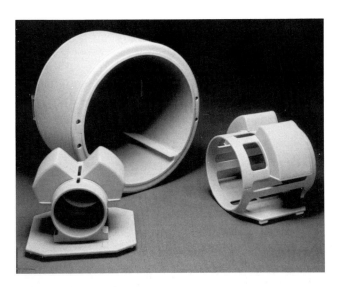

Figure 1-30

Surface coils. Typical send/receive surface coils are shown. The coil is located near the joint (*e.g.*, the knee for the coil in the lower left), which improves the filling factor and resultant image quality.

field strength of the MR imager (SNR increases with increasing magnetic field), electronic design, *EDDIE* current corrections, TR (an increase in TR is associated with an increase in SNR), TE (SNR decreases exponentially as TE increases), voxel—the volume of the smallest picture element in the image—size (SNR increases with the square root of voxel size), number of excitations (NEX; SNR increases with the square root of NEX), and efficiency of the receiving antenna. In extremity imaging, the efficiency of the receiving antenna can be markedly improved if properly designed surface coils are used.

The signal emanating from resonating nuclei are received as current in coils of wire, similar to the generation of current in an electric generator (see Fig. 1-11). The efficiency of this process is dependent on many factors, one of the most important of which is the "filling factor." This simply means that the wires of the coils should be placed as close as possible to the body part being examined. Thus, the design of surface coil is very much dependent on the anatomic area of interest.

IMAGE INTERPRETATION

An understanding of the basic principles of MR imaging can be helpful in image interpretation.[3,7] The multitude of parameters can be varied and adjusted in innumerable ways to produce images of differing contrast between soft tissues. Although the quality of this contrast is responsible for the remarkable success of MR imaging over the last 5 years, the complexity of differing param-

eters can be confusing to the novice and expert as well. This complex situation can be somewhat simplified for standard spin echo imaging by dividing the image contrast obtained into three broad categories.

The first category is a *T1-weighted image* that is obtained with a short TR and short TE spin echo pulse sequence (see p. 14) (Fig. 1-31). T1-weighted images can also be obtained using inversion recovery techniques. Tissues characteristically bright on a T1-weighted sequence include fat and paramagnetic substances (*e.g.*, gadolinium DTPA, subacute hemorrhage). Tissues with characteristic low signal intensity on T1-weighted images include tissues with a lack of mobile protons (*e.g.*, calcium, fibrous tissue), and liquids (*e.g.*, CSF, joint fluid, cysts). Tissues with intermediate signal intensity include muscle, solid organs, and hematopoietic bone marrow.

Figure 1-31

A T1-weighted image. T1-weighted images (short TR/TE spin echoes or inversion recovery) are characterized by bright signal intensity from fat (as seen in subcutaneous fat, *black curved arrow*) and low signal intensity from liquid collections *(straight arrow)*, unless associated with very high protein content or paramagnetic substances such as methemaglobin. Muscle is low to intermediate in signal intensity *(white curved arrow)*.

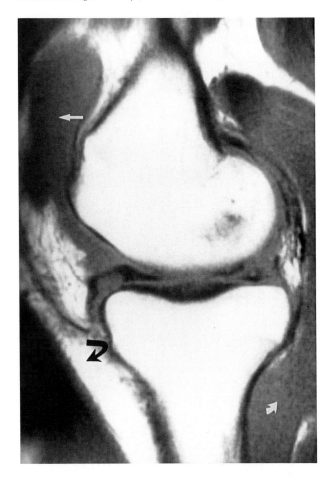

Intermediate-weighted images (balanced image, proton density image, density weighted image) are images acquired with a long TR and short TE (see p. 15; Fig. 1-32). These images typically have excellent SNR and, consequently, are excellent for depicting basic anatomy. Intermediate-weighted images have similar contrast to T1-weighted images in that fat and paramagnetic substances typically have high signal. However, collections of liquid, such as cysts, may not possess the characteristic low signal intensity seen on T1-weighted images and may be more variable in appearance depending on exact parameters chosen and the field strength of the imager used. Substances that lack mobile protons continue to have low signal intensity, as on T1-weighted images, and most solid organs including muscles have intermediate signal intensity similar to that on a T1-weighted image.

T2-weighted images are images obtained with a long TR and long TE (see p. 15; Fig. 1-33). The major advantage of T2-weighted images is that areas containing

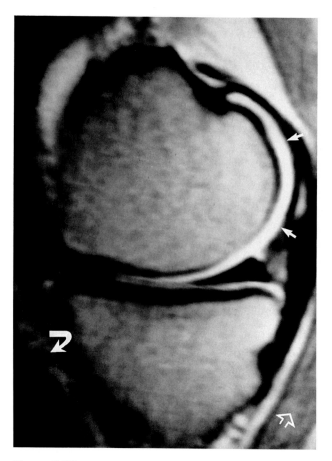

Figure 1-33

T2-weighted images (long TR/TE) are characterized by high signal intensity from liquid *(straight arrows)* and low signal intensity from fat *(curved arrow)*. Muscle and other soft tissues are typically intermediate to low in signal intensity *(open arrow)*. T2-weighted images are especially useful in detecting neoplasia, inflammation, and liquid collections because free water has high signal intensity on T2-weighted images. (See text for details.)

Figure 1-32

Intermediate-weighted images. Intermediate-weighted images (long TR, short TE) are characterized by contrast, not unlike that of T1-weighted images. The subcutaneous fat is again bright. However, liquid collections *(straight arrows)* can be more intermediate in signal intensity rather than uniformly low. Muscle and other soft tissues are usually intermediate in signal intensity on these images *(curved arrow)*.

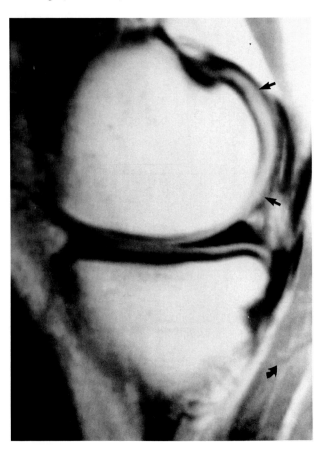

liquid or excess free water are bright in signal intensity. Many neoplasms and regions of inflammation are bright on T2-weighted images. T2-weighted images are also helpful in depicting anatomy in the region of liquid collections, such as joints with joint effusions, abscesses, and cysts. Fat has a relatively decreased signal intensity on T2-weighted images. As on intermediate and T1-weighted images, regions containing a paucity of free mobile protons, including calcium deposits and fibrous tissue, tend to have low signal intensity on T2-weighted images. Muscle and many other solid tissues have an intermediate signal intensity on T2-weighted images.

To a great degree, contrast in musculoskeletal imaging is from fat (fatty planes and marrow space of bones) highlighted against tissues of low signal intensity, including muscle and cortical bone. Therefore, T1- and intermediate-weighted images are often useful in depicting musculoskeletal anatomy. T1-weighted images have an additional advantage of shorter acquisition time and improved throughput, since imaging time is proportional to TR, which is short for T1-weighted images. However, T1-weighted images alone can be insensitive to the detection of certain important disease processes including neoplasia, inflammation, joint effusions, and cysts. Therefore, a balanced approach to imaging in the musculoskeletal system is generally taken. T1-weighted images are used for anatomic depiction, and a long TR sequence, with both short and long TE echoes, is used to obtain additional tissue characterization with intermediate and T2-weighted images of the area of interest.

Recently, much interest in the use of *gradient echo imaging* has been displayed (Fig. 1-34).[11] Gradient echoes have the advantage of shorter acquisition time for a given slice than standard spin echo imaging. Tissue contrast with the gradient echoes, however, is somewhat

Table 1-1
TR and TE pulse parameters for variously weighted images.

	T_1-W	Mixed[(2)]	T_2*-W	D-W
	*	†	‡	
TR (ms)	200-400	20-50	200-400	200-400
TE (ms)	12-15	12-15	30-60	12-15
Θ (deg.)	45-90	30-60	5-20	5-20

* T_1-W = T_1-Weighted; T_2*-Weighted; D-W = Density-Weighted.

† Steady-State Free Precession (SSFP) Regime: Signal Proportional to T_2 T_1.

‡ T_2*-Weighted.

(Wehrli FW, Shaw D, Kneeland B. Signal-to-noise, resolution, and contrast. In Principles, Methodology and Applications of Biomedical Magnetic Resonance Imaging. New York, VCH Publishers, 1987)

Figure 1-34

Gradient echo images. Contrast in gradient echo images can vary markedly depending on the TR, TE, and excitation flip angles used. In general, flow (such as CSF or vascular flow) is high in signal intensity due to flow-related enhancement. Soft tissue contrast is usually less prominent than on spin echo images. T2* gradient echo images are characterized by bright signal intensity from fluid *(solid arrow),* high signal intensity hyaline cartilage *(solid curved arrow),* and low signal intensity (dark) marrow *(open curved arrow).* Muscle and fat *(open straight arrow)* are decreased in signal intensity compared to conventional T2-weighted images. (See text for details.)

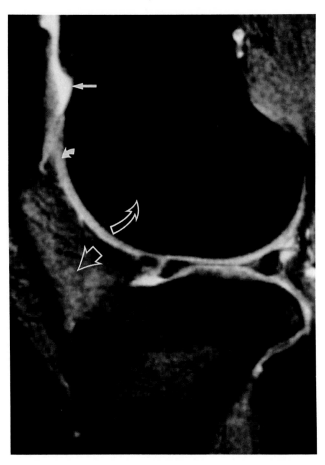

complicated by the multiple parameters utilized in gradient echo imaging (TR, TE, and flip angle). Gradient echoes, in general, are very sensitive to laminar flow with marked flow related enhancement. This is very helpful in vascular imaging (*e.g.,* the evaluation of deep vein thrombosis)[12] and evaluation of CSF (in spine imaging).[13] Parameters can also be selected to provide contrast that is somewhat similar to standard spin echo imaging (Table 1-1).[14] However, as already discussed, gradient echo contrast is less dependent on the intrinsic physical–chemical properties of a given tissue and is more dependent on extraneous field inhomogeneities than is standard spin echo imaging. Therefore, in general, soft tissue contrast is not as good with gradient echo techniques as with standard spin echo techniques.

REFERENCES

1. Damadian R: Tumor detection by nuclear magnetic resonance. Science 171:1151, 1971

2. Lauterbur PC: Image formation by induced local interactions: Examples employing nuclear magnetic resonance. Nature 242:190, 1973

3. Crues JV III, Shellock FG: Technical considerations. In Mink JR, et al (eds): Magnetic Resonance Imaging of the Knee. New York, Raven Press pp 3–27, 1987

4. Block F: Nuclear induction. Phys Rev 70: 460, 1946

5. Mitchell D, et al: The biophysical basis of tissue contrast in extracranial MR imaging. AJR 149:831, 1987

6. Fullerton GD: Basic concepts for nuclear magnetic resonance imaging. Magnetic Resonance Imaging 1:39, 1982

7. Bradley WG Jr, Tsuruda JS: MR sequence parameter optimization: An algorithmic approach. AJR 149:815, 1987

8. Gomori JM, et al: Variable appearances of subacute intracranial hematomas on high-field spin-echo MR. AJR 150:171, 1988

9. Bradley WG Jr: Flow phenomena. In Stark DD, Bradley WG (eds): Magnetic Resonance Imaging, pp 108–137. St. Louis, CV Mosby, 1987

10. Wehli FW: Principles of magnetic resonance. In Stark DD, Bradley WG (eds): Magnetic Resonance Imaging, pp 3–23. St. Louis, CV Mosby, 1987

11. Winkler ML, et al: Characteristics of partial flip angle and gradient reversal MR imaging. Radiology 166:17, 1988

12. Spritzer CE, et al: Deep venous thrombosis evaluation with limited flip angle, gradient-refocused MR imaging: Preliminary experience. Radiology 166:371, 1988

13. Enzmann DR, Rubin JB: Cervical spine: MR imaging with a partial flip angle, gradient-refocused pulse sequence, Part I: General considerations and disc disease. Radiology 166:467, 1988

14. Wehrli FW, et al: Signal-to-noise, resolution, and contrast. In Principles, Methodology and Applications of Biomedical Magnetic Resonance Imaging. New York, VCH Publishers, 1987

Sheila G. Moore
David W. Stoller

Chapter 2
PEDIATRIC MUSCULOSKELETAL MAGNETIC RESONANCE IMAGING

OUTLINE

Magnetic resonance (MR) imaging is becoming increasingly useful in the evaluation of pediatric musculoskeletal disease. It has no known deleterious biologic effects, does not require intravenous contrast agents, and utilizes no ionizing radiation. Spatial and contrast resolution of soft tissue and muscle is increased with MR. Bone marrow can be directly imaged, which is not possible with computed tomography (CT), ultrasound, or conventional radiography. The potential for tissue identification, evaluation of extent of marrow involvement, and visualization of disease processes in multiple planes using a smaller field of view (FOV) makes MR the imaging modality of choice in many pediatric bone and joint diseases.

Pediatric patients with orthopedic fixation devices and hardware (pins, screws, rods, and joint prostheses) can be safely imaged. Even at high field strengths there is no significant heating of orthopedic appliances. Most orthopedic materials (high-grade stainless steel, titanium, and cobalt-chromium) are not ferromagnetic, although local signal voids are produced. Metal artifacts commonly image with low signal intensity bordered by a rim of bright signal intensity and vary with the size, shape, number, and orientation of the metallic components. There is no artifact in children who are wearing plaster or fiberglass casts. This is especially useful in the evaluation of a child on whom an abduction cast has been applied for treatment of congenital dislocation of the hip.

IMAGING PROTOCOLS FOR PEDIATRIC MUSCULOSKELETAL DISEASE

Sedation

Sedation is usually required for any patient over the age of 2 months and under the age of 6 years. In general, 75 to 100 mg/kg of chloral hydrate is given orally one half hour prior to the examination. When this is not effective, or the child is known to have an adverse reaction to chloral hydrate, an intramuscular injection of demerol/phenergan/thorazine (DPT) or an intravenous injection of ketamine may be substituted. With low field-strength magnets (less than 0.5 Tesla), general inhalation anesthesia can be used, but at present there are no anesthesia machines that can be used near a high field-strength magnet.

When sedated with chloral hydrate or DPT, the patient should be monitored by ECG gating (which can be provided by the peripheral gating available with most commercial MR scanners), an apnea monitor, and close observation by a person in the room with the patient. We usually have at least one parent stay in the room. During general anesthesia, monitoring should include ECG gating, a capnometer, an apnea monitor, and a pulse oximeter, whenever possible.[1,2] Even with sedation, it is often desirable to swaddle the child to prevent motion; the chest, however, should not be swaddled. Although it occurs only rarely in children, any feeling of claustrophobia can be alleviated by placing the child in a prone position.

Imaging Parameters

The smallest coils possible should be used to image the extremities of a child. The head coil can usually be used in babies and infants, especially when it is desirable to compare the opposite extremity and larger FOVs are required (Fig. 2-1). Extremity and surface coils are useful in evaluating a single joint or anatomic region of interest.

Joint disease is evaluated using the guidelines established in adult patients. Thinner slice sections (3 mm) are frequently required in order to gain comprehensive joint coverage in an infant or child. An increased number of signal averages (excitations) optimizes signal-to-noise ratio (SNR) when scanning at a higher spatial resolution using small pixel volumes. Pediatric appendicular joints are usually imaged with FOVs less than 16 cm using a 256 × 256 acquisition matrix.

Routine T1-weighted protocols are supplemented with T2-weighted sequences in selected cases of acute trauma, arthritis, and neoplasia. Short TI inversion recovery (STIR) imaging sequences in at least one plane (usually coronal or sagittal) may be useful in characterizing marrow disease and tumor extension.

Figure 2-1

Head coil used in imaging pediatric patients (infants). Both extremities can be placed in the diameter of this coil.

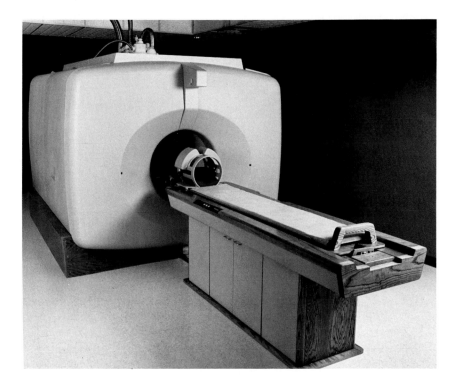

NORMAL MUSCULOSKELETAL ANATOMY IN CHILDREN

Specific knowledge of developmental changes in the immature skeleton is key to understanding the differences in MR imaging characteristics in adult and pediatric patients. Changes in marrow distribution and growth center anatomy present with unique imaging characteristics, important in evaluating the pediatric musculoskeletal system.

Marrow

A knowledge of the normal distribution of hematopoietic (red) and fatty (yellow) marrow is necessary before a complete evaluation of the marrow in the pediatric patient can be undertaken.[3–5] Fetal hematopoietic activity is seen first in the yolk sac. During the second trimester it is evident in the liver and spleen, and in the lymph nodes and marrow during the third trimester. At birth, the majority of hematopoietic activity occurs in the marrow. After birth, hematopoietic marrow is replaced by fatty marrow, beginning first peripherally and advancing centrally. By the age of 6 years the bones of the hands and feet, tibia, fibula, radius, and ulna are primarily yellow marrow, whereas hematopoietic activity remains in the femur and the axial skeleton (Fig. 2-2). The amount of red marrow decreases in these areas until, by adulthood, only 75% of the spine and 20% of the flat bones contain red marrow.

On MR examination red marrow images with low signal intensity on T1-weighted sequences and with low to intermediate signal intensity on T2-weighted sequences. In contrast, yellow marrow images with bright signal intensity on T1-weighted sequences, and with intermediate to bright signal intensity on T2-weighted sequences. With T2* gradient echo sequences, separation of red and yellow marrow is difficult. With STIR imaging sequences yellow marrow images with low signal intensity when marrow fat is set at the signal null point.

Yellow and red marrow signal intensities change with marrow involvement in inflammatory or neoplastic conditions. Familiarity with the normal imaging properties of marrow is important in evaluating underlying disease processes.

Ephiphyses

The normal ossified epiphyses, which are primarily yellow marrow, image with high signal intensity on T1- and T2-weighted sequences. The physeal plate is visualized as a low signal intensity line between the metaphysis and epiphysis on T1- and T2-weighted images (Fig. 2-3). In children, a chemical shift artifact of bright signal in-

Figure 2-3

Low signal intensity physeal plate separating bright signal intensity epiphyseal yellow marrow from low signal intensity metaphyseal red marrow *(arrow).* T1-weighted sagittal image; TR = 600 msec, TE = 20 msec.

Figure 2-2

Normal red marrow of femoral metaphysis *(open arrows)* shown in contrast to yellow marrow of epiphyseal centers and tibial diaphysis *(curved arrows).* T1-weighted coronal image; TR = 600 msec, TE = 38 msec.

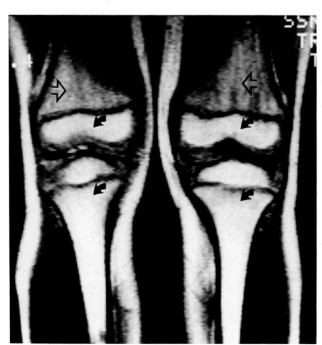

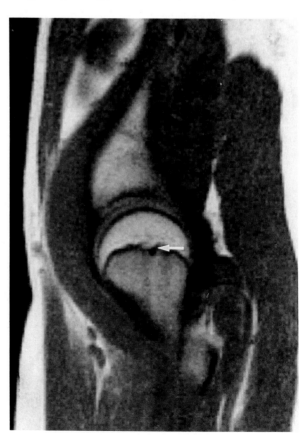

tensity may be seen paralleling the physis. This is not seen in the adult physeal scar. The cartilaginous epiphyses, such as the femoral epiphyses, are seen at birth and correspond to the size and contour of the fully formed ossified epiphyses (Fig. 2-4). In general, the signal intensity of the normal cartilaginous epiphyses is intermediate on both T1- and T2-weighted images. Occasionally, epiphyses in newborns, especially in the femoral head, may image with bright signal intensity. Clinical followup of these patients has revealed normal development of the ossified femoral epiphyses.

MUSCULOSKELETAL PATHOLOGY IN CHILDREN

Musculoskeletal Neoplasia

MR has demonstrated superior contrast discrimination in the evaluation of bone and soft tissue tumors.[6-10] A variety of malignant tissue types have prolonged T1 and T2 relaxation times, so that malignant change tends to image with low to intermediate signal intensity on T1-weighted images, and with bright signal intensity on T2-weighted images. Although CT may afford superior evaluation of cortical detail, MR is much more sensitive to marrow involvement by edema or tumor and provides superior soft tissue definition of the surrounding musculature, fascial planes, and neurovascular bundles without artifact from cortical bone. Direct multiplanar imaging facilitates improved preoperative and pretherapy evaluation of the exact extent of the lesion. Since there is minimal artifact from nonferromagnetic implants with MR, it is often possible to identify postoperative and posttreatment fibrous tissue not visualized on CT. A tu-

mor bed with postoperative scarring will image with low signal intensity on both T1- and T2-weighted images (Fig. 2-5). If, however, T1- and T2-weighted images show intermediate and high signal intensity, respectively, the possibility of recurrent tumor is more likely. With CT evaluation, this distinction often cannot be made.

MR may not be as sensitive to cortical disruption, fine periosteal reactions, and small calcifications as CT, although the sensitivity of MR versus CT needs further documentation. With proper imaging planes and resolution, we have been able to distinguish early endosteal and cortical erosions, as well as periosteal changes on MR.

In the evaluation of tumors, a combination of both T1 weighting (*e.g.*, inversion recovery [IR] or partial saturation) and T2 weighting (spin echo or gradient echo) is essential. In STIR imaging sequences, T1 and T2 contrast are additive.[11] T1-weighted images provide excellent contrast for the identification of marrow, cortical, and soft tissue involvement. In particular, T1-weighted images are important in differentiating between fat and tumor and for defining muscular planes in separate anatomic compartments. T2-weighted images are valuable in distinguishing muscle from tumor and can increase the diagnostic specificity in evaluating marrow infiltration, visualized as areas of low signal intensity on T1-weighted images.

Although each MR examination must be tailored to the patient and pathology in question, certain general guidelines can be followed. The longitudinal extent of tumors can be displayed on T1-weighted coronal or sagittal images. If the lesion is difficult to differentiate from (*i.e.*, isointense with) adjacent tissues, either a conventional spin echo or a fast-scan gradient echo T2-weighted scan should be obtained. T1- and T2-weighted

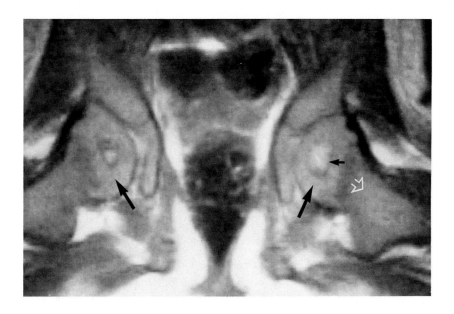

Figure 2-4

Intermediate signal intensity epiphyseal cartilage *(large arrows)* with high signal intensity ossific nucleus *(small arrow)*. Red marrow images with low signal intensity *(open arrow)*. T1-weighted coronal image; TR = 600 msec, TE = 20 msec.

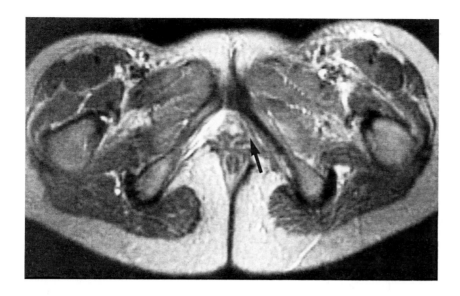

Figure 2-5

Postoperative rhabdomyosarcoma. Postoperative fibrous scarring of the pelvis *(arrow)* images with low to intermediate signal intensity. T2-weighted axial image; TR = 2000 msec, TE = 60 msec.

sequences in the axial plane provide the most important images in delineating the relationship of tumor to adjacent neurovascular structures and compartments—essential information in preoperative limb salvage planning. In addition, proximal and distal extent can be assessed by observing the extent of tumor involvement on multiple axial sections. The region of abnormality should be positioned as close to the center of the coil as possible. The patient's position, prone or supine, is determined by the area of abnormality. Prior to imaging the particular region of interest, a large FOV localizer, using an increased diameter surface coil or body coil may be necessary to exclude skip lesions or to determine accurately the proximal and distal extension in a large mass.

It is often not possible to distinguish benign from malignant lesions of bone and soft tissue on the basis of MR signal characteristics. Both benign and malignant lesions may image with low signal intensity on T1-weighted images and with bright signal intensity on T2-weighted images. Malignant lesions tend to be more extensive, involving marrow, cortical bone, and soft tissues, but these criteria cannot always be depended on to distinguish benign from malignant lesions. If the neurovascular bundle is involved, the lesion is likely to be malignant. In a recent study,[6] a low signal intensity margin surrounding a lesion was seen in 33% of patients with osteomyelitis and benign neoplasms. This margin is rarely seen in malignant lesions, and may be useful in differentiating the two.

Bone Tumors

Benign Lesions of Bone

Osteocartilaginous exostosis (osteochondroma) is one of the most common bone tumors in children. An exostosis has spongiosa and cortex that are continuous with

the adjacent shaft, with the exception of a proliferative cartilage cap. Malignant transformation into osteosarcoma is rare, but has been reported with increased frequency in cases of multiple exostoses (Fig. 2-6). The thickness and irregularity of the cartilage cap are associated with the potential for malignant degeneration. On MR examination, benign osteochondromas are isointense with normal marrow.[12] The intact cartilage cap images with intermediate signal intensity on T1-weighted images and high signal intensity on T2-weighted images. With malignant degeneration, the

Figure 2-6

Under-tubulation of the knee and exostosis *(arrows)* are imaged in multiple hereditary exostosis. T1-weighted coronal image; TR = 600 msec, TE = 20 msec.

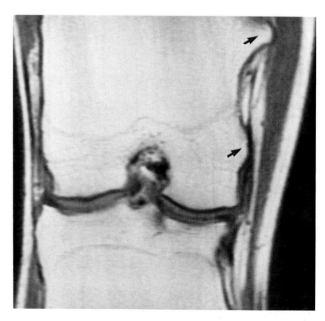

signal intensity of the exostosis is decreased on T1-weighted images and increased on T2-weighted images. Disruption of the high signal intensity cartilaginous cap may also be observed with aggressive tumor invasion.

A solitary *unicameral bone cyst* enters into the differential diagnosis for benign bone lesions. Bone cysts in pediatric patients less than 16 years of age commonly occur in the proximal humerus or femur in close proximity to the cartilaginous growth plate, and it may recur following surgical removal. Malignancy in a solitary unicameral bone cyst has been reported, but it is extremely rare. The unicameral bone cyst has a characteristic appearance on MR examination (Fig. 2-7). On T1-weighted images, it is well defined and images with low signal intensity secondary to simple fluid within the cyst. On T2-weighted images, the fluid contents image with uniform increased signal intensity. A low signal intensity peripheral border representing reactive sclerosis often demarcates this lesion.[13]

Nonossifying fibromas are frequently found in the long bones of children and are thought to represent one end of the spectrum of benign cortical defects.[14] On T1-weighted MR images these lesions are low in signal intensity and have a lobulated contour with an eccentric epicenter (Fig. 2-8).

Fibrous and *osseous fibrous dysplasia* of children image with low signal intensity on T1-weighted images and increased signal intensity on T2-weighted images (Fig. 2-9). The intracortical cystic lesions of osseous fibrous dysplasia may mimic an adamantinoma and demonstrate heterogeneity on T2-weighted images.

Aneurysmal bone cysts occur in children and young adults. The neural arches of the vertebrae and the shafts of the long bones are the most common sites. These cysts contain varying amounts of blood, fluid, and fibrous tissue. On MR examination, the lesions tend to be well circumscribed but heterogeneous, with both low and high signal intensity areas (Fig. 2-10). The expansile lesion may have internal septations, a fluid-fluid level, and areas of bright signal intensity on both T1 and T2-weighted images, depending on the chronicity of associated hemorrhage.[15]

Osteoid osteomas are benign tumors of bone, composed of osteoid and trabeculae of newly formed osseous tissue embedded in a substrate of highly vascularized osteogenic connective tissue. They are common during the first two decades of life, rarely exceed 1 cm in diameter, and are located in either the spongiosa or the cortex of the bone. On MR images the area of reactive sclerosis visualizes with low signal intensity (Fig. 2-11). Focal thickening of low signal intensity cortex may be identified. The nidus demonstrates intermediate signal intensity on T1-weighted images and intermediate to high signal intensity on more heavily

Figure 2-7

Unicameral bone cyst. **(A)** AP radiograph with lytic lesion in tibial metaphysis *(arrows)*. **(B)** T2-weighted coronal image shows uniform increased signal intensity within cyst fluid contents *(arrows)*. TR = 2000 msec, TE = 60 msec.

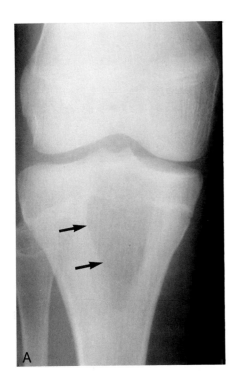
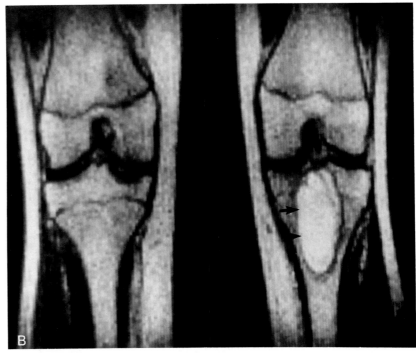

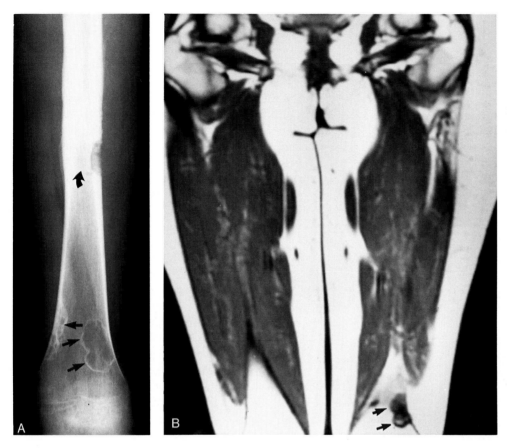

Figure 2-8

Nonossifying fibroma. *(A)* AP radiograph with sclerotic border *(arrows)*. Incidental biopsy site for Ewing sarcoma can also be seen *(curved arrow)*. *(B)* T1-weighted image shows lobulated low signal intensity in distal femoral metaphysis *(arrow)*. TR = 600 msec, TE = 20 msec.

T2-weighted images. [13,16] Associated joint effusions are not uncommon when location is intracapsular.

The solitary and diffuse lesions of *eosinophilic granuloma* (Fig. 2-12) may be confused with osteomyelitis or Ewing sarcoma on MR images. Subperiosteal new bone and high signal intensity peritumoral edema have been identified on T1- and T2-weighted images. The site of histiocytic proliferation will demonstrate increased signal intensity on T2-weighted images.

The *benign chondroblastoma* is an epiphyseal or epiphyseal-equivalent cartilage tumor occurring in the second decade. This tumor demonstrates a well-defined area of low signal intensity on T1-weighted images and heterogeneity with increased signal intensity in noncalcified chondroid matrix on T2-weighted images (Fig. 2-13).

Benign/Malignant Lesions of Bone

The *giant cell tumor* of bone originates in the distal metaphysis of the long bones and abuts the physeal plate. It does not occur in or cross the physis prior to fusion of the epiphysis and metaphysis, at which time it occupies a subchondral position. These lesions can be aggressive with malignant potential in 20%, and are usually treated by surgical removal. Metastatic disease, especially to the lungs, has been described. On MR images the giant cell tumor is visualized with low to intermediate signal intensity on T1-weighted images and high signal intensity on T2-weighted images (Fig. 2-14).[17] Heterogeneity on T2-weighted images may represent central areas of liquification, hemorrhage, or necrosis. We have used gradient refocused images to identify areas of tumor recurrence after excision and packing with methylmethacrylate (Fig. 2-15).

Malignant Lesions of Bone

Since the primary component of most malignant bone tumors has prolonged T1 and T2 tissue relaxation times, these tumors image with low signal intensity on T1-weighted images and bright signal intensity on T2-weighted images.[6] Nonuniformity of signal intensity is most evident on T2-weighted images in areas of necrosis or hemorrhage. Neurovascular bundle encasement, peritumoral edema, and irregular margins are second-

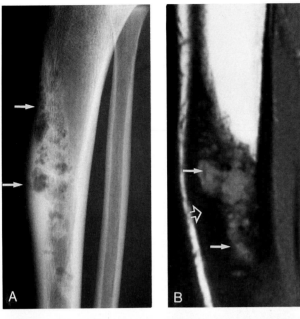

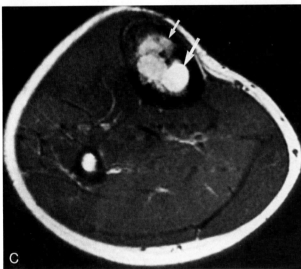

Figure 2-9
Osseous fibrous dysplasia. **(A)** Lateral radiograph showing sclerotic, bubbly lesion in the anterior tibial shaft *(arrows)*. **(B)** T1-weighted sagittal image with intermediate signal intensity fibrous dysplasia *(closed arrows)* and low signal intensity thickened cortical tissue *(open arrow)*. TR = 600 msec, TE = 20 msec. **(C)** T2-weighted axial image with increased signal intensity observed within fibrous dysplasia *(small arrow)* separate from tibial shaft *(large arrow)*. TR = 2000 msec, TE = 60 msec.

ary evidence of the malignant nature of the lesions. Except in cases of postradiation marrow edema, extensive marrow involvement by edema or tumor is highly suggestive of either a malignancy or an infection.

When there is marrow involvement in neoplastic or inflammatory disease, the MR signal characteristics depend on whether the marrow in the affected limb is yellow or red. On T1-weighted images, neoplastic or inflammatory involvement of yellow marrow visualizes

with low signal intensity within or adjacent to bright marrow fat and demonstrates increased signal intensity with progressive T2-weighting. When the affected limb is primarily red marrow, however, lesions often appear isointense with normal hematopoietic marrow on T1-weighted images, and brighten on T2-weighted images.

In the postoperative evaluation of malignant neoplasms, there may be some initial edema and inflammatory changes that image with low signal intensity on T1-weighted images and bright signal intensity on T2-weighted images. This bright signal intensity on T2-weighted images is feathery, infiltrative, and conforms to the contour of the muscle. With increasing time, the surgical field is replaced with fibrous tissue that images with low to intermediate signal intensity on both T1- and T2-weighted images (Fig. 2-16). Postoperative hematomas and seromas are well marginated, confined to the region of surgery, and demonstrate uniform increased signal intensity with long TR and TE settings (Fig. 2-17). Chronic hemorrhage with hemosiderin deposits will remain dark on T1- and T2-weighted images, because of the paramagnetic effect of iron.

Certain changes, when seen on MR followup evaluation, strongly suggest recurrence of tumor. These include (1) the reappearance of edema (characterized by low signal intensity on T1-weighted images and bright signal intensity on T2-weighted images); (2) a new area of increased signal intensity on T2-weighted images with a corresponding area of intermediate signal intensity on T1-weighted images; and (3) a change in the contour of

Figure 2-10
Aneurysmal bone cyst. Hemorrhagic fluid-fluid level *(arrow)* images with high and low signal intensity, characteristic of bone cysts. T1-weighted coronal image; TR = 1000 msec, TE = 40 msec.

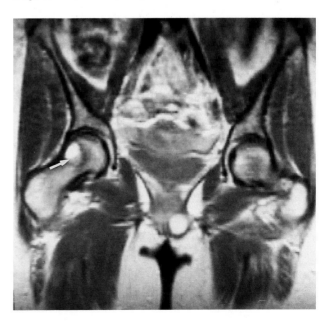

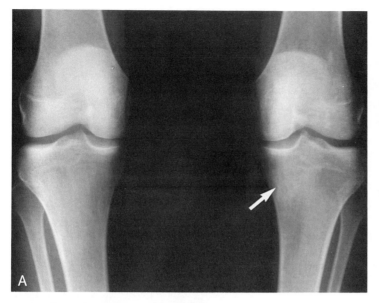

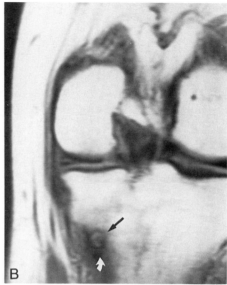

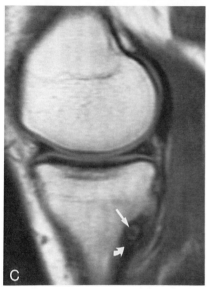

Figure 2-11

Osteoid osteoma. *(A)* AP radiograph showing focal sclerosis of the medial tibial metaphysis *(arrow)*. T1-weighted coronal *(B)* and sagittal *(C)* images demonstrate osteoid osteoma nidus *(straight arrow)* and thickened cortex *(curved arrow)*. TR = 600 msec, TE = 20 msec.

a muscle or postoperative surgical field, such that the margins are convex instead of concave.

Osteosarcoma is the most common primary malignant bone tumor in childhood.[18] It usually occurs during the second decade of life, and there is slight preponderance in males. In 96% of cases, the tumor develops in the long bones and limbs. The tumor is usually metaphyseal, destroys trabecular and cortical bone, invades the soft tissues, and may extend into the epiphysis. In numerous cases, evidence of tumor crossing the physis, not evident on conventional radiographs, has been demonstrated with MR (Fig. 2-18). Although osteosarcomas tend to image with low signal intensity on T1-weighted sequences and high signal intensity on T2-weighted sequences, specific cellular constituents can modify signal characteristics (*e.g.,* fibrous, chondroid, blastic, or telangiectatic components). There is excellent correlation between the MR appearance of the extent of marrow, cortical bone, and soft tissue involvement with the gross pathologic specimen. Lesions that are primarily blastic (and therefore sclerotic on plain films) image with low signal intensity on both T1- and T2-weighted sequences (Fig. 2-19). Even in lesions with extensive sclerosis, areas of increased signal intensity may be identified on T2-weighted images. Hemorrhagic components within telangiectatic osteosarcoma image with focal areas of high signal intensity on T1- and T2-weighted images.

Skip lesions and multiple sites of involvement are common in multicentric osteosarcoma which affects a younger age group (Fig. 2-20). In cases of parosteal osteosarcoma, the precise involvement of cortex and marrow can be assessed using sagittal plane images (Fig. 2-21). Both edema and tumor extension may encase

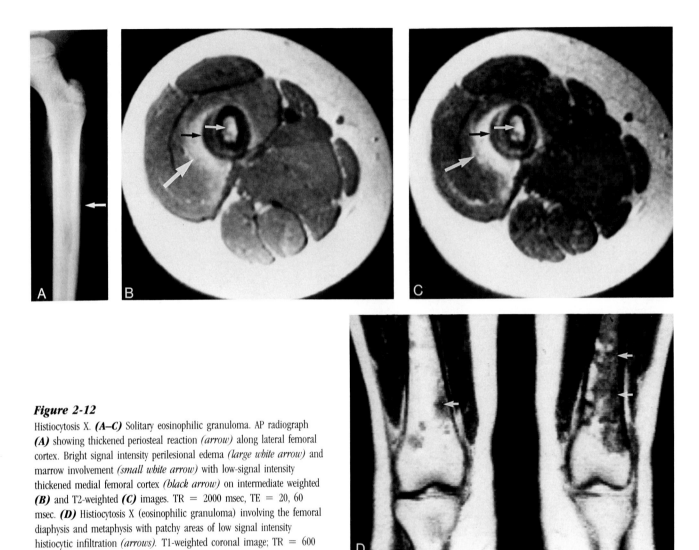

Figure 2-12

Histiocytosis X. *(A–C)* Solitary eosinophilic granuloma. AP radiograph *(A)* showing thickened periosteal reaction *(arrow)* along lateral femoral cortex. Bright signal intensity perilesional edema *(large white arrow)* and marrow involvement *(small white arrow)* with low-signal intensity thickened medial femoral cortex *(black arrow)* on intermediate weighted *(B)* and T2-weighted *(C)* images. TR = 2000 msec, TE = 20, 60 msec. *(D)* Histiocytosis X (eosinophilic granuloma) involving the femoral diaphysis and metaphysis with patchy areas of low signal intensity histiocytic infiltration *(arrows).* T1-weighted coronal image; TR = 600 msec, TE = 20 msec.

vessels, and multiple axial images are usually required to distinguish edema that conforms and tracks along specific muscle groups. MR is superior to CT in determining the exact extent of marrow involvement by tumor and edema, particularly important in limb salvage procedures (Fig. 2-22). Interval response of tumor and edema to chemotherapy can be monitored by serial MR scans prior to surgery (Fig. 2-23). In addition, radiation therapists often find direct coronal or sagittal images of the tumor helpful in planning pre- or postoperative therapeutic regimens.

Ewing sarcoma is seen primarily during the last part of the first decade and the first half of the second decade of life. It is the second most common malignant bone tumor in childhood, and although any bone in the body may be affected, the femur, ilium, humerus, and tibia are the most common sites. Ewing sarcoma images with low signal intensity on T1-weighted sequences and bright signal intensity on T2-weighted sequences (Fig.

2-24).[19] Marrow involvement is clearly delineated, with the involved marrow being hypointense with normal marrow on T1-weighted images and hyperintense with normal marrow on T2-weighted images (Fig. 2-25). MR is superior to CT or plain film radiography in the evaluation of Ewing sarcoma because the soft tissue component, which is usually substantial, is better evaluated with MR, especially in the distal extremities. Since MR provides excellent delineation of soft tissues, the extent of muscular and neurovascular involvement in extraosseous Ewing sarcoma can also be evaluated (Fig. 2-26). Ewing sarcoma originates in the bone marrow and can be identified in the early stages, before cortical erosion and periostitis have developed (Fig. 2-27).

Although extremely rare in childhood, *chondrosarcoma* arising from malignant transformation of an enchondroma in Ollier's disease has been noted (Fig. 2-28). On MR examination of a 6-year-old child, two separate sites of chondrosarcoma were imaged. On T2-

weighted images these visualized with greater signal intensity than surrounding enchondromas, with evidence of periosteal reaction and cortical transgression.[20,21]

Metastatic Disease

MR imaging is very sensitive in the evaluation of metastatic disease.[22] In general, metastatic bone disease appears as focal lesions involving both cortical bone and marrow, and images with low signal intensity on T1-weighted sequences and bright signal intensity on T2-weighted sequences. Neuroblastoma has a high frequency of metastasis to both bone and soft tissue (*e.g.,* paraspinal lesions; Fig. 2-29). Nuclear scintigraphy has produced false-positive scans and may be negative in very aggressive lesions. Metastatic deposits may be identified on MR scans in patients with negative conventional radiographs.

Soft Tissue Lesions

In the evaluation of soft tissue tumors, MR offers distinct advantages over CT[9,10,23]: both cortical and marrow involvement can be evaluated; there is improved visualiza-

tion of tissue planes surrounding the lesions; and neurovascular involvement can be evaluated without the use of intravenous contrast.

Benign soft tissue tumors are usually homogeneous, clearly marginated, and do not involve neurovascular structures. Malignant soft tissue lesions tend to be inhomogeneous, with irregular margins and surrounding muscle edema. On long TR/TE sequences (TR $\geq$ 2500 msec and TE $\geq$ 80 msec) a tumor may demonstrate higher signal intensity than associated edema.

Lipomas of the soft tissue are homogeneous and clearly marginated, with or without internal fibrous septations. They image with the signal intensity of subcutaneous fat—bright on T1-weighted images and intermediate to high on T2-weighted images (Fig. 2-30).[9]

Liposarcomas are more inhomogeneous than lipomas.[24] Those with a greater cellular component may image with lower signal intensity on T1-weighted images. Focal areas of malignant change within a lipomatous matrix visualize with intermediate signal intensity on T1-weighted images, and high signal intensity on T2-weighted images (see also Chap. 4).

Hemangiomas can occur in bone or soft tissues.

Figure 2-13

Chondroblastoma. **(A)** Chondroblastoma of the tibial epiphysis *(arrow)* images with intermediate signal intensity on T1-weighted coronal image. TR = 600 msec, TE = 20 msec. **(B)** On T2-weighted sagittal image chondroblastoma *(large arrow)* images with nonuniform increased signal intensity *(small arrow)*. TR = 2000 msec, TE = 60 msec.

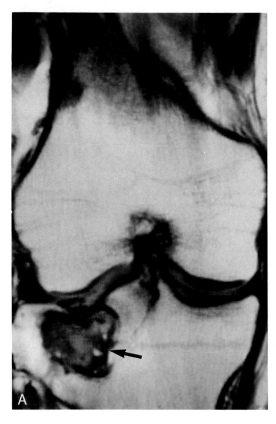
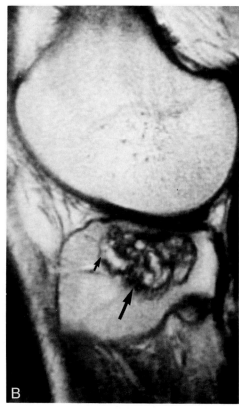

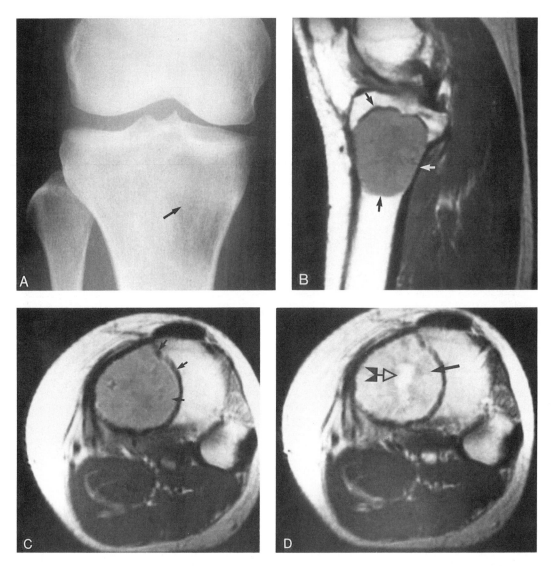

Figure 2-14

Giant cell tumor. **(A)** Lytic focus on medial tibial metaphysis and epiphysis *(arrow)*. T1-weighted sagittal **(B)** and axial **(C)** images demonstrating well-circumscribed low signal intensity tumor *(black arrows)*, with intact overlying cortex *(white arrow)*. TR = 600 msec, TE = 20 msec. **(D)** T2-weighted coronal image identifying central necrosis *(flagged arrow)* within high signal intensity lesion *(solid arrow)*. TR = 2000 msec, TE = 60 msec.

Hemangiomas generate low to intermediate signal intensity on T1-weighted images and high signal intensity on T2-weighted images (Fig. 2-31). Because of the paramagnetic effect, central hemorrhage with hemosiderin deposits or peripheral hemosiderin laden macrophages image with low signal intensity on T1- and T2-weighted images.[25]

Arteriovenous malformations of the soft tissues are visualized as an irregular tangle of vessels with low signal intensity on T1- and T2-weighted images in areas of rapidly flowing blood.[26]

Juvenile fibromatosis is a locally invasive tumor that demonstrates low signal intensity on T1- and T2-weighted images (Fig. 2-32). This tumor resembles the fibrous desmoid tumor and may recur after initial excision.

Cystic hygromas, usually found in the neck, image with the signal intensity of fluid on T1- and T2-weighted images.[27] In a case of cystic hygroma involving the axilla, recurrence after initial resection was identified on MR examination (Fig. 2-33).

Neurofibromatosis is a hereditary, hamartomatous disorder involving neuroectoderm, mesoderm, and endoderm. MR is useful, not only to evaluate the soft tissue extent of neurofibromatosis, but also to assess spinal canal, adjacent cortical bone, and marrow involve-

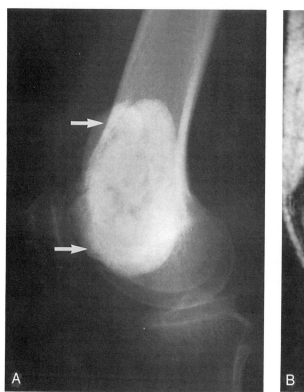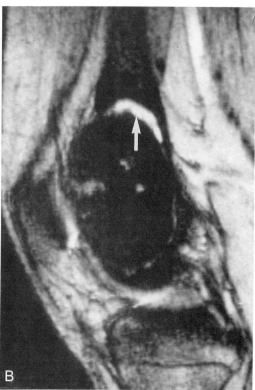

Figure 2-15

Recurrent giant cell tumor. *(A)* Lateral radiograph of methylmethacrylate packed cavity in postoperative resection of giant cell tumor *(arrows)*. *(B)* Corresponding T2* gradient echo image identifying recurrent giant cell tumor imaging with bright signal intensity *(arrow)*. Methylmethacrylate generates dark signal intensity. TR = 400 msec, TE = 30 msec, flip angle = 30°.

Figure 2-16

Postoperative osteosarcoma. *(A)* AP radiograph of limb salvage with total knee prosthesis. *(B)* Corresponding intermediate-weighted axial image identifying postoperative fibrous tissue *(solid white arrow)*, surgical incision site *(black arrow)*, and prosthesis signal artifact *(open arrow)*. TR = 1500 msec, TE = 40 msec.

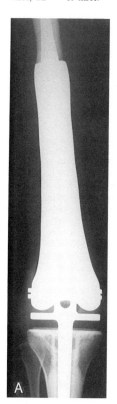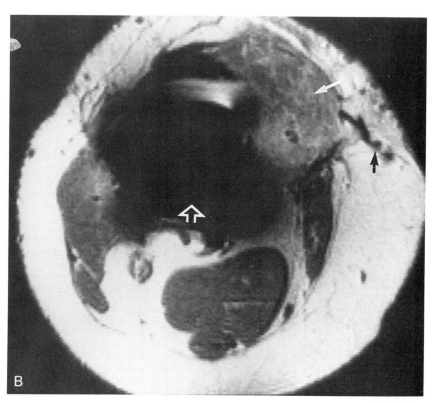

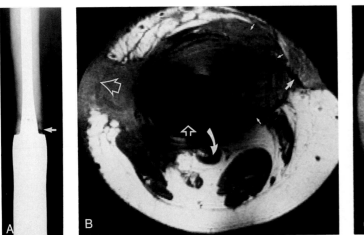
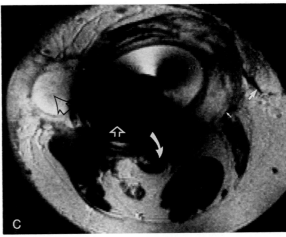

Figure 2-17

Interval postoperative osteosarcoma with infection. (See also Fig. 2-16). **(A)** AP radiograph showing cortical irregularity at prosthesis–bone interface *(arrow)*. Axial images demonstrate abscess *(large open arrow)* formation in lateral soft tissues as low signal intensity on T1-weighted images **(B)** and high signal intensity on T2-weighted images. **(C)** Metallic artifact *(small open arrow)*, fibrous tissue *(small solid arrow)*, surgical incision site *(large solid arrow)*, and popliteal vessels *(curved arrows)* are indicted. **(B)** TR = 600 msec, TE = 20 msec; **(C)** TR = 2000 msec, TE = 60 msec.

Figure 2-18

Osteosarcoma. **(A)** AP radiograph showing lytic metaphyseal-based osteosarcoma with aggressive cortical destruction *(white arrow)*. No extension of tumor is seen proximal to the physeal line *(black arrow)*. **(B)** Corresponding T1-weighted coronal image demonstrating low signal intensity marrow infiltration involving the epiphysis, metaphysis, and proximal diaphysis *(arrowheads)*. Soft tissue mass with cortical breakthrough involves the medial tibial metaphysis *(open arrow)*. Biopsy site packed with gelfoam is shown as a dark focus of low signal intensity *(curved arrow)*. TR = 800 msec, TE = 25 msec.

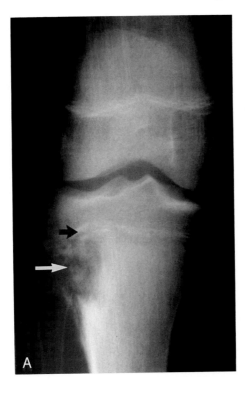
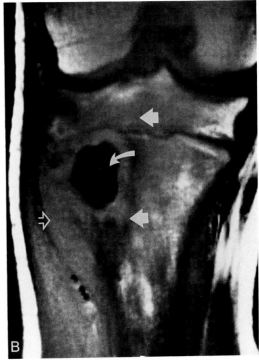

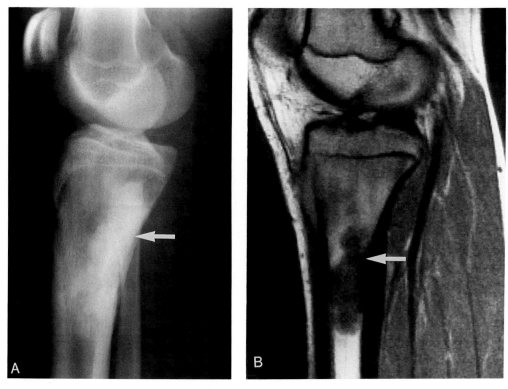

Figure 2-19

Osteoblastic osteosarcoma. *(A)* Lateral radiograph with sclerotic response *(arrow)*. *(B)* Corresponding T1-weighted sagittal image demonstrating low signal intensity in blastic tumor *(arrow)*. TR = 600 msec, TE = 20 msec.

ment.[28] Neurofibromas image with low to intermediate signal intensity on T1-weighted sequences and uniform, bright signal intensity on T2-weighted images. Plexiform may be distinguished from nonplexiform neurofibromas by the presence of longitudinal tracking along neural fasicles (Fig. 2-34).

The development of *neurofibrosarcoma* may be characterized by irregular areas of necrosis that visualize with increased heterogeneity on T1- and T2-weighted images.

Marrow Disorders

In addition to understanding the normal, age-related conversion of red to yellow marrow discussed earlier, it is also important to recognize the conversion of yellow marrow back to red marrow that appears with different disease states.[3] For instance, in diffuse hematopoietic disease, the replacement of normal hematopoietic cells in the spine with abnormal cells or marrow causes reconversion of yellow to red marrow in the femurs, ribs, sternum, and peripheral extremities. This reconversion to red marrow will visualize as a change from the normally bright signal intensity seen in fatty marrow to a low to intermediate signal intensity associated with hematopoietic marrow.

Malignant Diseases of Marrow

Several reports describing the efficacy of MR in the evaluation of *leukemia* have been published.[29,30] In children with leukemia, vertebral marrow images with diffuse low signal intensity on T1-weighted images (Fig. 2-35). With progressive T2-weighting, the affected marrow will image with increasing signal intensity. Since normal children can have low signal intensity marrow on T1-weighted images, this imaging characteristic alone cannot be used as a criterion for leukemic infiltration. Because T1 and T2 contrast properties are additive, and signal intensity from yellow or fatty marrow is nulled on STIR imaging, these sequences may provide additional diagnostic potential for identifying areas of red marrow conversion and yellow marrow replacement. By also measuring T1 relaxation time, it is possible to differentiate patients without bone marrow disease from patients with: (1) newly diagnosed acute lymphocytic leukemia (ALL), (2) ALL in relapse, and (3) ALL in remission. The T1 relaxation time is prolonged in patients with acute leukemia and with leukemia in relapse,

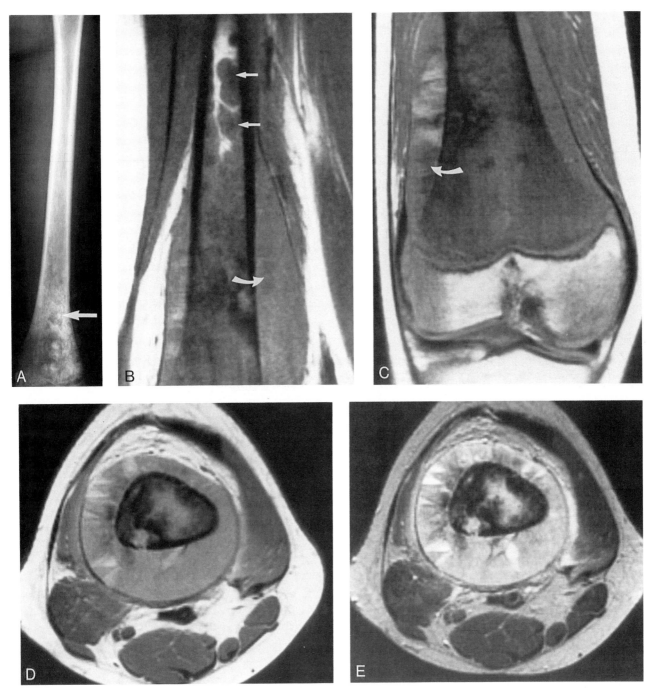

Figure 2-20

Multicentric osteosarcoma. *(A)* AP radiograph identifying distal femoral lytic sclerotic reaction. Skip lesions *(straight arrows)* identified on sagittal image *(B)* proximal to primary tumor focus on coronal image *(C)* Soft tissue mass identified *(curved arrow).* T1-weighted images; TR = 600 msec, TE = 20 msec. Intermediate *(D)* and T2-weighted *(E)* axial images demonstrating increased signal intensity in marrow and surrounding soft tissue. TR = 2000 msec, TE = 20, 60 msec.

whereas normal relaxation times are observed in patients whose disease is in remission.

Prolongation of the T1 relaxation time has also been found in patients with diffuse marrow involvement by non-Hodgkin's lymphoma, Hodgkin's lymphoma, hairy cell leukemia, acute myelogenous leukemia, and polycythemia vera. In addition, patients with reactive bone marrow (*i.e.,* a nonspecific reaction of bone marrow cells to external stimuli resulting in an increased cellularity and slight disturbance of maturation of one

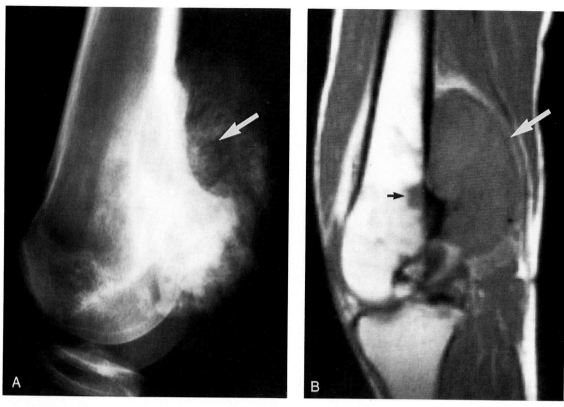

Figure 2-21

Parosteal osteosarcoma. **(A)** Lateral radiograph showing posterior sclerosis and soft tissue osteoid *(arrow).*
(B) Soft tissue parosteal osteosarcoma *(white arrow)* images with low signal intensity on T1-weighted
sagittal image. The focus of marrow involvement *(black arrow)* was not appreciated on plain film.
TR = 600 msec, TE = 20 msec.

Figure 2-22

CT and MR scans of osteosarcoma. **(A)** Axial CT scan identifying cortical breakthrough and soft tissue
mass *(arrow).* **(B)** Coronal T1-weighted image defines proximal and distal tumor extent across the physis
(black arrow), soft tissue involvement *(curved arrow),* and cortical destruction *(small white arrows),*
on a single section. TR = 600 msec, TE = 20 msec.

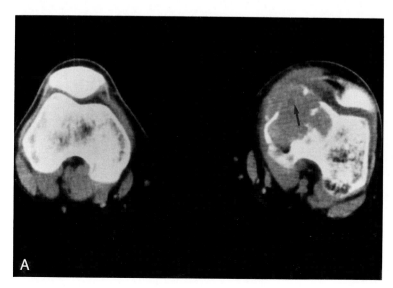
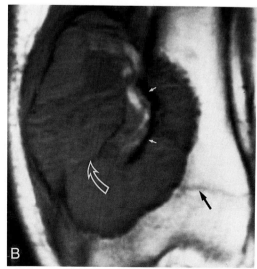

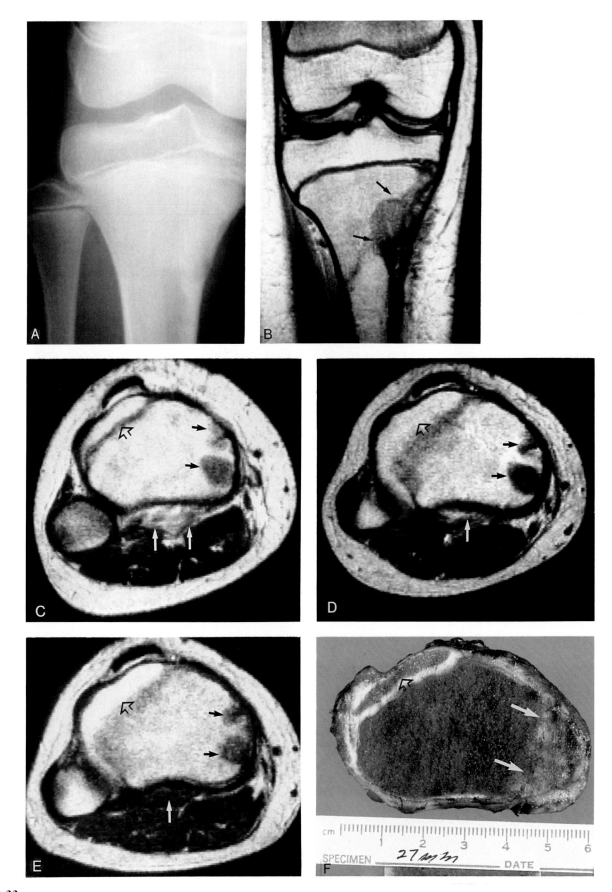

Figure 2-23

Blastic osteosarcoma. **(A)** Appearance as a sclerotic metaphyseal focus on AP radiograph **(B)** Appearance as a low signal area of marrow replacement *(arrows)* on T1-weighted coronal image. TR = 1000 msec, TE = 40 msec. **(C–E)** Interval response to monthly chemotherapy as seen on T2-weighted images. First **(C)**, second **(D)**, and third **(E)** months of treatment. While blastic foci of tumor *(black arrows)* remain unchanged, popliteus muscle edema *(white arrows)* decreases with continued chemotherapy. Unfused tibial apophysis is demarcated *(open arrow)*. TR = 2000 msec, TE = 60 msec. **(F)** Anatomic gross section identifying blastic tumor *(white arrows)* and tibial apophysis *(open arrow)*.

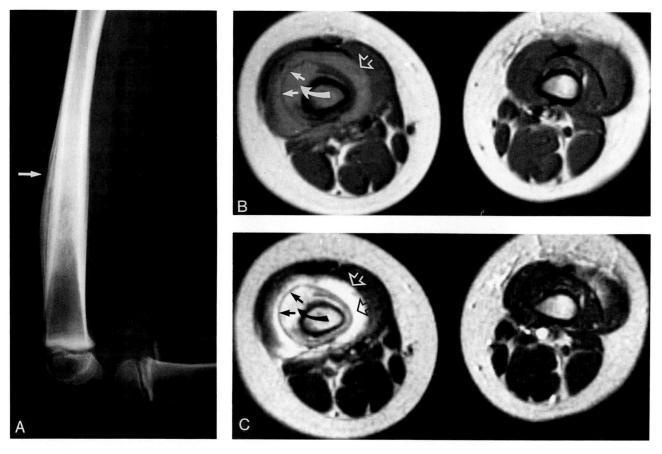

Figure 2-24

Ewing sarcoma. *(A)* Lateral radiograph showing "onion skin" type periosteal reaction in Ewing sarcoma of the femur *(arrow)*. T1-weighted *(B)* and T2-weighted *(C)* axial images defining low signal intensity periosteal reaction *(solid arrows)*, peritumoral edema *(open arrows)*, and marrow and soft tissue components *(curved arrow)*. Edema, marrow, and soft tissue components image with low signal intensity on T1-weighted image and with bright signal intensity on T2-weighted image. *(B)* TR = 600 msec, TE = 20 msec; *(C)* TR = 2000 msec, TE = 60 msec.

or several of the bone marrow cell lines) also shows a prolongation of the T1 relaxation time.[31] However, no statistically significant difference in relaxation time between marrow replaced with malignant cells, abnormal hematopoietic cells, or reactive marrow has been discovered.

In *lymphoma,* bone marrow involvement is usually focal and patchy, with low signal intensity on T1-weighted images and increased signal intensity on T2-weighted images (Fig. 2-36).[32]

Nonmalignant Diseases of Marrow

The MR appearance of bone marrow in nonmalignant diffuse hematopoietic disease depends on the predominant cell type present. In *sickle cell anemia,* the marrow shows diffuse, low intensity signal on T1-weighted images, indicating an increased population of hematopoietic precursors (Fig. 2-37). On T2-weighted images,

therefore, no significant increase in signal intensity is observed. An acute infarct in a patient with sickle cell anemia images with a low signal intensity serpiginous border, with or without associated edema.[33]

In patients with *hemolytic anemia* and diffuse deposition of iron in the marrow, there is an overall decrease in signal intensity due to the paramagnetic effect of deposited iron.

Infection

MR can be useful in the evaluation of both soft tissue and skeletal infections.[34,35] Acute pyogenic hematogenous *osteomyelitis* is primarily a disease of childhood, although adults can be affected. Most commonly, Staphylococcus is the etiologic agent, with blood-borne bacteria most frequently lodging in the terminal capillary

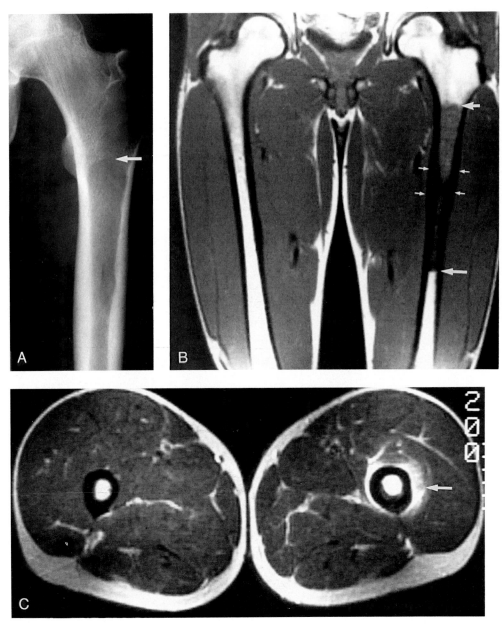

Figure 2-25

Ewing sarcoma. **(A)** AP radiograph demarcating proximal extent of medullary involvement *(arrow)*. **(B)** Corresponding T1-weighted coronal MR image identifying both proximal *(medium arrow)* and distal *(large arrow)* marrow extension and periosteal thickening *(small arrows)*. **(C)** T2-weighted axial image with high signal intensity peritumoral edema *(arrow)* without associated soft tissue mass. TR = 2000 msec, TE = 60 msec.

loops of the spongiosa near the end of the shaft. This results in the early infection of the metaphyseal marrow adjacent to the physis, and less frequent infection in the epiphysis (Fig. 2-38). Seeding in the epiphysis is caused by bacteria borne through the articular and cortical arteries or in periosteal vessels of the shaft. Following infection of the marrow, the cortical bone is soon invaded. MR imaging in acute osteomyelitis reveals marrow of low signal intensity on T1-weighted images and bright signal intensity (presumably secondary to edema) on T2-weighted images. When the acute infection extends into the surrounding soft tissues, T2-weighted images often demonstrate a subtle area of intermediate to high signal intensity in cortical bone, with increased signal intensity in surrounding muscles. Periosteal reaction may be visualized as an area of low signal intensity, lift-

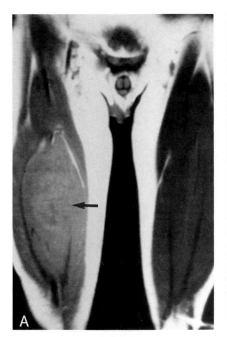

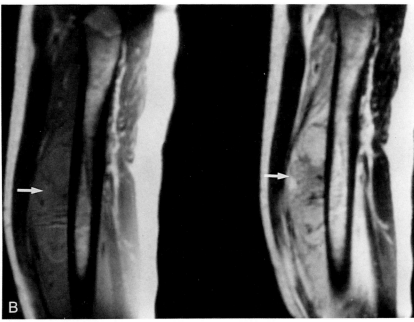

Figure 2-26

Extraosseous Ewing sarcoma *(arrow)*. *(A)* Extraosseous Ewing sarcoma images with intermediate signal intensity on balanced weighted image. TR = 1500 msec, TE = 40 msec. *(B)* Signal intensity is low on T1-weighted image *(left)* and high on T2-weighted image *(right)*. *Left,* TR = 600 msec, TE = 20 msec; *right,* TR = 2000 msec, TE = 60 msec.

Figure 2-27

Ewing sarcoma. *(A)* Early marrow involvement *(arrow)* images as a focus of decreased signal intensity on T1-weighted image. TR = 600 msec, TE = 20 msec. *(B)* On STIR image, focus of involved marrow *(arrow)* shows increased signal intensity. TR = 1400 msec, TI = 125 msec, TE = 40 msec.

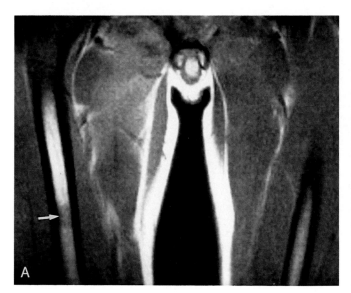

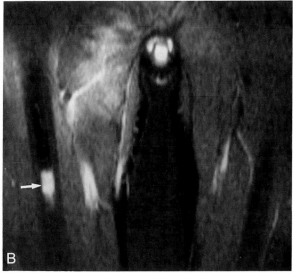

Figure 2-28

Ollier's disease. **(A)** AP forearm radiograph demonstrating proximal and distal radius lesions *(arrows)*. **(B)** T1-weighted coronal image of distal radius lesions shows satellite enchondromas *(black arrow)* and larger low signal intensity chondrosarcoma *(white arrows)*. TR = 600 msec, TE = 20 msec. Chondrosarcoma *(open arrow)* on axial T1-weighted **(C)** and T2-weighted **(D)** images demonstrating low and high signal intensity, respectively, with disruption of cortical bone *(arrows)*. **(C)** TR = 600 msec, TE = 20 msec; **(D)** TR = 2000 msec, TE = 60 msec; respectively.

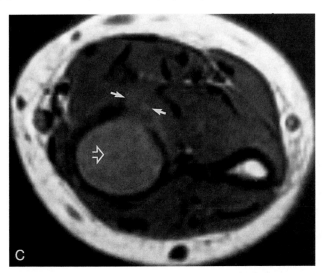

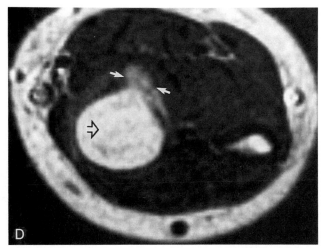

ing or extending from adjacent cortical bone. As many as one third of patients with osteomyelitis may have a low signal intensity marginated focus representing reactive bone.

Acute purulent hematogenous *joint infection* is much more common during infancy and childhood than during adult life. It can develop as a complication of bacteremias due to infections elsewhere in the body. Staphylococcal infections predominate in the hip at all ages. For children less than 6 months old or more than

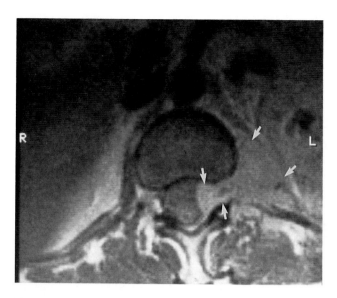

Figure 2-29

Metastatic neuroblastoma infiltrating the left neural foramina *(arrows)* on intermediate-weighted image. TR = 2000 msec, TE = 28 msec.

2 years old, Staphylococcus is the most common offending organism in all joints. Between 6 months and 2 years of life, however, Hemophilus influenzae is commonly found.

MR evaluation is useful in determining the extent of the complex joint fluid, presence of cartilaginous destruction, cortical invasion, and resultant osteomyelitis. On T1-weighted images, infected fluid is heterogeneous and of low to intermediate signal intensity that increases on T2-weighted images. Joint debris (detritus) and epiphyseal marrow inhomogeneity may be associated in the setting of a septic joint (Fig. 2-39). Often, septations and locations separate bright signal intensity pockets of

fluid. The exclusive use of signal intensity to distinguish infected from noninfected fluid, however, is not possible.

MR is sensitive to soft tissue infection and muscle inflammation. *Acute fasciitis* in a 3-year-old boy was detected as a diffuse increase in signal intensity conforming to the involved muscle group on T2-weighted images (Fig. 2-40). Corresponding gallium scintigraphy and CT were negative in this case. Soft-tissue edema in infection demonstrates low signal intensity on T1-weighted images and increased signal intensity on T2-weighted images. If soft tissue infection is suspected, MR evaluation may be the examination of choice.

Joint Diseases

Hip

MR can be used for a variety of joint disorders in the pediatric patient. In the hip, MR is a sensitive examination for the identification of *avascular necrosis (AVN)*.[36,37] In children, AVN may be secondary to steroid therapy (frequently a part of chemotherapy protocols), Cushing's syndrome, hypothyroidism, Meyer's dysplasia of the femoral head, the mucopolysaccharidoses, sickle cell anemia, or Gaucher's disease.

Legg–Calvé–Perthe's disease of the hip develops in children between the ages of 4 and 8 years, is more common in boys, and has a bilateral incidence of about 10%. The principal clinical signs are a painful limb with limitation of hip motion. Low signal intensity is visualized within the epiphyseal marrow center on T1- and T2-weighted images (Fig. 2-41). Associated findings that can be identified on MR images include: intraarticular effusion and a small, laterally displaced ossification nucleus.[38,39] Revascularization of the necrotic portion of

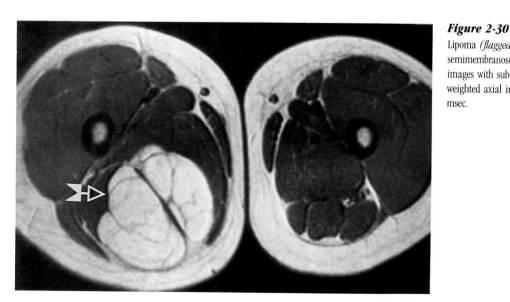

Figure 2-30

Lipoma *(flagged arrow)* located between the semimembranosus and semitendinosus muscles images with subcutaneous fat signal intensity on T1-weighted axial image. TR = 600 msec, TE = 20 msec.

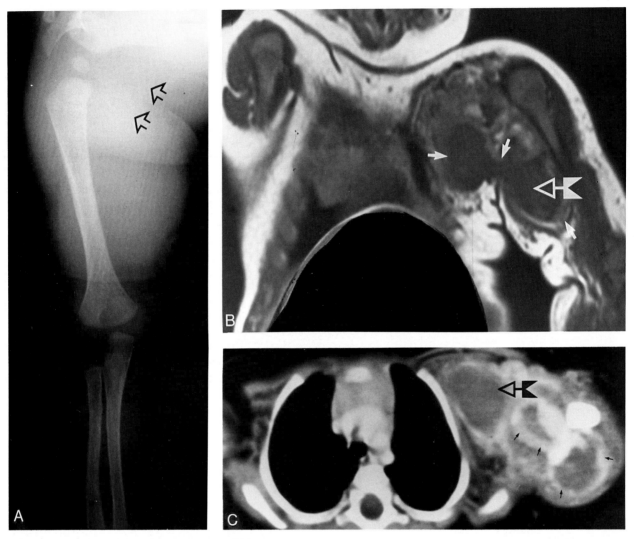

Figure 2-31
Hemangioma with hemorrhage in a 6-month-old infant. **(A)** Axillary soft tissue density seen on conventional radiograph *(open arrows)*. **(B)** Low signal intensity bilobed central hemorrhagic component *(flagged arrow)* and intermediate signal intensity wall *(solid arrows)* are visualized on T1-weighted coronal image. TR = 800 msec, TE = 20 msec. **(C)** Corresponding axial CT with contrast demonstrating vascular rim enhancement *(solid arrows)* surrounding lower attenuation hemorrhage *(flagged arrow)*.

the femoral epiphysis has been shown in a case of Legg–Calvé–Perthe's disease treated with varus osteotomy. The initial low signal intensity focus was replaced with high signal intensity marrow fat. Coxa plana and coxa magna can occur with later remodeling.

MR may also be useful in the evaluation of *physeal fractures.* We recently used MR to diagnose a case of fractured physis in the newborn (Fig. 2-42). On plain film, the metaphysis was noted to be laterally displaced, and the patient was thought to have congenital dislocation of the hip. On MR examination, the intermediate signal intensity cartilaginous femoral epiphysis was

identified and was well seated within the acetabulum. With MR, a physeal fracture was demonstrated as the cause of the laterally displaced femoral metaphysis. Had this not been noted, a coxa vara deformity of the hip would have resulted.

Slipped capital femoral epiphysis generally occurs in children and adolescents, is more frequent in boys, and is bilateral in about 20% to 25% of cases. The widened growth plate and epiphyseal slippage are clearly demonstrated on MR images (Fig. 2-43). MR may be useful in identifying early associated osteonecrosis reported in up to 15% of children.[40]

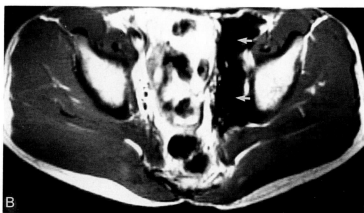

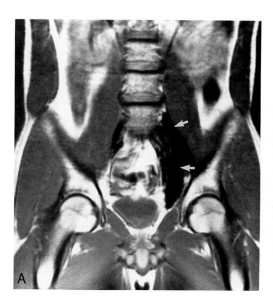

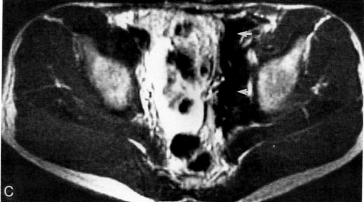

Figure 2-32

Juvenile fibromatosis. Fibrous tissue images with uniform low signal intensity *(arrows)* on T1-weighted coronal *(A)* and axial *(B)* images and on T2-weighted axial image *(C). (A and B)* TR = 800 msec, TE = msec; TR = 2000 msec, TE = 80 msec.

Figure 2-33

Cystic hygroma. *(A)* Areas of inhomogeneous low signal intensity *(small black arrows)* can be seen in the axillary subcutaneous fat on T1-weighted coronal image. TR = 500 msec, TE = 40 msec. *(B)* Fluid filled cystic structures *(arrows)* image with high signal intensity on T2-weighted axial image through the upper arm. TR = 2000 msec, TE = 60 msec.

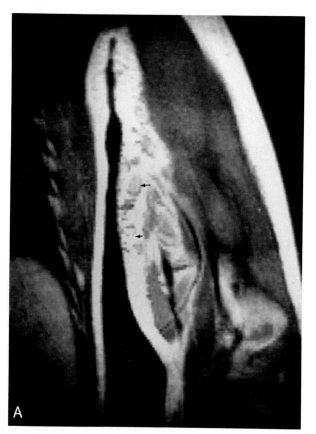

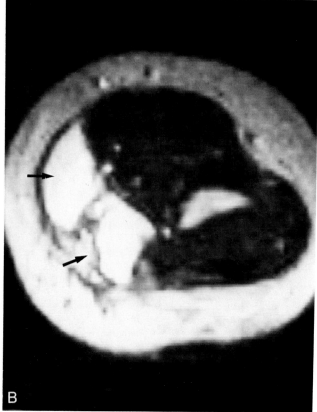

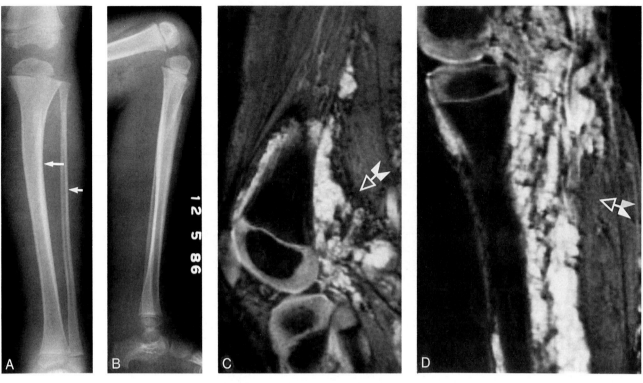

Figure 2-34

Neurofibromatosis. AP *(A)* and lateral *(B)* radiographs in a 5-year-old child with neurofibroma. Tibial dysplasia-bowing *(A, large arrow),* and a gracile fibula are shown. *(A, small arrow)* High signal intensity plexiform neurofibromas *(flagged arrow)* tracking from the popliteal fossa *(C)* to the soft tissue posterior to the tibia *(D),* as imaged on T2* gradient echo images. TR = 400 msec, TE = 30 msec, flip angle = 30°.

Figure 2-35

Marrow infiltration in acute leukemia (ALL) images with low signal intensity *(left)* compared to spine in normal age-matched control with high signal intensity fatty marrow *(right).* T1-weighted sagittal image; TR = 500 msec, TE = 28 msec.

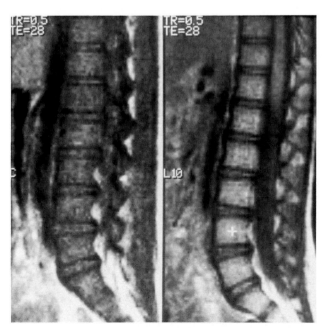

MR has been used in the evaluation of *congenital dislocation of the hip (CDH;* Fig. 2-44). T1-weighted coronal and axial images display the exact position of the intermediate signal intensity cartilaginous femoral head. This is important when the position of the femoral head is uncertain on plain film radiography and when serial followup examinations, in or out of plaster casts, are required, and obviates the need to expose the child to ionizing radiation. T2-weighted images are helpful when evaluating complications associated with CDH, such as ischemic necrosis and associated effusions.

With MR imaging, the etiology of CDH and failure to achieve adequate reduction can be determined without the use of invasive arthrography.[41] In these patients, an hourglass configuration of the acetabulum or inverted, hypertrophied limbus must be excluded. With inversion, the intermediate signal intensity limbus is often visualized in the lateral aspect of the joint, with increased fat (high signal intensity on T1-weighted images) noted medially. An interposed iliopsoas tendon crossing the joint space will prevent reduction of the femoral head in the acetabulum and can create an hourglass configuration of the joint capsule. While superolateral subluxation or dislocation is identified on coronal

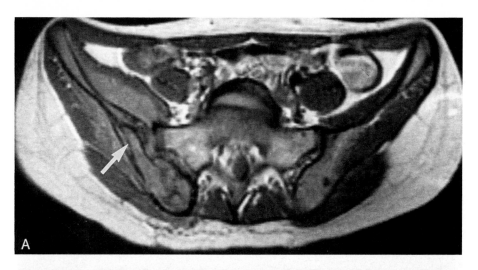

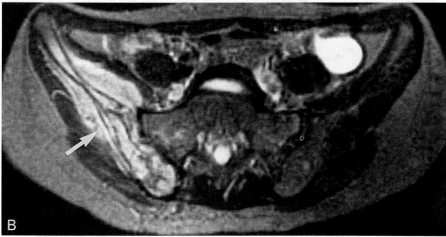

Figure 2-36

Lymphoma. **(A)** Asymmetric pattern of lymphoma involving the right ilium *(arrow)* images with low signal intensity on intermediate weighted image. TR = 2000 msec, TE = 20 msec. **(B)** Lesion images with high-signal intensity *(arrow)* on T2-weighted image. TR = 2000 msec, TE = 60 msec.

Figure 2-37

Sickle cell anemia. Diffuse low signal intensity *(arrows)* in the humeri **(A)** and pelvis **(B)** in two patients with sickle cell disease having persistent red marrow hypercellularity. T1-weighted coronal images; TR = 800 msec, TE = 20 msec.

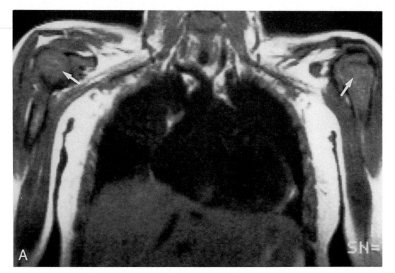

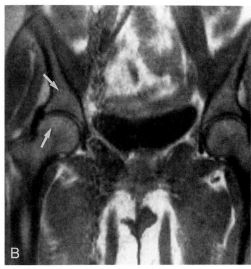

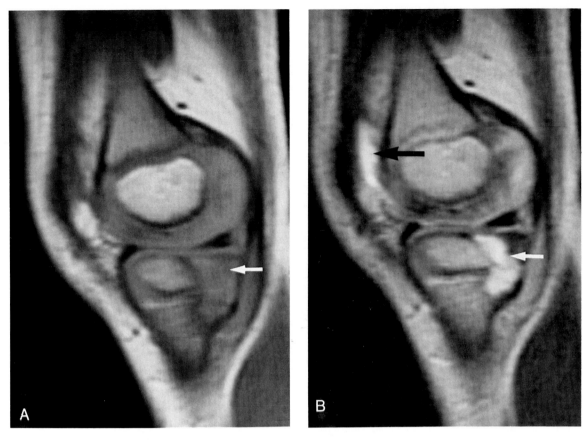

Figure 2-38

Osteomyelitis. Infection involves the metaphysis and epiphysis crossing the physeal plate *(white arrows)*.
(A) Staphylococcal osteomyelitis *(white arrow)* images with low signal intensity on T1-weighted image.
(B) On T2-weighted image osteomyelitis images with high signal intensity. Associated joint effusion
visualizes with bright signal *(black arrow)*.

Figure 2-39

Septic joint. **(A)** Joint effusion visualized on lateral radiograph. **(B)** Low signal intensity intraarticular
debris *(solid arrow)* and high signal intensity joint effusion *(open arrow)* are identified in a patient with
juvenile rheumatoid arthritis with a staphylococcal infected joint. T2-weighted sagittal image; TR = 2000
msec, TE = 60 msec.

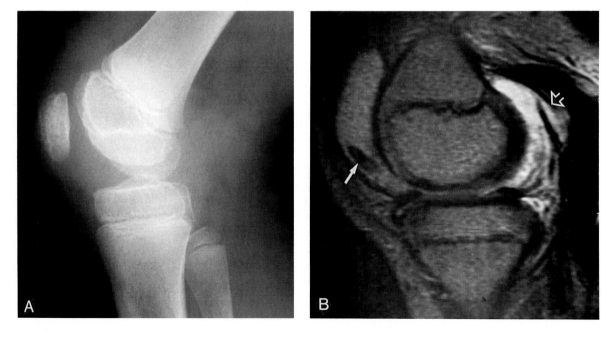

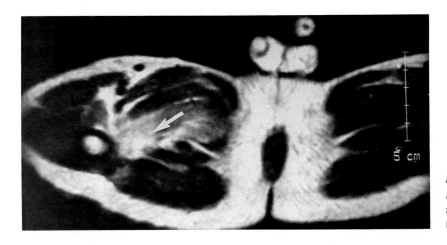

Figure 2-40

Acute fasciitis. High signal intensity edema *(arrow)* along muscle fascial plane on T2-weighted axial image. TR = 2000 msec, TE = 60 msec.

Figure 2-41

The spectrum of Legg-Calvé-Perthes disease is shown from early *(A–B)* to late advanced *(C–D)* disease on T1-weighted coronal images. TR = 600 msec, TE = 20 msec. *(A)* Small laterally displaced ossific nucleus with loss of yellow marrow signal intensity *(large black arrow)*. Normal contralateral epiphyseal cartilage *(curved arrow)* and high signal intensity marrow *(small black arrow)* are labeled. *(B)* Complete loss of right femoral epiphyseal marrow signal intensity *(arrow)*. *(C)* Low signal intensity osteonecrotic foci in the femoral epiphysis bilaterally *(arrows)*. Articular cartilage is thinner in the older child. *(D)* Advanced remodeling in Legg-Calvé-Perthes disease with coxa plana and coxa magna of the femoral heads *(arrows)*.

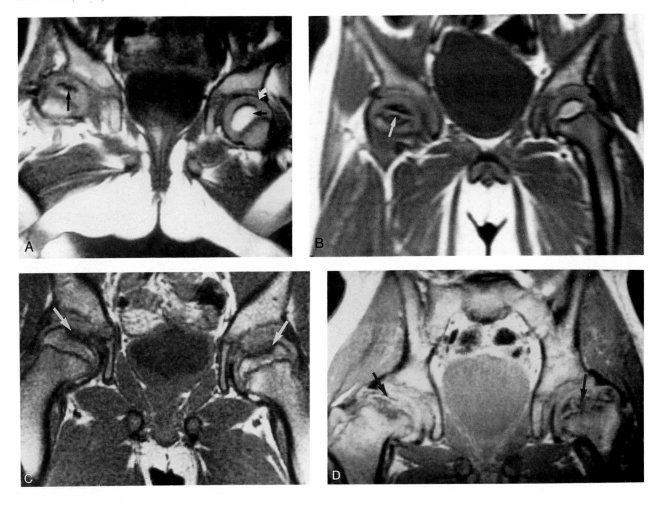

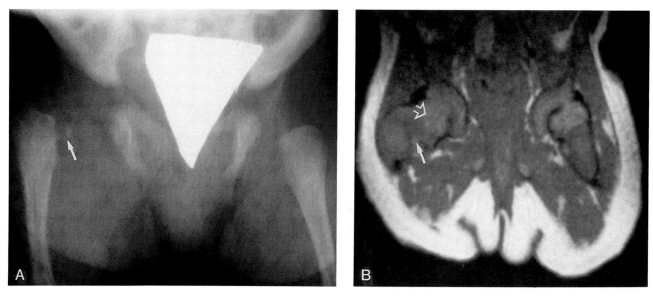

Figure 2-42

Physeal fracture. **(A)** Physeal fracture *(white arrow)* simulating congenital dislocation of the right hip on AP radiograph. **(B)** Corresponding T1-weighted coronal image identifying fracture site *(solid arrow)* and normally seated cartilaginous epiphyseal center *(open arrow)*. TR = 500 msec, TE = 30 msec.

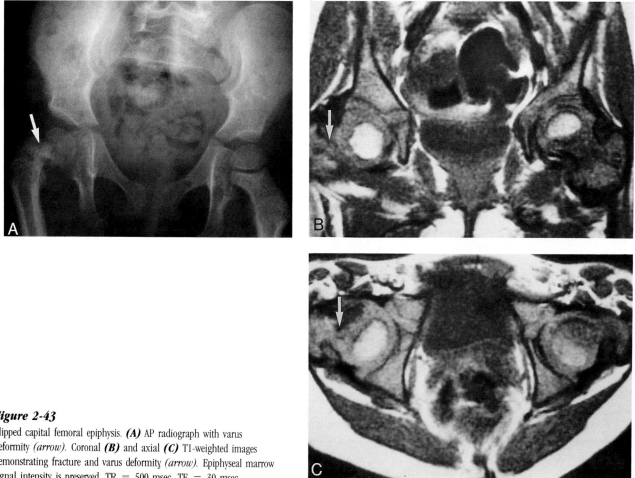

Figure 2-43

Slipped capital femoral epiphysis. **(A)** AP radiograph with varus deformity *(arrow)*. Coronal **(B)** and axial **(C)** T1-weighted images demonstrating fracture and varus deformity *(arrow)*. Epiphyseal marrow signal intensity is preserved. TR = 500 msec, TE = 30 msec.

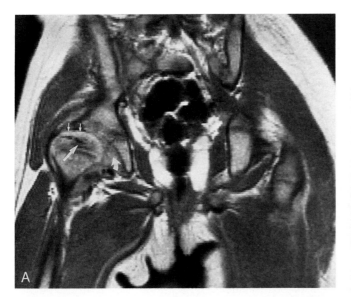

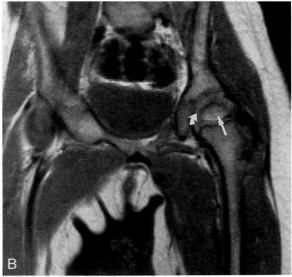

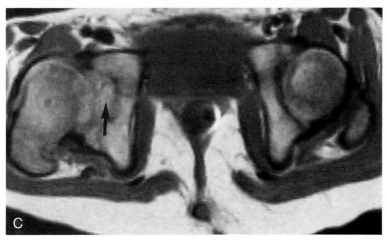

Figure 2-44

Congenital dislocation of the hip (CDH). **(A)** Superolateral subluxation of the right femoral head and interposed soft tissue *(curved arrow)* within the acetabulum. Osteonecrosis *(large straight arrow)* and flattening of the cartilaginous epiphysis *(small straight arrows)* are visualized. **(B)** Normal left hip shown for comparison with intact intermediate signal intensity articular cartilage *(curved arrow)* and bright signal intensity yellow marrow epiphyseal center *(straight arrow)*. **(C)** Axial image with interposed cartilage *(arrow)* resulting in lateral subluxation. Normal anteroposterior relationships are maintained. T1-weighted; TR = 600 msec, TE = 20 msec.

MR images, the axial plane will best demonstrate anteroposterior relationships and dysplasia of the acetabular wall (Fig. 2-45).

MR is useful in the long-term followup and postoperative evaluation of patients with CDH. There is no artifact from plaster or fiberglass abduction spica casts, allowing for noninvasive evaluations of the femoral head.

Multiple epiphyseal dysplasia is an autosomal dominant condition involving the epiphyseal chondrocyte of the growth plate with resultant joint incongruity and premature degenerative arthritis. MR demonstrates ir-

regularity of the femoral head and articular and cortical surfaces (Fig. 2-46). Joint space narrowing and secondary degenerative joint disease are present by the third or fourth decades of life.

Proximal femoral focal deficiency (PFFD) is a term used to describe the unilateral lack of or shortening of the proximal segments of the femur. A radiographic classification system (classes A–D) is based on whether or not a femoral head is present on acetabular dysplasia, and on the shape of the femoral segment.[42] We have used MR to evaluate pseudoarthrosis in subtrochanteric varus deformity (Fig. 2-47). On MR examina-

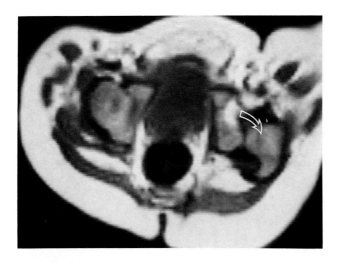

Figure 2-45

T1-weighted axial image demonstrating left posterior dislocation *(curved arrow)* in congenital dislocation of the hip. There is associated acetabular dysplasia. TR = 600 msec, TE = 20 msec.

tion, fibrous and osseous connection between the femoral head and shaft can be differentiated.

In *juvenile rheumatoid (chronic) arthritis (JRA)* of the hip, MR is useful in evaluating the contour of the femoral epiphysis, erosions, subchondral cysts, synovial proliferation, joint effusions, and subluxations (Fig. 2-48).[43] Early osteonecrosis in patients on steroids is visualized, even when plain radiographs are negative (Fig. 2-49). This is especially important when the clinical presentation is indistinguishable from joint sepsis. Early

stages of articular cartilage thinning are imaged prior to joint space narrowing on conventional radiographs (Fig. 2-50).

Diaphyseal sclerosis or *Engelman's disease* is characterized by long bone sclerosis involving both endosteal and cortical surfaces with relative sparing of the epiphysis and metaphysis. There is usually bilateral symmetry and varying degrees of pain associated with this condition. Although MR is not indicated as the initial study of choice, low signal intensity cortical thickening can be assessed without the use of ionizing radiation (Fig. 2-51).

Knee

As in the adult patient, MR of the knee in children is useful in the evaluation of trauma, arthritis, infection, and neoplasia.[44,45] Intact menisci, cruciate, and collateral ligaments can be identified in athletic injuries and congenital defects (Fig. 2-52). Degenerative changes and tears have been observed in the menisci of young children. On either sagittal or coronal MR images a discoid lateral meniscus is visualized as a slab of fibrocartilage without distinct anterior and posterior horn development. Associated cysts and tears of a discoid meniscus are commonly imaged (see also Chap. 4).

Developmental or congenital defects in the anterior cruciate ligaments are associated with a variety of conditions or syndromes. In *thrombocytopenia-absent radius (TAR) syndrome,* the lack of both cruciate ligaments, a known association, was identified with MR images obtained in the coronal and sagittal planes (Fig. 2-53).

Figure 2-46

Multiple epiphyseal dysplasia. Irregularity of the femoral head seen bilaterally *(arrows)* **(A)** AP radiograph. **(B)** T1-weighted coronal image. TR = 800 msec, TE = 20 msec.

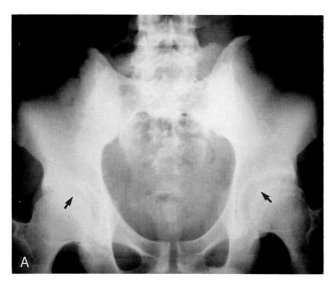

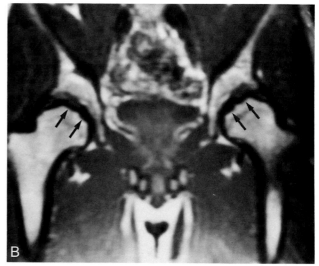

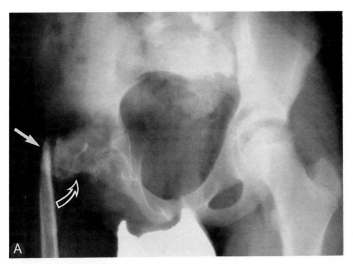
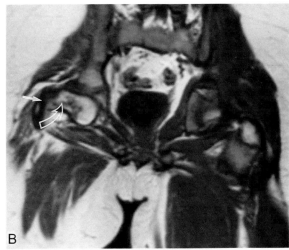
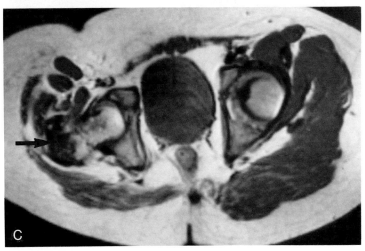

Figure 2-47
Proximal focal femoral deficiency (PFFD). AP radiograph **(A)** and T1-weighted coronal image **(B)** of
PFFD type 4, characterized by short, sharply tapered dysgenic femoral shaft *(straight arrow)* and resultant
coxa vara deformity *(curved arrow).* **(C)** T1-weighted axial image demonstrating region of low signal
intensity pseudoarthrosis *(arrow)* bridging femoral head and neck to the ossified diaphysis. TR = 600
msec, TE = 20 msec.

In *juvenile chronic arthritis* in the knee (see also
Chap. 4), early articular erosions, synovial hypertrophy,
hypoplastic menisci, effusions, synovial cysts, and osteonecrosis have been clearly identified on MR scans, when
only minimal changes were apparent on corresponding
plain radiographs (Fig. 2-54).

Hemosiderin deposits (of low signal intensity),
cartilage destruction, and intraosseous cysts are demonstrated in the spectrum of changes seen in MR examination of patients with *hemophilia* (Fig. 2-55).[46]

In a case of *Blount disease (tibia vara),* MR imaging of hypertrophy of the medial tibial plateau hyaline
cartilage, with depression of the adjacent tibial epiphysis, has been reported.[47]

PERSPECTIVE ON MR IMAGING IN MUSCULOSKELETAL DISEASE OF CHILDREN

MR offers superior imaging capabilities for studying the
immature or pediatric skeleton. Nonossified cartilaginous structures, not visible with standard radiographic
techniques, are easily identified in direct multiplanar
imaging with MR. Anatomic and pathologic assessments
of marrow disorders and neoplasia are possible in the
initial and treatment phases of these diseases. The
epiphysis and physis, unique to the growing skeleton,
are defined in normal and abnormal disease processes.

The cartilage, synovium, marrow, and cortex can be separately evaluated in infection and arthritis. In congenital and traumatic conditions, noninvasive imaging is possible in assessing ligaments, tendons, soft tissue, muscle, hyaline, and fibrocartilage structures. High spatial and contrast resolution, smaller FOVs, and shorter imaging times in examination of small and complex articulations will continue to promote the use of MR in the evaluation of pediatric musculoskeletal disease.

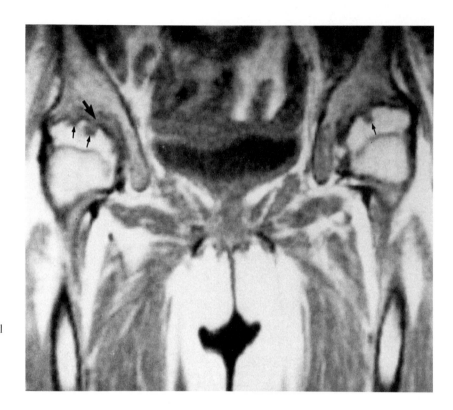

Figure 2-48
Juvenile chronic arthritis of the hips with low signal intensity subchondral cysts *(small arrows)* and denuded intermediate signal intensity hyaline articular cartilage *(large arrow)*. T1-weighted coronal image; TR = 800 msec, TE = 20 msec.

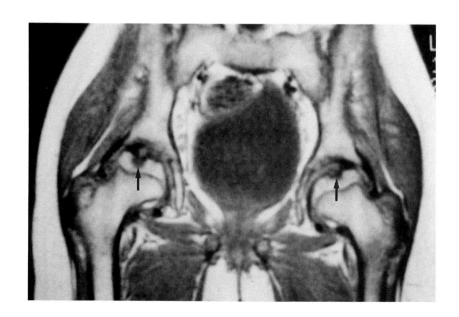

Figure 2-49
Bilateral osteonecrosis in a juvenile rheumatoid arthritic patient on steroid therapy. Necrotic foci image with low signal intensity on weight-bearing surface *(arrows)*. T1-weighted image; TR = 600 msec, TE = 20 msec.

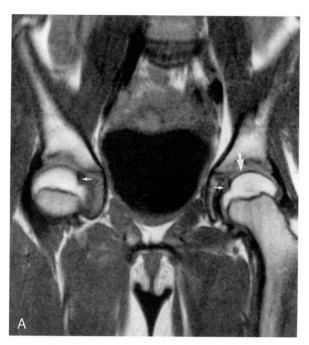
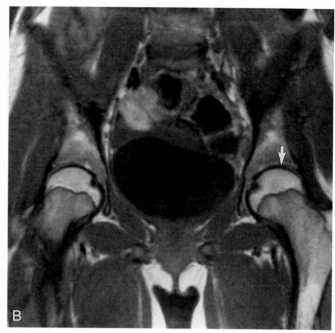

Figure 2-50

Early juvenile chronic arthritis. *(A)* Normal age-matched control hips in a 9 year old with intact, intermediate signal intensity articular cartilage *(large arrow)*. Normal low signal intensity fovea are indicated *(small arrows)*. T1-weighted coronal image; TR = 600 msec, TE = 20 msec. *(B)* Attenuated articular cartilage in the early states of juvenile rheumatoid arthritis *(arrow)*. T1-weighted coronal image; TR = 600 msec, TE = 20 msec.

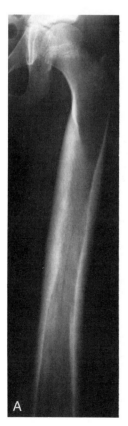
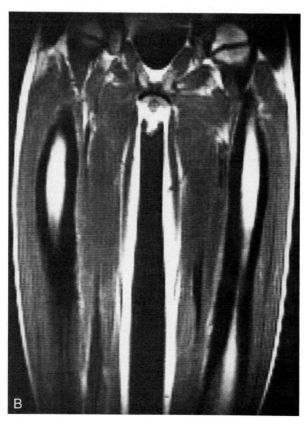

Figure 2-51

Engleman's disease. *(A)* Diaphyseal sclerosis on AP radiograph of the femur. *(B)* T1-weighted coronal MR image with low signal intensity cortical thickening. TR = 500 msec, TE = 40 msec.

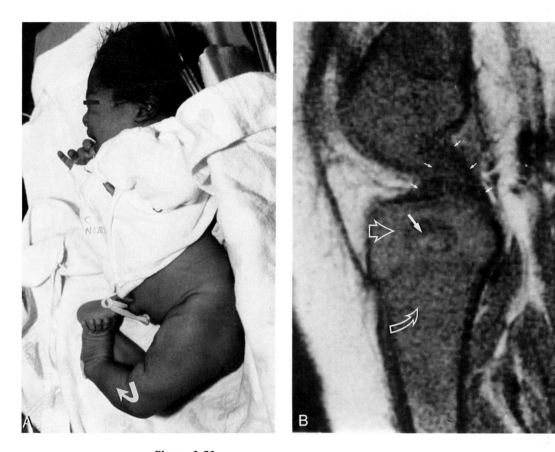

Figure 2-52

Anterior cruciate injury. **(A)** Anterior subluxation of the knee joint *(curved arrow)* in a newborn. **(B)** Corresponding T1-weighted sagittal image after closed reduction demonstrates intact posterior cruciate ligament *(three small arrows)* and tibial attachment of the anterior cruciate *(two small arrows)*. Intermediate signal intensity articular cartilage *(open straight arrow)*, low signal intensity red marrow *(curved open arrow)*, and ossific nucleus with central yellow marrow with bright signal intensity *(large solid arrow)* are visualized. T1-weighted sagittal image; TR = 600 msec, TE = 20 msec.

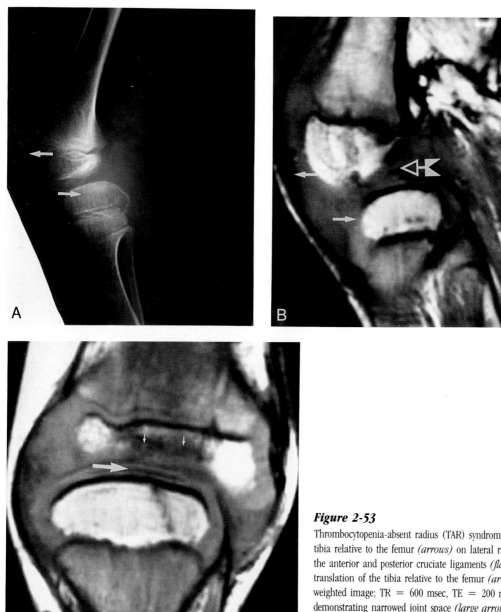

Figure 2-53

Thrombocytopenia-absent radius (TAR) syndrome. *(A)* Posterior translation of the
tibia relative to the femur *(arrows)* on lateral radiograph. *(B)* Complete absence of
the anterior and posterior cruciate ligaments *(flagged arrow)* with posterior
translation of the tibia relative to the femur *(arrows)* in the sagittal plane. T1-
weighted image; TR = 600 msec, TE = 200 msec. *(C)* Coronal image
demonstrating narrowed joint space *(large arrow)* without cruciate ligaments or an
intercondylar notch. Subchondral low signal intensity is observed within epiphyseal
yellow marrow of high signal intensity *(small arrows)*. T1-weighted image; TR =
600 msec, TE = 20 msec.

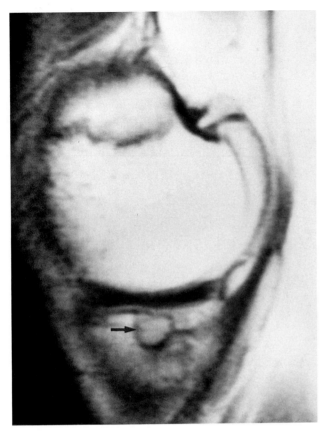

Figure 2-54

Subarticular cyst *(arrow)* in juvenile rheumatoid arthritis. T1-weighted sagittal image; TR = 800 msec, TE = 20 msec.

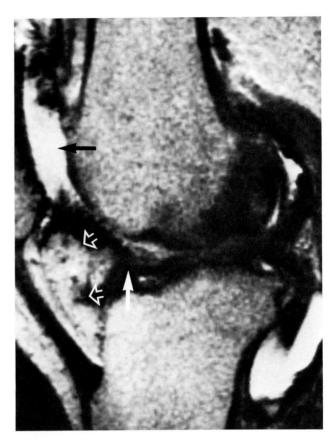

Figure 2-55

Hemophiliac with bright signal intensity joint effusion *(black arrow).* Low signal intensity hemosiderin *(closed white arrow)* is deposited in a thickened synovium, overlying an irregular infrapatellar fat pad *(open white arrows).*

REFERENCES

1. McArdle CB, et al: Monitoring of the neonate undergoing MR imaging: Technical considerations. Radiology 159:223, 1986

2. Roth JL, et al: Patient monitoring during magnetic resonance imaging. Anesthesiology 145:903, 1985

3. Cohen MD, et al: Magnetic resonance imaging of bone marrow in children. Radiology 151:715, 1984

4. Moore SG, et al: Bone marrow in children with acute lymphatic leukemia: MR relaxation times. Radiology 160:237, 1986

5. Kangarloo H, et al: MR imaging of bone marrow in children. JCAT 10:205, 1986

6. Zimmer WD, et al: Magnetic resonance imaging of bone tumors: Comparison with CT. Radiology 155:709, 1985

7. Bloem JL, et al: Magnetic resonance imaging of primary malignant bone tumors. RadioGraphics 7:425, 1987

8. Wetzel LH, et al: A comparison of MR imaging and CT in the evaluation of musculoskeletal masses. RadioGraphics 7:851, 1987

9. Petasnick JP, et al: Soft-tissue masses of the locomotor system: Comparison of MR imaging with CT. Radiology 160:125, 1986

10. Totty WG, et al: Soft-tissue tumors: MR imaging. Radiology 160:135, 1986

11. Porter B, et al: Magnetic resonance imaging of bone marrow disorders. Radiol Clin North America June, 1986

12. Lee JK, et al: MR imaging of solitary osteochondromas: Report of eight cases. AJR 149:557, 1987

13. Harms SE: MRI of the musculoskeletal system. In Scott WW, et al (eds): CT of the Musculoskeletal System, pp 171–206. New York, Churchill Livingstone, 1987

14. Resnick D, Niwayama, G: Diagnosis of Bone and Joint Disorders, 2nd ed, Vol 6, pp 3739–3746. Philadelphia, WB Saunders, 1988

15. Beltran J, et al: Aneurysmal bone cysts: MR imaging at 1.5T. Radiology 158:689, 1986

16. Glass RBJ, et al: MR imaging of osteoid osteoma. JCAT 10:1065, 1986

17. Brady TJ, et al: NMR imaging of forearms in healthy volunteers and patients with giant-cell tumors of bone. Radiology 144:549, 1982

18. Sundaram M, et al: Magnetic resonance imaging of osteosarcoma. Skeletal Radiol 16:23, 1987

19. Boyko OB, et al: MR imaging of osteogenic and Ewing's sarcoma. AJR 148:317, 1987

20. Berquist TH, et al: Magnetic Resonance of the Musculoskeletal System, pp 85–107. New York, Raven Press, 1987

21. Hudson TM et al: Magnetic resonance imaging of bone and soft tissue tumors: Early experience in 31 patients compared with computed tomography. Skeletal Radiol 13:134, 1985

22. Moon KL, et al: Musculoskeletal applications of nuclear magnetic resonance. Radiology 147:161, 1983

23. Sundaram M, et al: Soft-tissue masses: Histologic basis for decreased signal (short T2) on T2-weighted MR images. AJR 148:1247, 1987

24. Dooms GC, et al: Lipomatous tumors and tumors with fatty component: MR imaging potential and comparison of MR and CT results. Radiology 157:479, 1985

25. Levine E. et al: MR imaging and CT of extrahepatic cavernous hemangiomas. AJR 147:1299, 1986

26. Cohen JM, et al: Arteriovenous malformations of the extremities: MR imaging. Radiology, 158:475, 1986

27. McCarthy SM, et al: Magnetic resonance imaging of fetal anomalies in utero: Early experience. AJR 145:677, 1985

28. Levine E, et al: Malignant nerve-sheath neoplasms in neurofibromatosis: Distinction from benign tumors by using imaging techniques. AJR 149:1059, 1987

29. Moore SG, et al: Magnetic resonance relaxation times of the marrow in children with acute lymphocytic leukemia. Radiology 160:237, 1986

30. Olson DO, et al: Magnetic resonance imaging of the bone marrow in patients with leukemia, aplastic anemia, and lymphoma. Presented at the annual Meeting of Society Magnetic Resonance Medicine, London, August 1985.

31. Nyman R, et al: Magnetic resonance imaging in diffuse malignant bone marrow diseases. Acta Radiologica 28:199, 1987

32. Shields AF, et al: The detection of bone marrow involvement by lymphoma using magnetic resonance imaging. J Clinical Oncology 5:225, 1987

33. Rao BM, et al: Painful sickle cell crisis: Bone marrow patterns observed with MR imaging. Radiology 161:211, 1986

34. Beltran J, et al: Infections of the musculoskeletal system: High field strength MR imaging. Radiology 164:449, 1987

35. Modic MR, et al: Magnetic resonance imaging of musculoskeletal infections. Radiol Clin North America 24:247, 1986

36. Mitchell DG, et al: Avascular necrosis of the femoral head: Morphologic assessment by MR imaging, with CT correlation. Radiology 161:739, 1986

37. Mitchell MD, et al: Avascular necrosis of the hip: Comparison of MR, CT, and scintigraphy. AJR 147:67, 1986

38. Easton EJ Jr, et al: MR imaging and scintigraphy in Legg-Perthes disease: Diagnosis, treatment, and prognosis, Radiology 165(P):35, 1987

39. Heuck A, et al: MR imaging in the evaluation of Legg-Perthes disease. Radiology 165(P):83, 1987

40. Resnick D, Niwayama, G: Diagnosis of Bone and Joint Disorders, 2nd ed, Vol 5, pp 2962–2964. Philadelphia, WB Saunders, 1988

41. Lang P, et al: Three-dimensional CT and MR imaging in congenital dislocation of the hip: Technical considerations. Radiology 165(P):279, 1987

42. Hillmann JS, et al: Proximal femoral focal deficiency: Radiologic analysis of 49 cases. Radiology 165:769, 1987

43. Stoller DW, et al: MRI in juvenile rheumatoid (chronic) arthritis. Presented to the Association of University Radiologists, Charleston, South Carolina, March 22–27, 1987

44. Reicher MA, et al: MR imaging of the knee, part I: Traumatic disorders. Radiology 162:547, 1987

45. Hartzman S, et al: MR imaging of the knee, part II: Chronic disorders. Radiology 162:553, 1987

46. Stoller DW, Genant HK: MR imaging of knee arthritides. Radiology 165(P):233, 1987

47. Reicher MA: Osteonecrosis, osteochondrosis, and osteochondritis. In Mink JH, et al (eds): Magnetic Resonance Imaging of the Knee, pp 113–122. New York, Raven Press, 1987

David W. Stoller

Chapter 3   THE ANKLE AND FOOT

Routine evaluation of the ankle joint is usually accomplished with anteroposterior (AP), lateral, and mortise radiographs. In patients with foot trauma, an additional oblique view may be obtained. Less frequently, arthrography and tenography may be used, primarily in the evaluation of ligamentous tears and articular cartilage defects. In tarsal coalitions and in sustentacular trauma, computed tomography (CT) scans have been used to delineate talocalcaneal, transverse tarsal, and tibiotalar joint anatomy.[1] CT is limited, however, to the specified plane of section (axial or modified coronal), and is dependent on reformatted images for visualization in the other orthogonal planes. With a surface coil, magnetic resonance (MR) imaging of the ankle provides high tissue contrast and excellent spatial resolution, affording superior depiction of complex soft tissue anatomy, including muscles, ligaments, and tendons. In addition, marrow and cortical bone definition permit increased sensitivity in the detection of fractures, cysts, infections, and trauma. The unique ability to image hyaline articular cartilage directly with MR has made MR valuable in assessing arthritis and transchondral fractures, and in identifying intraarticular loose bodies.

IMAGING PROTOCOLS FOR THE ANKLE AND FOOT

High resolution anatomic images of the ankle and foot are obtained with a dedicated extremity surface coil using a 12 to 16 cm field of view (FOV) and a 256 × 256 acquisition matrix (Fig. 3-1).

Routine T1-weighted axial, sagittal, and coronal images are obtained with a repetition time (TR) of 600 to 800 msec and an echo time (TE) of 20 msec. Thin (5 mm) sections—contiguous interleaved or with a 1mm

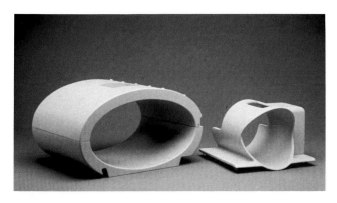

Figure 3-1

Extremity surface coil. Clam shaped coil *(left)* for bilateral evaluation of the ankles. Smaller extremity coil for unilateral imaging of the ankle or foot *(right)*.

interslice gap—are preferred. T2-weighted images are generated with a TR of 1500 to 2000 msec, and a TE of 20 and 60 to 80 msec. With the use of a proper extremity coil (providing an optimum signal-to-noise ratio), T1- and T2-weighted sequences can be performed at one excitation (NEX).

When a FOV less than 16 cm is used in either the coronal or sagittal plane, a wrap-around or aliasing artifact may occur. Use of a "no phase-wrap" technique may compensate for this artifact.

Gradient echo techniques can be used to generate effective T2 (T2*)-weighted contrast using a partial flip angle of less than 90°.[2] By placing both legs within the circular extremity coil, comparison with the contralateral ankle and foot can be achieved. Alternatively, when smaller FOVs are needed, the extremities may be imaged one at a time by repositioning the surface coil. The foot is usually placed in a neutral position, although partial plantar flexion may be useful when comparing MR images to a CT ankle exam that was performed with 45° tibiotalar orientation.

NORMAL MR ANATOMY OF THE ANKLE AND FOOT

Axial Images

In the axial plane, images of the neutral-positioned foot show the full-length display of the anterior and posterior talofibular ligaments.[3] It has been reported that the calcaneofibular ligament is optimally visualized in 40° of plantar flexion.[3] Superior to the lateral malleolus, the tendons of the extensor digitorum longus, extensor hallucis longus, and tibialis anterior occupy the anterior compartment. The tendons of the anterolateral peroneus longus and peroneus brevis are seen posterior to the distal fibula. At the level of the upper ankle, the pos-

terior ankle compartment is composed of the flexor hallucis longus muscle (laterally), the flexor digitorum longus tendon (medially), and the tibialis posterior tendon (anteriorly; Fig. 3-2).[4] The posterior talofibular ligament is best imaged at the level of the midankle joint proper (Fig. 3-3). The sural nerve, imaged with intermediate signal intensity, is located posteromedial to the peroneus brevis muscle (Fig. 3-4). The deltoid ligament can be visualized spanning the medial malleolus and talus. The Achilles tendon, the continuation of the more proximal gastrocnemius tendon, is identified in cross section as a thick structure of low signal intensity, posterior to the soleus muscle. In axial images through the foot, the tendons of the flexor hallucis brevis and longus muscles are seen posterior to the first metatarsal and cuneiform. The longitudinally oriented quadratus plantae and abductor hallucis muscles are seen medial to the calcaneus

Figure 3-2

Axial image through the upper ankle. Distal tibia *(1)*, fibula *(2)*, tibialis anterior tendon *(3)*, extensor hallucis longus tendon *(4)*, extensor digitorum longus *(5)*, flexor hallucis longus tendon and muscle *(6)*, soleus muscle *(7)*, calcaneal tendon *(8)*, tibialis posterior tendon *(9)*, flexor digitorum longus tendon *(10)*, posterior tibial artery and vein *(11)*, posterior talofibular ligament *(12)*. *Small arrow* marks the peroneus brevis muscle. T1-weighted image; TR = 600 msec, TE = 20 msec.

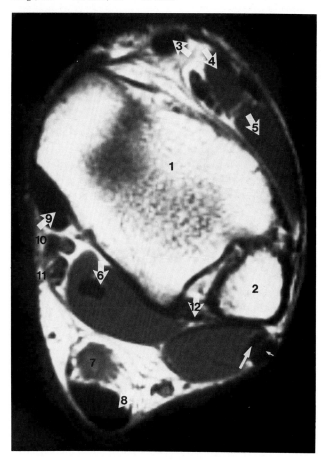

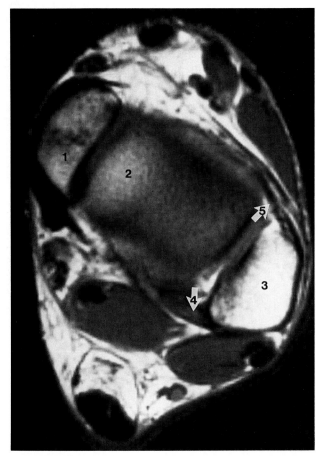

Figure 3-3
Axial image through the mid ankle joint. Medial malleolus *(1)*, talus *(2)*, lateral malleolus *(3)*, posterior talofibular ligament *(4)*, anterior talofibular ligament *(5)*. T1-weighted image; TR = 600 msec, TE = 20 msec.

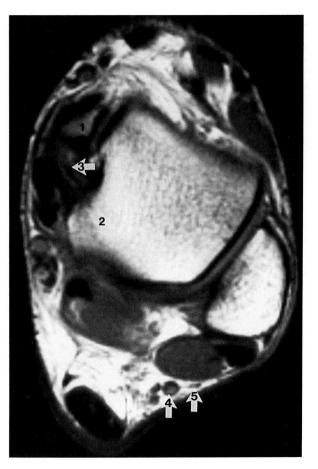

Figure 3-4
Axial image through the lower ankle joint. Medial malleolus *(1)*, talus *(2)*, deltoid ligament *(3)*, small saphenous vein *(4)*, sural nerve *(5)*. T1-weighted image; TR = 600 msec, TE = 20 msec.

Figure 3-5
Sagittal image of the medial ankle. Tibialis posterior tendon *(1)*, flexor digitorum longus tendon *(2)*, abductor digiti minimi muscle *(3)*, calcaneus *(4)*, tibia *(5)*. T1-weighted image; TR = 600 msec, TE = 20 msec.

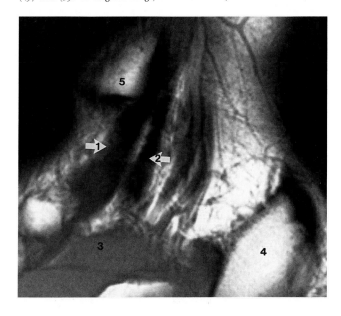

and cuboid. The anterior neurovascular bundle (the anterior tibial artery and vein and deep peroneal nerve) is visualized posterior to the extensor tendons, whereas the posterior neurovascular bundle (the posterior tibial artery and vein and tibial nerve) is situated posterior to the flexor digitorum and flexor hallucis longus tendons.[5]

Sagittal Images

On sagittal planar images the long axis of tendons crossing the ankle joint are displayed.[5] In the plane of the medial malleolus the tibialis posterior and flexor digitorum longus tendons track directly posterior to the medial malleolus (Fig. 3-5). The deltoid ligament (the tibiocalcaneal, tibionavicular, and anterior and posterior tibiotalar ligaments) appears as a wide band of low signal intensity radiating from the distal tibia (medial malleolus) to the tuberosity of the navicular, talus, and sustentaculum tali.[4] The flexor hallucis longus tendon courses inferior to the sustentaculum tali (Fig. 3-6). Separate hyaline articular surfaces of the distal tibia and

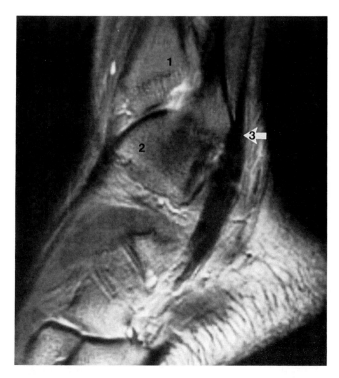

Figure 3-6
Sagittal image of the medial midankle. Tibia *(1)*, talus *(2)*, flexor hallucis longus tendon *(3)*. T1-weighted image; TR = 600 msec, TE = 20 msec.

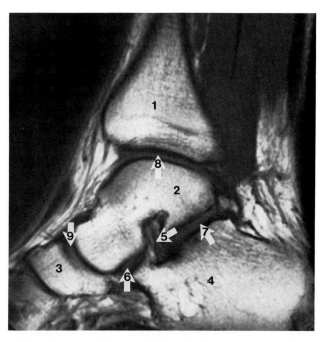

Figure 3-7
Sagittal image of the midankle. Tibia *(1)*, talus *(2)*, navicular *(3)*, calcaneus *(4)*, interosseous ligament *(5)*, midtalocalcaneal joint *(6)*, posterior talocalcaneal joint *(7)*, tibiotalar joint *(8)*, talonavicular joint *(9)*. T1-weighted image; TR = 600 msec, TE = 20 msec.

talar dome are optimally imaged in the plane of the midankle joint (Figs. 3-7 and 3-8). The hyaline articular cartilage surfaces of the tibiotalar, talonavicular, and subtalar joints image with intermediate signal intensity (on T1- or T2-weighted images) and are optimally visualized in the sagittal plane. The interosseous ligament is associated with fat that images with high signal intensity. On T1-weighted sequences, the pre-Achilles fat pad is visualized as an area of high signal intensity, anterior to the calcaneus tendon, that is of low spin density. The division of hyaline articular cartilage surfaces is less clearly defined in the mid- and posterior talocalcaneal joints. In the plane of the fibula, the peroneus brevis and longus tendons pass posterior to the lateral malleolus (Fig. 3-9). In medial sagittal sections through the foot, the insertion of the flexor hallucis tendon is demonstrated in profile, with attachment along the plantar surface of the distal phalanx of the great toe.

Coronal Images

The collateral ligaments of the ankle are visualized with low signal intensity on coronal images through the tibiotalar joint. The deltoid ligament and tibialis posterior (Fig. 3-10) can be visualized medially. On posterior coronal sections, the calcaneofibular ligament, along with the posterior talofibular components of the lateral collateral ligament, are defined (Fig. 3-11). The joint cap-

Figure 3-8
Sagittal image of the midankle. Tibia *(1)*, talus *(2)*, navicular *(3)*, calcaneus *(4)*, sinus tarsi *(5)*, flexor hallucis longus tendon and muscle *(6)*, calcaneus tendon *(7)*, pre-Achilles fat pad *(8)*. T1-weighted image; TR = 600 msec, TE = 20 msec.

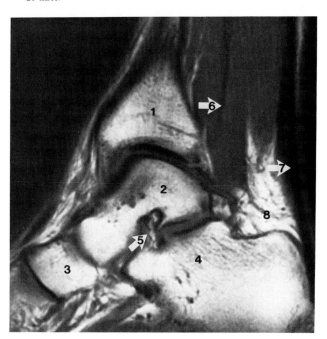

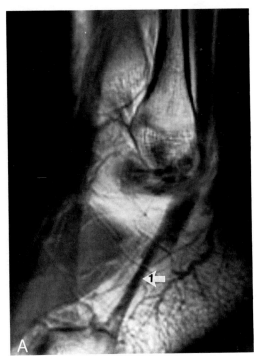
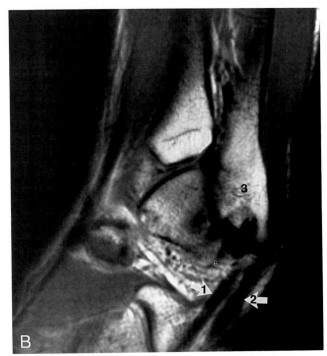

Figure 3-9

Sagittal images of the lateral ankle. Peroneus longus tendon *(1)*, peroneus brevis *(2)*, fibula (lateral malleolus) *(3)*. T1-weighted image; TR = 600 msec, TE = 20 msec.

sule can be visualized by using T2-weighting to create an arthrographic effect. (On T2-weighted sequences the high signal intensity of synovial fluid contrasts with the lower intensity of the joint capsule.[6]) The transverse tibiofibular ligament is seen posteriorly in the same coronal plane as the calcaneofibular ligament. Paraaxial visualization of the tibionavicular component of the deltoid ligament has been reported at 40° of plantar flexion.[3] The tibiospring and posterior tibiotalar ligaments are displayed in 15° of plantar flexion. The flexor tendons and retinaculum are defined medially, whereas the peroneus longus and brevis tendons can be distinguished laterally. The interosseous talocalcaneal ligament and sinus tarsi are additionally identified in coronal plane images.[6]

Anatomic Variants

There are a number of normal variants in MR imaging of the ankle that may be misleading. These have been characterized in studies of asymptomatic patients.[7] In the posterior tibiotalar joint, low signal intensity cortical irregularity may mimic the appearance of osteonecrosis. On occasion, the intact posterior talofibular ligament may appear as an attenuated structure with signal inhomogeneity. Less commonly, fluid in the peroneal tendon sheath may be confused with a longitudinal tendon tear. In one patient, axial planar images revealed marked

asymmetry and hypertrophy of the peroneus brevis muscle and tendon as a normal anatomic variant (Fig. 3-12).

PATHOLOGY OF THE ANKLE AND FOOT

Transchondral Fractures

Transchondral fracture is the accepted term for several osteochondral lesions including osteochondral fracture, osteochondritis dessicans, and talar dome fracture. Transchondral fractures of the medial or lateral talar dome involve the articular cartilage and subchondral bone, and have a high association with antecedent trauma.

The ability, with MR imaging, to delineate marrow in cancellous bone, cortex, and hyaline cartilage, makes this modality well suited to the evaluation of osteochondral lesions of the talus.[8] Conventional radiographs and CT scans cannot assess the integrity of hyaline articular cartilage surfaces in osteocartilaginous defects. Berndt and Harty have developed a four-part staging system for characterizing transchondral fractures based on plain radiographs.[9] In Stage I there is compression fracture of the talus with no ligamentous sprain. Stage II and III lesions represent partial and complete nondisplaced osteochondral fractures, respectively. Detachment with a loose osteochondral fragment characterizes Stage IV. Al-

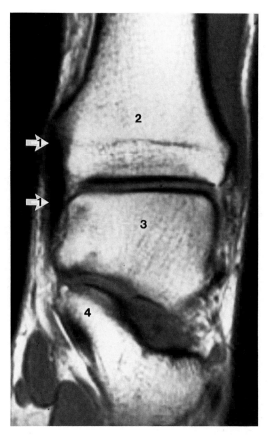

Figure 3-10

Coronal image of the midankle. Tibialis posterior tendon *(1)*, distal tibia *(2)*, talus *(3)*, sustentaculum tali *(4)*. T1-weighted image; TR = 600 msec, TE = 20 msec.

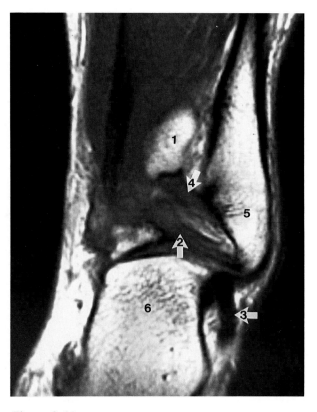

Figure 3-11

Coronal image of the posterior ankle. Tibia *(1)*, talofibular ligament *(2)*, calcaneofibular ligament *(3)*, posterior tibiofibular ligament *(4)*, fibula *(5)*, calcaneus *(6)*. T1-weighted image; TR = 600 msec, TE = 20 msec.

Figure 3-12

Asymmetric hypertrophy of the peroneus brevis muscle. Normal anatomic variant *(black arrows)*. Contralateral normal size peroneus brevis shown for comparison *(open arrow)*. Associated Achilles tendinitis images with a central area of intermediate signal intensity within enlarged, low signal intensity tendon *(white arrow)*. T1-weighted image; TR = 800 msec, TE = 20 msec.

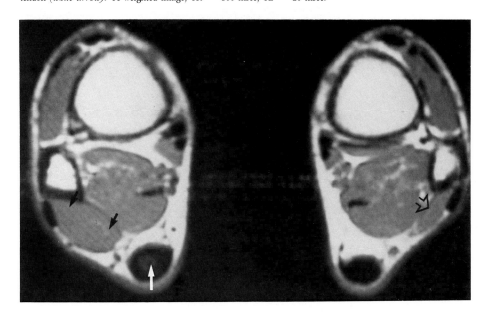

though Stage II–IV lesions are themselves painless, they may be associated with a painful sprain or rupture of the collateral ankle ligaments.

Treatment protocols for transchondral fracture vary depending on the stage of the lesion. Immobilization with conservative treatment is usually employed, except in lateral Stage II and Stage IV fractures that often require free fragment excision, curettage, and drilling. Complications include locking of the joint (with larger bone fragments), degenerative arthritis (more likely to occur with lateral lesions that have been reported to be more symptomatic), and nonunion of the fracture, leading to traumatic osteoarthritis.

Early x-rays of transchondral fracture may be negative until a necrotic focus is demarcated. With MR imaging, however, tibiotalar anatomy can be displayed in the coronal, axial, or sagittal plane to identify the talar defect and presence of an avulsed bony fragment.

The hyaline articular cartilage surface of the talar dome images with intermediate signal intensity on T1- or T2-weighted images, whereas a detached cortical fragment will remain low in signal intensity. Adherent hyaline articular cartilage, reparative fibrocartilage, or associated fibrous tissue is imaged with intermediate signal intensity. On T1-weighted images the bony defect of the talus demonstrates low or intermediate signal intensity, depending on the composition of synovial fluid and fibrous tissue, respectively. (On T2-weighted images, synovial fluid contents generate increased signal intensity.) Peripheral areas of low signal intensity within the subchondral bone on T1- and T2-weighted images have been correlated with reactive bone sclerosis on plain radiographs.

Abnormalities of the articular surface include regions of cartilage thinning, bowing, nodularity, or disruption.[8] The accumulation of high intensity joint fluid, within or undermining the cartilage surface, indicates small fissures or breaks in articular cartilage (Fig. 3-13).

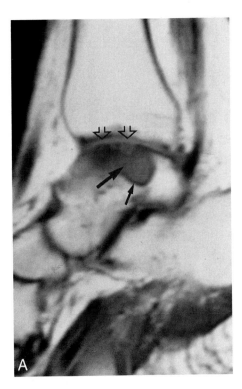

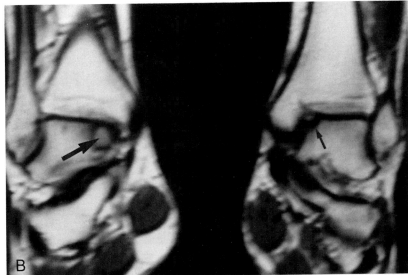

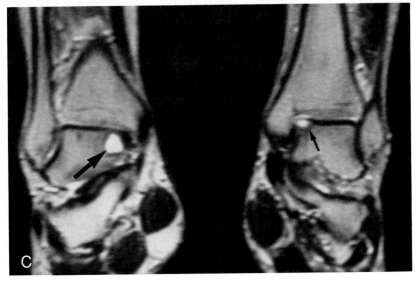

Figure 3-13

Transchondral fracture. *(A)* Medial talar osteochondral defect with low signal intensity periphery of reactive bone *(small solid arrow)* and intermediate signal intensity viscous synovial fluid contents *(large solid arrow)*. Overlying hyaline articular cartilage is intact *(open arrows)*. T1-weighted sagittal image; TR = 600 msec, TE = 20 msec. Corresponding T2-weighted coronal spin echo sequence with talar cavity *(large arrow)* identified with intermediate signal intensity on balanced weighted image *(B)* and with uniform high signal intensity fluid on second echo *(C)*. Contralateral smaller talar defect shown *(small arrow)*. TR = 2000 msec, TE = 20, 60 msec.

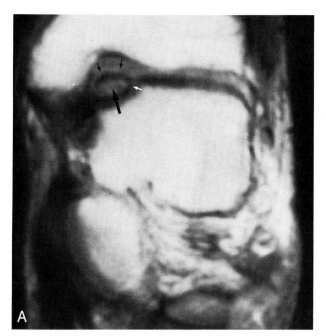 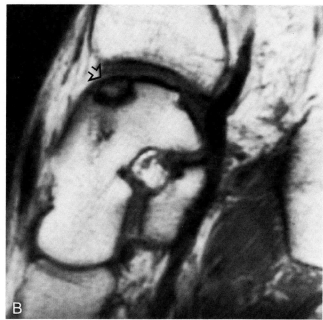

Figure 3-14

Transchondral fracture. **(A)** Osteochondral talar lesion *(large black arrow)* with upward bowing of the medial talar hyaline articular cartilage surface *(small black arrows)*. Intermediate signal intensity fluid is seen undermining transchondral defect *(white arrow)*. TR = 800 msec, TE = 20 msec. **(B)** Sagittal image demonstrating attenuated articular cartilage overlying transchondral fracture *(open arrow)*. TR = 800 msec, TE = 20 msec.

On sagittal or coronal images, a focal, upward bowing of the hyaline cartilage overlying the bony defect may be demonstrated (Fig. 3-14). The cartilage may be deformed or bowed without disruption, frequently showing softening at surgery. A postsurgical fibrocartilaginous scar may appear as a focal area of thickening, imaging with intermediate signal intensity, bridging a cartilaginous defect. With gradient echo—effective T2*-weighting—hyaline cartilage images with high signal intensity, and these images are useful for the identification of small areas of cartilage disruption (Fig. 3-15).[2]

Although conventional radiographic techniques should remain the basis for the initial evaluation of patients with suspected osteochondral defects, MR imaging offers the ability to assess both the talar defect and the integrity of overlying cartilage surfaces. The presence of an intact articular surface could obviate the need for surgical excision and curettage, in favor of the more conservative treatments such as drilling.

Injuries to the Tendons and Ligaments

Preliminary investigations have shown potential application of MR imaging in the evaluation of tendinous and ligamentous structures about the ankle.[10] Intact tendons and ligaments image with low signal intensity on all pulsing sequences. The thicker tendons of the ankle can be studied in multiple planes, while smaller ligamentous bands may be visualized in only one orthogonal plane.

Achilles Tendon

The Achilles tendon represents the largest tendon in the body and is formed from the confluence of the gastrocnemius and soleus muscle complexes. Injuries to this tendon, secondary to athletic activity, are frequent in middle-age males.[11,12] There may be a predisposition to disruption of the Achilles tendon in the already weakened connective tissue and collagen fibers of patients with disorders such as rheumatoid arthritis, systemic lupus erythematosus, diabetes mellitus, and gout.

Clinical examination alone has missed rupture of the Achilles tendon in up to 25% of cases. The tendon is most susceptible to rupture 2 to 6 cm superior to the os calcis, with acute rupture associated with forced dorsiflexion of the foot against a contracting force generated by the triceps surae group.

Lateral radiography and xerography have not been effective in identifying abnormalities in the Achilles tendon. Although tendon thickening in inflammation and discontinuities in tears have been visualized with some success using real time ultrasonography, this technique is limited in soft tissue contrast discrimination, FOV, and inability to accurately evaluate both adjacent soft tissue and bony structures.

The Achilles tendon is clearly demonstrated on

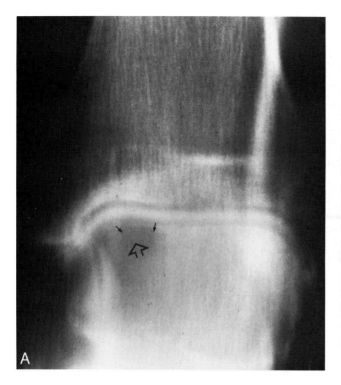

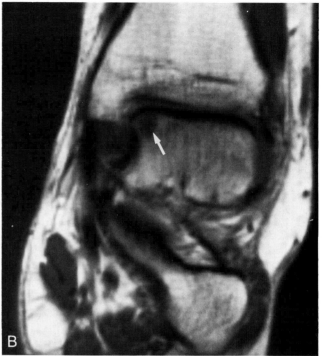

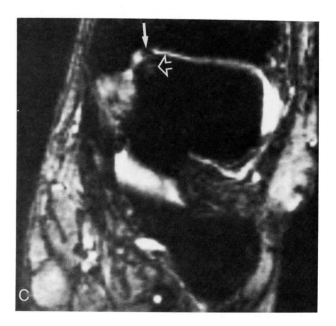

Figure 3-15

Osteochondritis dessicans (transchondral fracture). *(A)* AP tomogram showing medial talar lucency *(open arrow).* Superior outline is defined *(small arrows).* *(B)* T1-weighted coronal image identifies low signal intensity osteochondral defect *(arrow).* TR = 600 msec, TE = 20 msec. *(C)* T2* gradient echo image demonstrating fluid-filled osteochondral cavity *(open arrow)* and overlying cartilage disruption *(solid arrow).* TR = 400 msec, TE = 30 msec, flip angle = 30°.

sagittal and axial MR images.[13] A routine examination of the tendon uses a 16-cm field of view, and 5-mm-thick sections. A T1-weighted acquisition should be performed in both sagittal and axial planes. T2-weighted images are necessary in only one plane to document fluid, edema, hemorrhage, or inflammatory changes.

The normal Achilles tendon images with uniform low signal intensity. Axial images show the tendon in cross section with a mildly flattened anterior surface and convex posterior surface. In ruptures of the Achilles tendon, the relationship of the proximal and distal portions of the torn tendon can be seen in either pre- or post-plastercasting MR studies (Fig. 3-16). Associated hemorrhage within the tendon sheath is best appreciated on axial sections (Fig. 3-17). Subacute hemorrhage generates high signal intensity on T1-weighted images. Areas

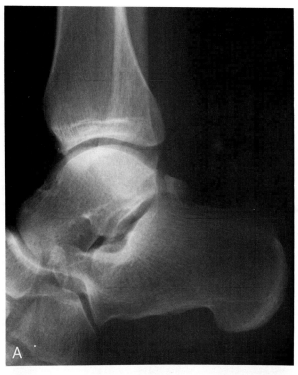

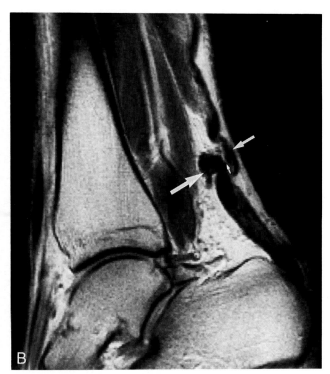

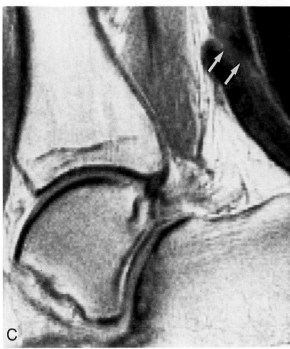

Figure 3-16

Achilles tendon rupture. *(A)* AP radiograph performed after acute injury to the Achilles tendon. Minimal posterior soft tissue swelling is present. *(B)* Complete rupture of the Achilles tendon with proximal *(medium arrow)* and distal *(large arrow)* tendon fibers identified in close approximation *(small arrow)*. T1-weighted sagittal image; TR = 1000 msec, TE = 40 msec. *(C)* Complete fibrous healing with apposition of torn tendon after 4 months of cast treatment *(arrows)*. T1-weighted sagittal image; TR = 1000 msec, TE = 40 msec.

of edema or inflammation will show increased signal intensity on T2-weighted images.

As more patients with tendon tears are conservatively managed with serial casting, MR has become invaluable in documenting the degree of apposition in the disrupted proximal and distal tendon fragments. Retracted tendon sections are less likely to heal with conservative management, and MR evaluation allows early identification of these patients, who are candidates for surgical intervention (Fig. 3-18). Fibrous bridging also appears to be more tenuous with increased tendon separation. A bulbous contour may be demonstrated in the proliferating ends of a torn Achilles tendon, and it increases with greater tendon diastasis. Fibrous healing, with approximation of torn fibers, can be evaluated with MR imaging performed at monthly intervals. With this

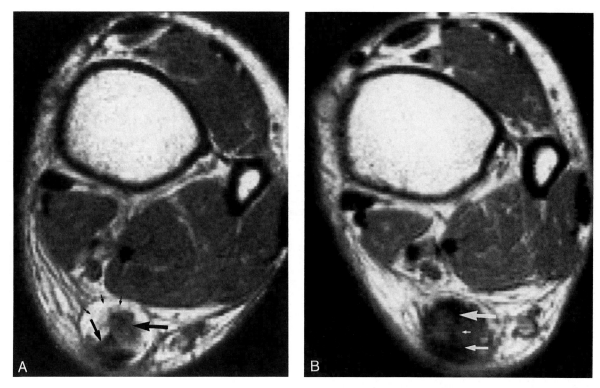

Figure 3-17

Achilles tendon rupture. (See also corresponding sagittal image, Fig. 3–16.) **(A)** T1-weighted axial image demonstrates high signal intensity subacute hemorrhage *(small arrows)* in rupture of Achilles tendon. Proximal tendon *(large arrow)* is shown anterior to the distal portion of the tendon *(medium arrow)*. TR = 1000 msec, TE = 40 msec. **(B)** Intermediate signal intensity fibrous union *(small arrow)* between proximal *(large arrow)* and distal *(medium arrow)* tendon ends indicated. T1-weighted axial image; TR = 1000 msec, TE = 40 msec.

information, those patients best suited for conservative therapy can be selected, improving the present statistics for rerupture with conservative treatment (10%), as compared with surgical treatment (4%).[14,15]

Partial tendon tears are also defined on MR images in the sagittal and axial planes (Fig. 3-19). Without inflammatory reaction, tendinitis—a common affliction among joggers—can be recognized by a thickening of the tendon complex.

Other Tendon Injuries

Partial ruptures of the posterior tibial tendon are seen either as hypertrophied regions with heterogeneous signal intensity or as areas of attenuation.[16] Complete tears are delineated by a tendinous gap (Fig. 3-20). When MR findings were correlated with CT scans and with surgical exploration, MR was shown to be superior to CT in detecting the spectrum of early partial tendon ruptures, longitudinal tearing, and presence of synovial fluid. Subtle areas of associated periostitis were more readily delineated with CT. Tears in the flexor hallucis longus and flexor digitorum longus tendons have been documented

by MR as fraying and irregularity at the ends of the ruptured tendons.[17]

Ligaments

The normal ligamentous anatomy of the ankle can be demonstrated on MR images, although extensive experience or indications for the use of MR imaging in evaluation of patients with ligament sprains or ruptures has not been established. In a report of a subtalar dislocation, torn talocalcaneal (interosseous) and calcaneofibular ligaments were documented on MR studies and later confirmed at surgery.[5] The tears were seen as widening of the posterior subtalar joint, secondary to interposition of torn calcaneofibular ligament fibers. On T2-weighted images of acute ligament ruptures, subcutaneous edema, hemorrhage, and joint effusions appeared as high signal intensity.[3] In evaluation of chronically unstable ankles, placing the ligament under study in a position of stress was effective in showing ligament rupture, thinning, and lengthening. MR imaging of a patient with a Watson Jones reconstruction of the lateral ligaments (anterior

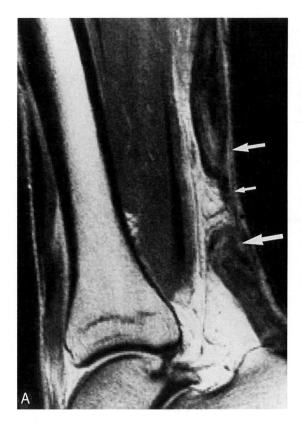

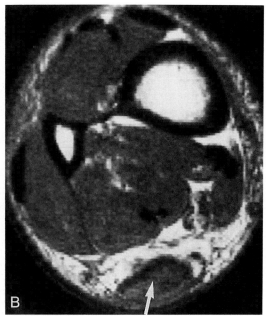

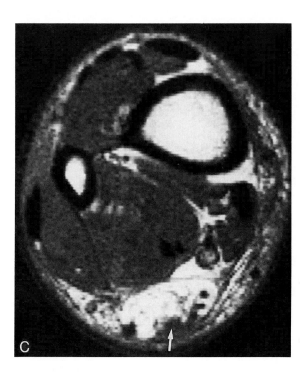

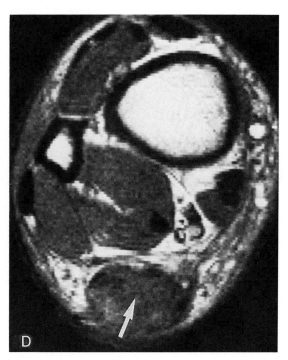

Figure 3-18

Suboptimal Achilles tendon union. Sagittal *(A)* and corresponding superior *(B)*, mid *(C)*, and inferior axial images *(D)* demonstrate healing Achilles tendon with enlarged proximal end *(medium arrow)*, tenuous union *(small arrow)* and bulbous distal tendon *(large arrow)*. TR = 1000 msec, TE = 40 msec.

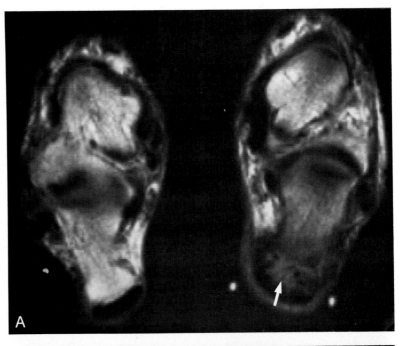

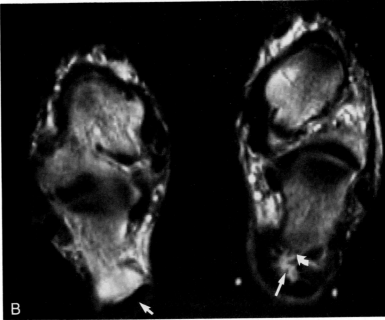

Figure 3-19

Achilles tendon tear. Partial tear of the left Achilles tendon *(large arrow)* images with low signal intensity on T1-weighted images *(A)* and with high signal intensity on T2-weighted images *(B)*. Intact right Achilles tendon *(small arrow)* shown for comparison. Erosion of posterior calcaneal surface indicated *(curved arrow)*. TR = 500 msec, TE = 40 msec; and TR = 2000 msec, TE = 80 msec, respectively.

talofibular), showed the mobilized peroneus brevis tendon that was rerooted through the fibula to be intact (Fig. 3-21).

Infection

Early detection and treatment of osteomyelitis and joint sepsis is critical in preserving joint function before cartilage breakdown and local or hematagenous spread occurs.[18] Changes on conventional radiographs are frequently nonspecific, with effusion (capsular distension) or disruption of soft tissue planes as the only findings. Often there is no evidence of cortical destruction until

there is extensive marrow involvement that may involve a lag time of 10 to 14 days. MR imaging has been shown to have potential in the early detection of musculoskeletal infections. Although applications in the ankle and foot are preliminary, new clinical indications are under development. The capability to detect skip lesions, to obtain high soft tissue contrast in a multiplanar format, and to evaluate marrow, cartilage, and cortex separately, shows great potential for the further use of MR as a tool to detect and monitor infection, targeting the foot and ankle.

Since infection causes an alteration in the ratio of free to bound water (prolonging T1 and T2 tissue relax-

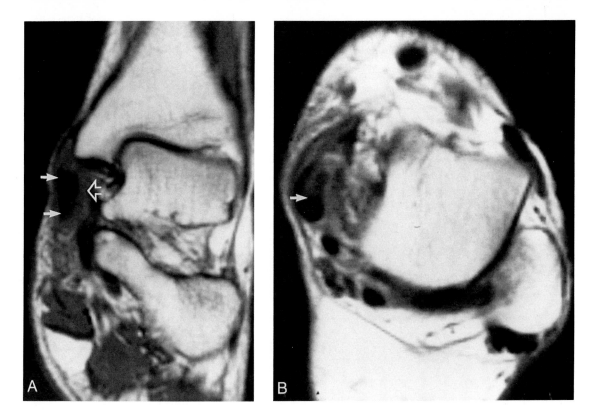

Figure 3-20

Torn tibialis posterior tendon. T1-weighted coronal *(A)* and axial *(B)* images of torn tibialis posterior tendon (solid white arrows).
Adjacent edema is imaged with low to intermediate signal intensity *(open arrow).* TR = 600 msec, TE = 20 msec.

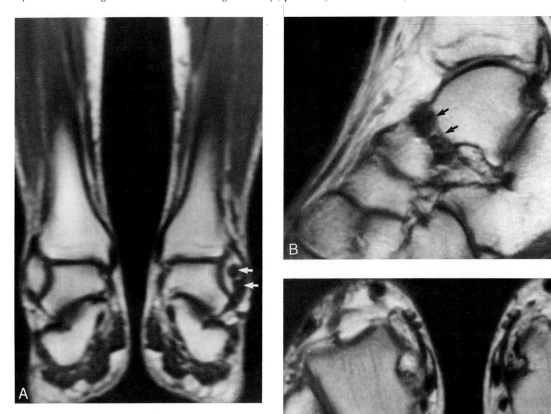

Figure 3-21

Reconstruction of the anterior talofibular and the calcaneofibular
ligaments. Tunneling of the peroneus brevis tendon through the
neck of the talus *(black arrows)* and the fibula are shown
(white arrows). T1-weighted coronal *(A),* sagittal *(B),* and
axial *(C)* images. TR = 600 msec, TE = 20 msec.

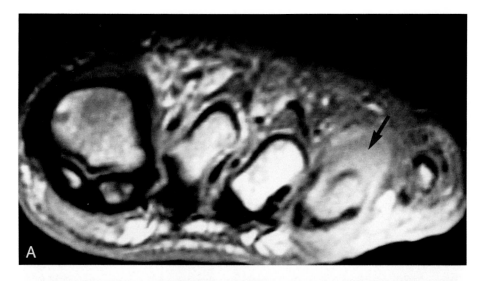

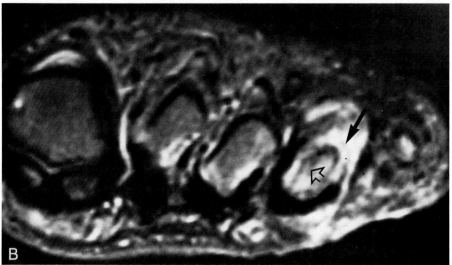

Figure 3-22

Osteomyelitis. Staphylococcal osteomyelitis of the fourth metatarsal *(closed arrow)*, visualized with intermediate signal intensity on a balanced weighted axial image *(A)*, and with high signal intensity on a T2-weighted axial image *(B)*. Marrow involvement is appreciated on the T2-weighted image *(open arrow)*. TR = 2000 msec, TE = 20, 60 msec.

ation times), infected regions image with low signal intensity on T1-weighted images and high signal intensity on T2-weighted images. Although this provides the basis for diagnostic sensitivity, neoplastic tissue undergoes similar T1 and T2 relaxation changes. Therefore, secondary characteristics such as location, distribution, extent, and morphology of signal intensity assume an important role in improving diagnostic specificity.

Osteomyelitis

Early osteomyelitis images with low signal intensity on T1-weighted images, and with high signal intensity on T2-weighted images (Fig. 3-22). Acute and chronic osteomyelitis has been studied in the calcaneus, cuboid, metatarsals, and distal tibia and fibula.[19] On T2-weighted

sequences, in the acute or subacute phase, a diffuse or patchy increase of signal intensity in the medullary bone indicates marrow involvement (Fig. 3-23). A peripheral rim of low signal intensity, representing reactive bone, may demarcate the focus, over time. Alterations in signal intensity may also be seen at sites of cortical transgression, periosteal reaction, soft tissue mass, and sequestra.

In the case of staphylococcal osteomyelitis involving the distal tibial metaphysis, a stellate pattern of signal change, mimicking the MR appearance of a stress fracture, was observed (Fig. 3-24). Infected material in serpiginous tracts was visualized on T2-weighted images as linear segments of high signal intensity.

In a case report of osteomyelitis of the tarsal navicular caused by *Nocardia,* there was complete replace-

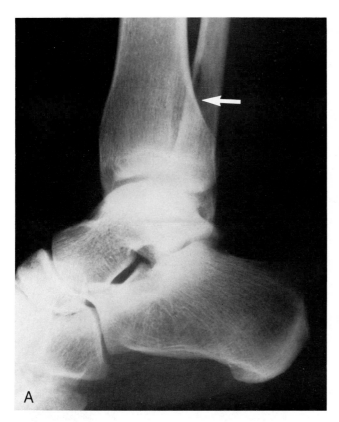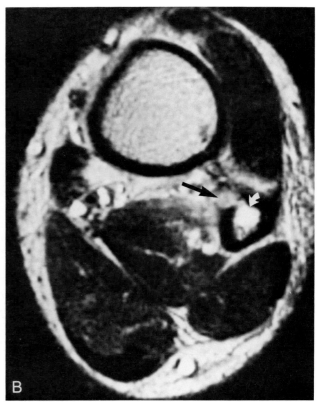

Figure 3-23
Osteomyelitis of the fibula. **(A)** Lateral radiograph showing localized osteopenia in the distal fibula
(arrow). **(B)** T2-weighted axial image demonstrating high signal intensity infectious tract *(straight
arrows)* and marrow *(curved arrow)*. TR = 2000 msec, TE = 60 msec.

ment of yellow marrow signal with homogeneous low
signal intensity on T1-weighted images, and high signal
intensity edema on T2-weighted images.[20] A radionuclide bone scan in this case was positive, but plain radiographs and CT scan were negative.

Other Infections

MR evaluation of a 5-month-old child detected chronic
granulomatous involvement of the ankle joint and surrounding tendons (Fig. 3-25). Synovial sheath distension and pockets of fluid visualized with increased signal intensity on T2-weighted images, while necrotic
granulomatous areas of involvement were imaged with
intermediate signal intensity. Subsequent surgical exploration failed to confirm a septic etiology, although
nonspecific giant cells were found on histologic examination.

In selected cases, MR may be indicated to identify
the location and composition of foreign bodies. In one
case, a foreign body (toothpick) with a surrounding inflammatory capsule was identified by MR (Fig. 3-26).
This lesion was missed both on radiography and surgical exploration.

MR has also been used to distinguish between soft
tissue cellulitis and bone involvement in a diabetic foot,
although changes of diabetic neuropathy could poten-

tially simulate marrow infection. In recent work, chemical shift imaging has been used to assess the water content of the sural nerve, and this technique may help to
identify patients with active neuropathic changes.[21]

Neoplasms

MR images provide superior soft tissue contrast and anatomic delineation for the staging of osseous and soft
tissue neoplasms.[22–25] The capability for direct multiplanar imaging (coronal, sagittal, axial, or oblique) is
particularly advantageous in imaging tumors about the
ankle and foot. As in other appendicular sites, axial
planar images with T1- and T2-weighting are the most
important for detecting the presence of a tumor and for
determining its relationship to adjacent muscle groups,
neurovascular bundles, and fascial planes in separate anatomic compartments. Direct T1-weighted coronal or
sagittal images are appropriate for depiction of longitudinal marrow extension, although sagittal images are
most accurate in demonstrating the longitudinal axis of
adjacent muscles and tendons crossing the ankle joint.
Low spin density cortical bone images with low signal
intensity, regardless of pulsing parameters. The signal
intensity of yellow marrow in the ankle or foot, however, can be manipulated to optimize contrast resolution

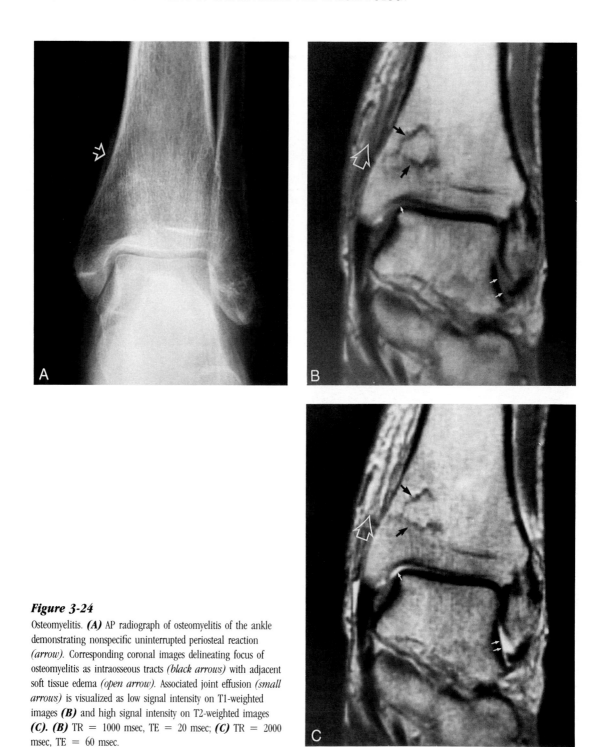

Figure 3-24

Osteomyelitis. *(A)* AP radiograph of osteomyelitis of the ankle demonstrating nonspecific uninterrupted periosteal reaction *(arrow)*. Corresponding coronal images delineating focus of osteomyelitis as intraosseous tracts *(black arrows)* with adjacent soft tissue edema *(open arrow)*. Associated joint effusion *(small arrows)* is visualized as low signal intensity on T1-weighted images *(B)* and high signal intensity on T2-weighted images *(C)*. *(B)* TR = 1000 msec, TE = 20 msec; *(C)* TR = 2000 msec, TE = 60 msec.

in displaying neoplastic tissue. Yellow marrow, usually bright on T1-weighted images and intermediate on T2-weighted images, images with low signal intensity when gradient echo or short TI inversion recovery (STIR) techniques are used.

Benign Lesions

In the benign tumor category, osteoid osteomas and enchondromas occur frequently about the ankle and foot. *Osteoid osteoma,* with reactive sclerotic osteoid matrix,

images as an area of low signal intensity with a central nidus of increased signal intensity.[26] On T1-weighted images the central nidus is of intermediate signal intensity, but on T2-weighted images the amount of increased signal intensity may vary.

MR imaging is also useful for the identification of *enchondromas.* We have studied multiple enchondromas about the ankle in a patient with Olliers disease, and the foci of cartilaginous tissue image with low to intermediate signal intensity on T1-weighted images,

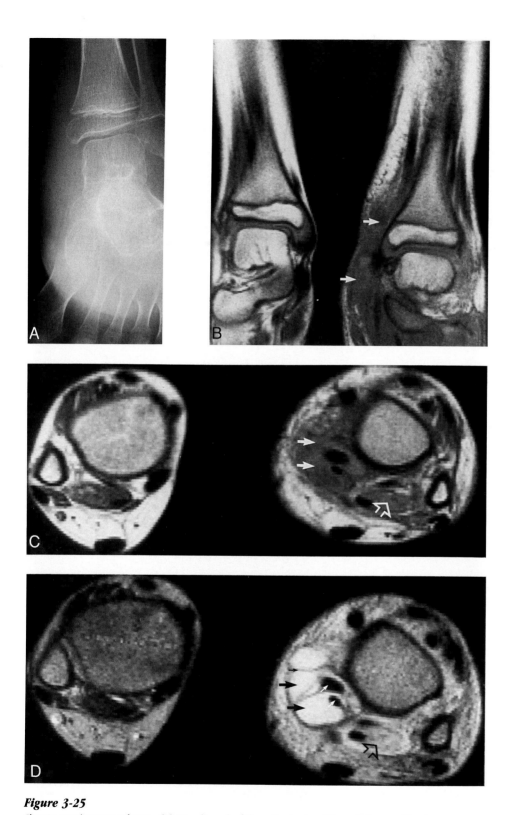

Figure 3-25

Chronic granulomatous infection. *(A)* AP radiograph of the ankle showing diffuse soft tissue swelling in a child with a chronic granulomatous infection. *(B)* Corresponding coronal image identifying low signal intensity fluid *(arrows)* distending the supporting capsule. TR = 500 msec, TE = 40 msec. Pockets of fluid *(large solid arrows)* that image with low signal intensity on T1-weighted images *(C)* and high signal intensity on T2-weighted images *(D)* are identified adjacent to thickened tendon sheaths of the tibialis posterior and flexor digitorum longus muscles *(small white arrows)*. Septations *(small black arrow)* and necrotic/granulomatous tissue *(open arrow)* are identified. *(C)* TR = 800 msec, TE = 40 msec; *(D)* TR = 2000 msec, TE = 80 msec.

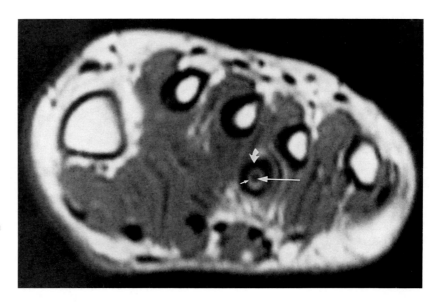

Figure 3-26

Foreign body. Low signal intensity toothpick *(long straight arrow)* inciting a foreign body reaction with intermediate signal intensity rim *(small straight arrow)* and fibrous periphery *(curved arrow).* T1-weighted axial image; TR = 1000 msec, TE = 20 msec.

and with high signal intensity on T2-weighted images (Fig. 3-27). Although differentiation from low-grade chondrosarcoma may be difficult on the basis of signal intensity alone, enchondromas can be differentiated from bone infarcts.

Bone infarcts (metaphyseal based) are circumscribed by a serpiginous low signal intensity border, that corresponds to the rim of reactive sclerosis that is often detected on plain radiographs (Fig. 3-28).[27] In the acute and subacute stages, signal from the central island of the infarct is isointense with fatty marrow signal. T2-weighting may demonstrate linear bright signal, paralleling the inner, low intensity signal from the periphery of the lesion. Except for location, the imaging characteristics of *subarticular degeneration* with necrotic bone are similar to those of bone infarction.

Axial and sagittal images may also be used to assess the fibrous lesions of *plantar fibromatosis.* These fibrous nodules, involving the plantar aponeurosis, image with low signal intensity on T1- and T2-weighted images. A *xanthofibroma* of the foot may also demonstrate low signal intensity on T1- and T2-weighted images (Fig. 3-29).

An expansile *aneurysmal bone cyst* of the distal tibia has been described with inhomogeneous cystic areas of hemorrhage.[20,28] These image with intermediate to high signal intensity on T1-weighted images, and high signal intensity on T2-weighted images. Cortical bowing and septation (trabeculation) may be observed in the low signal intensity contour of cortical bone.

We have also differentiated an *intraosseous lipoma* from a simple cyst of the calcaneus by the thick rind of adipose tissue (bright signal on T1-weighted images) circumscribing a central hemorrhagic component (low signal intensity on T1-weighted images and bright signal intensity on T2-weighted sequences; Fig. 3-30).

Synovial ganglion cysts projecting into the soft tissue are also well defined and image with low signal intensity on T1-weighted images and high signal intensity on T2-weighted images (Fig. 3-31). Septations, when present, are best seen on T2-weighted images, where they are outlined by the bright signal intensity of fluid.

Intramuscular hemorrhage (Fig. 3-32) and venous or arterial *thrombosis* (Fig. 3-33) may present with pain and can simulate a soft tissue mass.[29]

Aggressive and Malignant Lesions

Osteosarcoma, chondrosarcoma, giant cell tumor, and Ewing sarcoma are statistically the primary bony neoplasms which are likely to involve either the foot or the ankle. With MR imaging, intramedullary marrow involvement, soft tissue extension, joint space integrity in the tibiotalar and subtalar articulations, skip metastasis, and postoperative recurrence have been accurately assessed.

In one case of *osteosarcomatosis,* distal tibial marrow infiltration was precisely mapped on MR, although plain film radiographs were negative. In a case of *chondrosarcoma,* malignant degeneration or transformation of an enchondroma was inferred by the presence of frank cortical disruption, soft tissue extension, periosteal reaction, and disproportionate size of the lesion relative to satellite enchondromas (see Fig. 3-27). Although these findings were confirmed on pathologic evaluation, reliable MR criteria have not been developed to characterize these aggressive cartilage lesions.[30,31]

In one report, a cystic *giant cell tumor* of the calcaneus was described as imaging with low to intermediate signal intensity on T1-weighted images, and high signal intensity on T2-weighted images. A fluid-fluid level in this lesion was identified on MR scans but was not seen on corresponding CT sections.[20]

In a series of *synovial sarcomas* involving the ankle and foot, MR imaging was used to stage intra- and

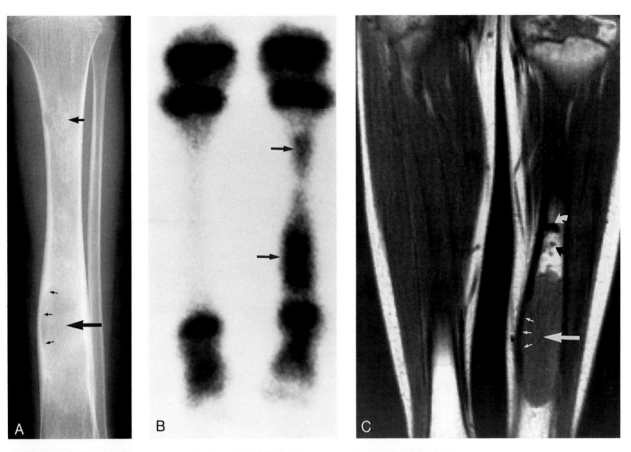

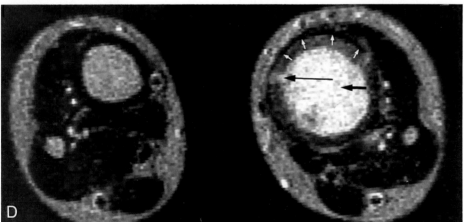

Figure 3-27

Enchondroma and chondrosarcoma. ***(A)*** AP radiograph showing multiple enchondromas *(medium arrow)* with a discrete lytic lesion in the distal femoral shaft representing transformation into a chondrosarcoma *(large arrow)*. Endosteal scalloping is identified *(small arrows)*. ***(B)*** Technetium bone scintigraphy identifies increased uptake in proximal femoral enchondromas and in larger distal lesion *(arrows)*. ***(C)*** T1-weighted coronal image displaying focus of malignant degeneration from an enchondroma to a chondrosarcoma *(large straight arrow)*. Endosteal scalloping with bowing of low signal intensity cortical bone *(small arrows)* and satellite enchondromas are shown *(curved arrows)*. TR = 500 msec, TE = 40 msec. ***(D)*** Chondrosarcoma visualized on corresponding T2-weighted axial image with uniform increased signal intensity *(short black arrow)*, cortical extension *(long black arrow)*, and periosteal reaction *(small white arrows)*. TR = 2000 msec, TE = 80 msec.

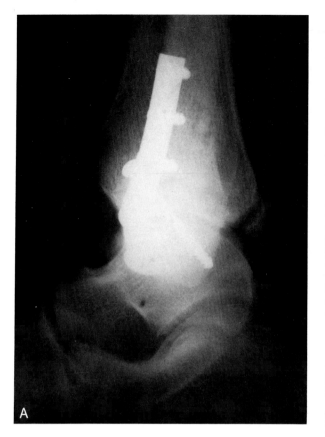

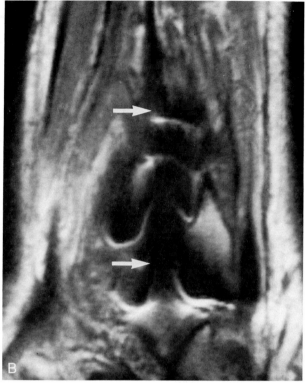

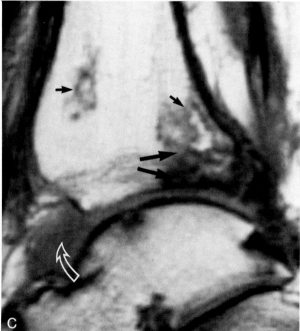

Figure 3-28

Ankle imaging with orthopedic hardware. *(A)* Fibular screw plate fixation device on lateral radiograph. *(B)* T1-weighted parasagittal image through the lateral ankle with localized metallic artifact *(arrows)*. TR = 600 msec, TE = 20 msec. *(C)* Midsagittal section in the same patient demonstrating subarticular degenerative changes *(large black arrow)* and metaphyseal bone infarcts *(small black arrows)*. Anterior capsular distention with ankle effusion is identified *(open arrow)*.

extraarticular involvement. The propensity for synovial sarcoma to track along tendon sheaths and to invade adjacent bone allowed for prospective MR diagnosis in four of the five cases studied (Fig. 3-34). These lesions imaged with low to intermediate signal intensity on T1-weighted images and were homogeneously bright on T2-weighted images.[32] Small areas of central necrosis were imaged as regions of higher signal intensity. Focal calcifications, although detected with MR, were better delineated on CT images.

Patients with lower extremity *neurofibromas* have been evaluated with T1, T2, and gradient echo imaging. Neurofibromas image with low to intermediate signal intensity on T1-weighted images and are bright on T2-

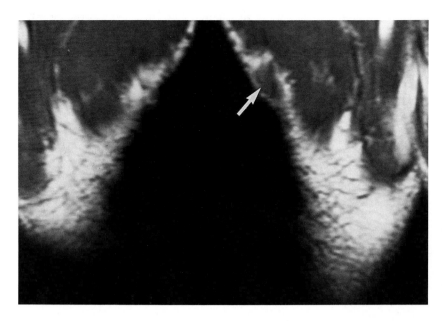

Figure 3-29

Xanthofibroma. Low signal intensity xanthofibroma seen scalloping the subcutaneous tissue on the medial plantar surface of the foot *(arrow)*. T1-weighted axial image; TR = 600 msec, TE = 20 msec.

weighted images.[33] Plexiform histology could be differentiated from nonplexiform lesions by the intensity, morphology, and distribution of MR signal. Plexiform lesions were uniformly bright on T2-weighted images and frequently tracked along neural bundles in a lobulated fashion (Fig. 3-35). The nonplexiform lesions that did not involve multiple fascicles were more likely to infiltrate into adjacent tissues and imaged with greater signal inhomogeneity (Fig. 3-36). Although the imaging properties of benign and malignant neurofibromas may be similar, neurofibrosarcomas have been reported to have increased signal inhomogeneity.

Leiomyosarcoma of the posterolateral calf imaged isointense with muscle tissue on T1-weighted images and showed uniform increase in signal intensity on T2-weighted images (Fig. 3-37).

A metastatic *malignant melanoma* of the calf generated high signal intensity on a STIR sequence that canceled out the high signal intensity from normal adjacent marrow fat (Fig. 3-38).[34]

Arthritis

Early experience with MR imaging of ankle arthritis has been restricted to cases of osteo- and posttraumatic arthritis and to infectious and hemophiliac arthropathies.[5]

In *osteoarthritis,* including cases of posttraumatic etiology, thinning of the tibiotalar and subtalar hyaline cartilage surfaces can be appreciated on coronal and sagittal T1-weighted images. As discussed for transchondral fractures, identification of loose bodies, possible on T1-weighted images (Fig. 3-39), may require T2-weighting to create contrast with the surrounding synovial fluid (that images with high signal intensity on T2-weighted sequences). Osteophytic spurs with marrow contents image as areas of bright signal intensity (isointense with fat) with a cortical rim of low signal intensity (the anterior tibial border). Cortical and subchondral irregularities can be visualized in association with denuded articular cartilage (Fig. 3-40). Primary osteoarthrosis of the first metatarsophalangeal joint, secondary to excessive biomechanical loading in a springboard diver, showed early joint space narrowing (not appreciated on plain films) and subchondral low signal intensity on coronal MR images through the foot. The presence of an acute or chronic joint effusion (of low signal intensity on T1-weighted images and high signal intensity on T2-weighted images) can also be determined on MR scans (Fig. 3-41). Subchondral or juxtaarticular cysts, which possess gelatinous synovial fluid, demonstrate uniform increased signal intensity with progressive T2-weighting (Fig. 3-42).

On MR images *hemophiliac arthropathy* is indicated by low signal intensity synovial hypertrophy with paramagnetic hemosiderin deposits. With gradient echo techniques, hyaline cartilage can be imaged with high signal intensity, permitting identification of subtle cartilage irregularities.[5]

Tenosynovitis presents with thickening or increased fluid accumulation around the affected tendon sheath (Fig. 3-43). In the absence of tendinitis, no intrasubstance signal intensity is observed within collagen fibers.[10]

Further evidence with inflammatory and noninflammatory arthritides is required before routine use of MR imaging is indicated in the evaluation of ankle and foot articulations.

Text continues on p. 95

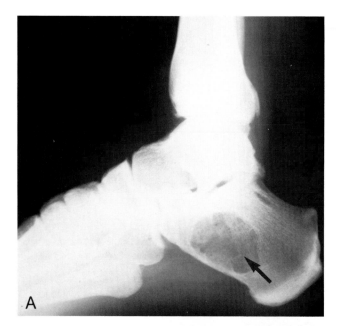

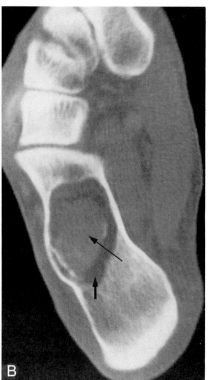

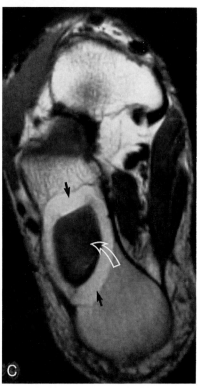

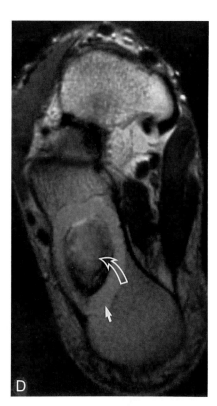

Figure 3-30

Intraosseous lipoma. ***(A)*** Lateral radiograph with intraosseous lipoma shown as a lytic area in the calcaneus *(arrow)*. ***(B)*** Corresponding axial CT scan identifying low attenuation periphery *(short arrow)* and higher attenuation central component *(long arrow)*. ***(C)*** High signal intensity fat *(closed arrows)* surrounding low signal intensity hemorrhagic fluid contents *(curved arrow)* on T1-weighted image. TR = 600 msec, TE = 20 msec. ***(D)*** Fat periphery shown with decreased signal intensity *(closed arrow)*, whereas central fluid contents *(curved arrow)* generate increased signal intensity on T2-weighted axial image. TR = 2000 msec, TE = 60 msec.

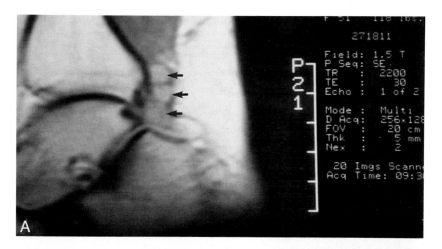

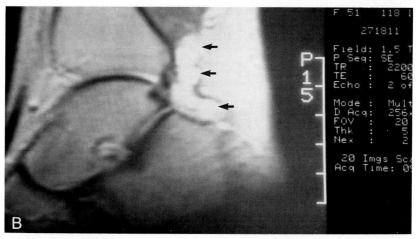

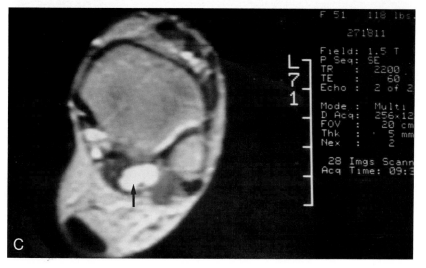

Figure 3-31

Juxtaarticular septated synovial cyst *(arrows)* posterior to the tibial-talar joint. Lesion images with low signal intensity on intermediate or proton weighted sagittal image *(A)* and high signal intensity on T2-weighted sagittal *(B)* and axial *(C)* images. TR = 2200 msec, TE = 30, 60 msec.

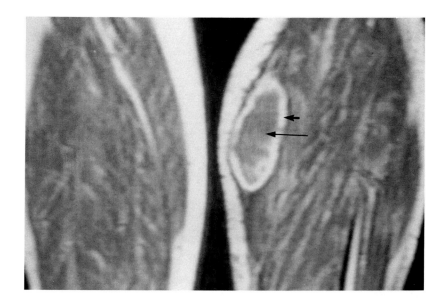

Figure 3-32

Intramuscular hemorrhage. Soleus muscle hemorrhage *(long arrow)* with subacute blood imaging with high signal intensity periphery *(short arrow)* on T1-weighted coronal image. TR = 800 msec, TE = 20 msec.

Figure 3-33

Arterial embolus. **(A)** Slow flow in posterior tibial artery *(solid straight arrow)* and vein *(curved arrow)* shown as high signal intensity on T2-weighted axial image. Surrounding muscle edema *(open arrow)* is visualized as high signal intensity. TR = 2000 msec, TE = 80 msec. **(B)** Lack of flow in the posterior tibial artery in an inferior axial image is visualized as signal void *(straight arrow)*, whereas the adjacent vein maintains high signal intensity *(curved arrow)*. Edema *(open arrow)* conforms to regional arterial supply. TR = 2000 msec, TE = 80 msec.

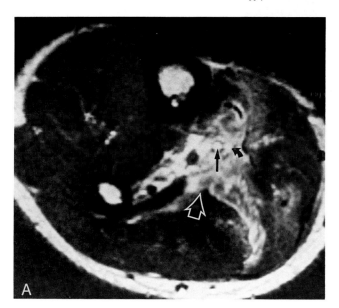

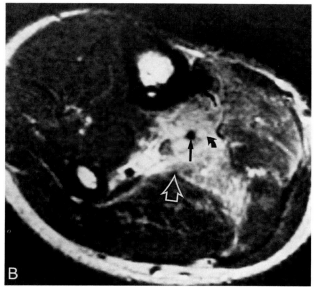

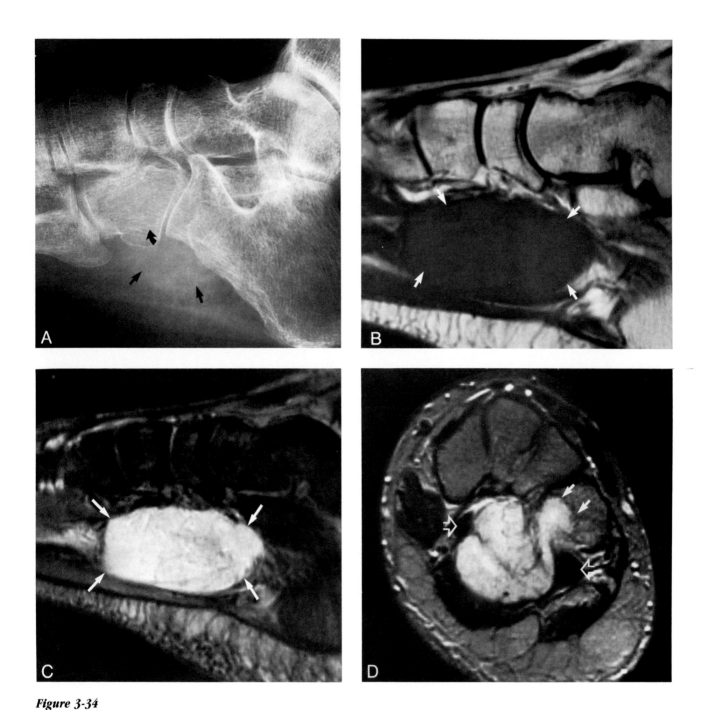

Figure 3-34

Synovial sarcoma. **(A)** Subtle plantar soft tissue mass *(straight arrows)* of synovial sarcoma on lateral radiograph. Localized osteoporosis and distortion of normal trabecular lawn is identified in the adjacent cuboid *(curved arrow)*. Corresponding sagittal images demonstrating large primary soft tissue synovial sarcoma *(arrows)*. The lesion images with low signal intensity on T1-weighted sequences **(B)** and with high signal intensity on T2* gradient echo sequence **(C)**. **(B)** TR = 600 msec, TE = 20 msec; **(C)** TR = 400 msec, TE = 30 msec, flip angle = 30°. **(D)** Documentation of cuboid bone invasion *(closed arrows)* and proximity of sarcoma to flexor and peroneal tendons *(open arrows)* on axial T2-weighted image. TR = 2000 msec, TE = 60 msec.

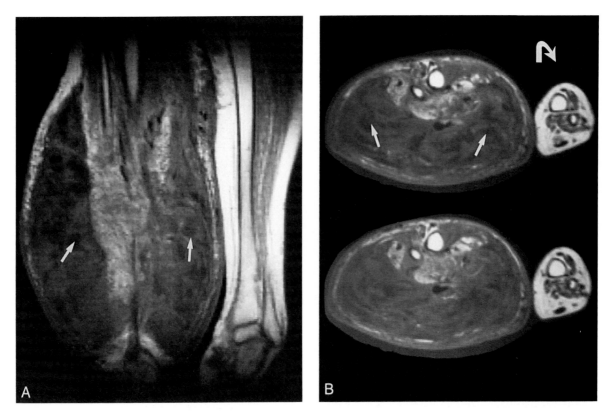

Figure 3-35

Neurofibroma. Large infiltrating nonplexiform neurofibroma invading and replacing soft tissue elements in the leg. Lower signal intensity areas of inhomogeneity represent fibrous components *(straight arrows)*. Opposite leg shown for comparison *(curved arrow)*. T1-weighted coronal *(A)* and axial *(B)* images; TR = 500 msec, TE = 40 msec.

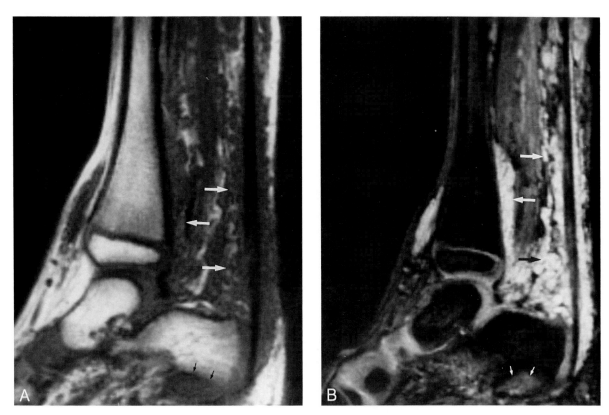

Figure 3-36

Neurofibromatosis. T1-weighted *(A)* and T2* gradient echo *(B)* images of the ankle demonstrating low and high signal intensity, respectively, in a plexiform neurofibroma tracking longitudinally along nerve bundles. Neurofibromas have a characteristic lobulated contour *(large arrows)*. Undercutting or erosion of the inferior calcaneal surface is shown *(small arrows)*. *(A)* TR = 600 msec, TE = 20 msec; *(B)* TR = 400 msec, TE = 30 msec, flip angle = 30°.

Figure 3-37

Leiomyosarcoma. *(A)* T1-weighted coronal image identifies posterolateral soft tissue mass isointense with muscle *(arrow)*. TR = 600 msec, TE = 20 msec. *(B)* Tumor displays uniform increase in signal intensity on T2-weighted axial image *(arrow)*.

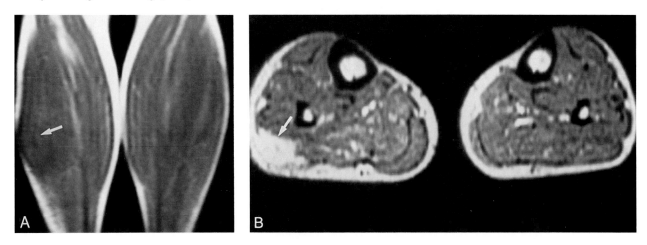

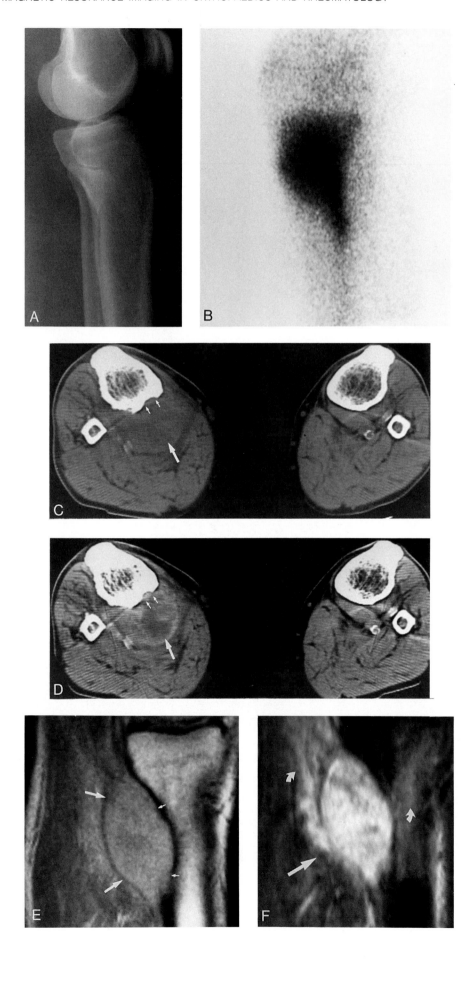

◄ *Figure 3-38*

Metastatic melanoma. *(A)* Lateral radiograph with subtle cortical irregularity along proximal posterior
tibial cortex. *(B)* Tc99-MDP bone scintograph with uptake of tracer in posterior tibia and soft tissues.
Axial CT scans before *(C)* and after *(D)* contrast enhancement showing hypervascularity of soft tissue
mass *(large arrow)*. Posteromedial cortical erosion is indicated *(small arrows)*. *(E)* T1-weighted sagittal
image identifying intermediate-signal intensity metastatic melanoma as an elliptical mass *(large arrows)*
invading low signal intensity posterior tibial cortex *(small arrows)*. *(F)* Corresponding STIR image
demonstrating high signal intensity contrast within metastatic melanoma *(straight arrow)* with reactive
marrow and soft tissue edema *(curved arrows)*.

Figure 3-39

Osteoarthritis. Degenerative subchondral (subarticular) cysts in the distal fibula *(curved black arrow)* and
lateral talus *(straight black arrow)*. Intraarticular chondral free fragment is identified *(straight white
arrow)*. Associated effusion is of intermediate signal intensity *(curved white arrow)*. *(A)* T1-weighted
coronal image. TR = 600 msec, TE = 20 msec. *(B)* T1-weighted axial image. TR = 600 msec, TE
= 20 msec.

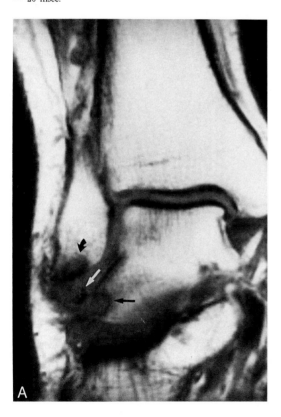 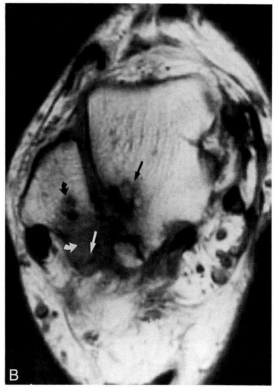

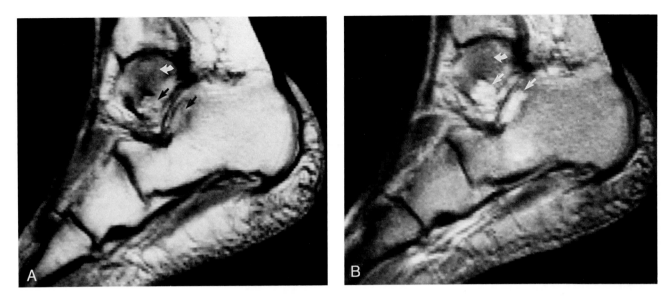

Figure 3-40

Osteoarthritis. **(A)** Degenerative cyst imaged on both sides of a narrowed subtalar joint with low signal intensity *(black arrows)*. T1-weighted sagittal image; TR = 1000 msec, TE = 400 msec. **(B)** On T2-weighted sagittal image the lesion images with high signal intensity *(straight white arrow)*. TR = 2000 msec, TE = 80 msec. Subchondral talar sclerosis images with low signal intensity on both T1- and T2-weighted images *(curved arrows)*.

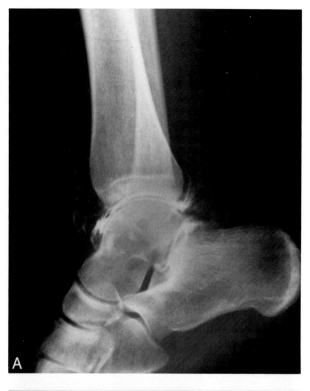

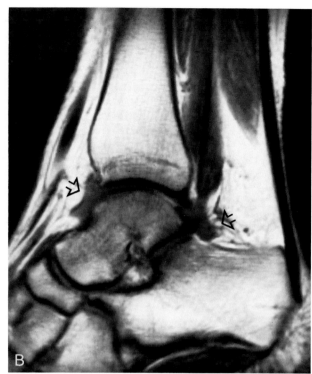

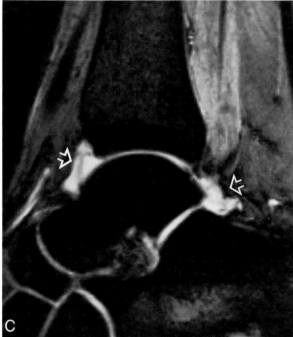

Figure 3-41

Ankle effusion. *(A)* Lateral radiograph showing distribution of arthrographic contrast within the tibiotalar joint. Corresponding sagittal images demonstrate the effusion *(open arrows)* as low signal intensity on T1-weighted image *(B)* and as high signal intensity on T2* gradient echo image *(C).* Anterior and posterior capsular distention is evident. *(B)* TR = 600 msec, TE = 20 msec; *(C)* TR = 400 msec, TE = 30 msec, flip angle = 30°.

Figure 3-42

Cyst. **(A)** Subarticular tibial cyst on AP ankle radiograph *(open black arrow)*. **(B)** Low signal intensity cyst *(open white arrow)* visualized on T1-weighted coronal image. TR = 1000 msec, TE = 40 msec. Increased signal intensity of synovial fluid contents demonstrated on T2-weighted axial image **(D)** *(black arrows)* compared with T1-weighted axial image **(C)** *(white arrows)*. Reactive sclerosis is best imaged on T2-weighted axial image *(small white arrow)*. **(C)** TR = 1000 msec, TE = 20 msec; **(D)** TR = 2000 msec, TE = 40 msec. **(E)** Corresponding axial CT scan defining sclerotic edge of the tibial cyst *(arrows)*.

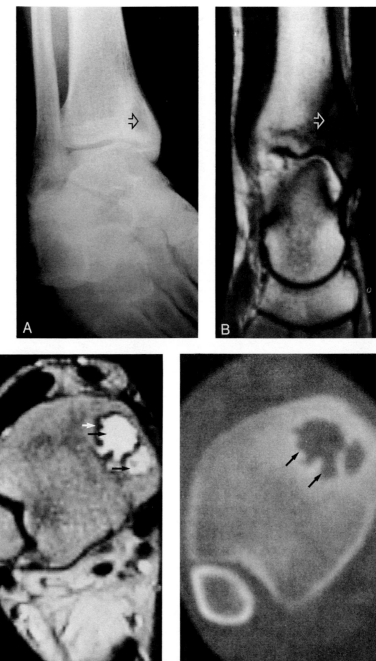

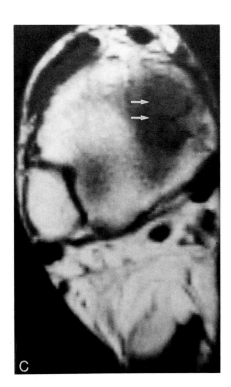

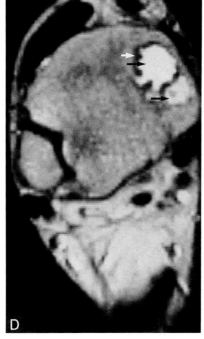

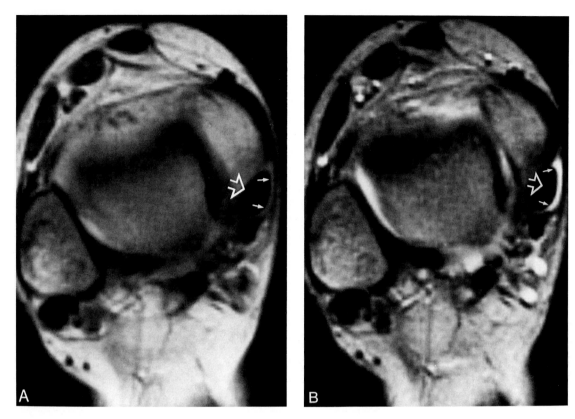

Figure 3-43

Tenosynovitis. Tenosynovitis of the tibialis posterior tendon *(open arrow)* with fluid-filled synovial sheath *(small arrows)* seen as low to intermediate signal intensity on intermediate-weighted image *(A)* and high signal intensity on T2-weighted image *(B)*. TR = 2000 msec, TE = 20, 60 msec.

PERSPECTIVE ON MR IMAGING OF THE ANKLE AND FOOT

MR visualization of hyaline articular cartilage and free fragments has made MR examination especially useful in the evaluation of transchondral fractures. Sagittal and axial plane MR assessment of the Achilles tendon (in inflammation and in tears) is excellent, and may facilitate evaluation of conservative orthopedic treatment. The routine use of MR in other tendon and ligamentous injuries needs further substantiation.

In infection and neoplasms, MR offers superior contrast resolution in identifying marrow, cortical, soft tissue, and compartmental disease involvement. Experience with MR imaging of ankle arthropathies in initial and in selective cases indicates that MR may provide more information than is possible with conventional radiography.

REFERENCES

1. Yousem DM, Scott WW Jr: The foot and ankle. In Scott WW, et al (eds): Computed Tomography of the Musculoskeletal System, pp 113–138. New York, Churchill Livingstone, 1987

2. Stoller DW, et al: Fast MR improves imaging of musculoskeletal system. Diagnostic Imaging, 1988, February:98

3. Schneck J: Optimization of MR imaging of the most commonly injured structures of the ankle. Radiology 165(P):149, 1987

4. Christoforidis JA: Atlas of Axial, Sagittal, and Coronal Anatomy with CT and MRI, pp 510–531. Philadelphia, WB Saunders, 1988

5. Beltran, J, et al: Ankle: Surface coil MR imaging at 1.5T. Radiology 161:203, 1986

6. Hajek PC, et al: High resolution magnetic resonance imaging of the ankle: Normal anatomy. Skeletal Radiol 15:536, 1986

7. Noto AM: MR imaging of the ankle: Normal variants. Radiology 165(P):148, 1987

8. Yulish BS, et al: MR imaging of osteochondral lesions of talus. JCAT 11:296, 1987

9. Berndt A, Harty M: Transchondral fractures (osteochondritis dessicans) of the talus. J Bone Joint Surg 41A:988, 1959

10. Beltran J, et al: Tendons: High-field-strength, surface coil MR imaging. Radiology 162:735, 1987

11. Hattrup SJ, Johnson KA: A review of ruptures of the Achilles tendon. Foot and Ankle 6:34, 1985

12. Willis CA, et al: Achilles tendon rupture: A review of the literature comparing surgical versus nonsurgical treatment. Clinical Orthopaedics and Related Research 1986 No. 207 (June), pp 156–163

13. Quinn SF, et al: Achilles tendon: MR imaging at 1.5T. Radiology 164:767, 1987

14. Beskin JL, et al: Surgical repair of Achilles tendon ruptures. American J Sports Medicine 15:1, 1987

15. Kellam JF, et al: Review of the operative treatment of Achilles tendon rupture. Clinical Orthopaedics and Related Research, 1985, No. 201 (December), pp 80–83

16. Rosenberg: Chronic tears of the posterior tibial tendon: A correlative study of CT, MR imaging, and surgical exploration. Radiology 165(P):149, 1987

17. Berquist TH, et al: Musculoskeletal trauma. In Berquist TH, et al (eds): Magnetic Resonance of the Musculoskeletal System, pp 127–161. New York, Raven Press, 1987

18. Tang JSH, et al: Musculoskeletal infection of the extremities: Evaluation with MR imaging. Radiology 166:205, 1988

19. Berquist TH: Musculoskeletal infection. In Berquist TH, et al (eds): Magnetic Resonance of the Musculoskeletal System, pp 109–125. New York, Raven Press, 1987

20. Stark DD, Bradley WG (eds): Magnetic Resonance Imaging, pp 1323–1433. St. Louis, CV Mosby, 1988

21. Griffey RH, et al: Correlation of magnetic resonance imaging and nerve conduction for the early detection of diabetic neuropathy in humans. Society of Magnetic Resonance in Medicine, (abstr) p 125. New York City, August 17–21, 1987

22. Bloem JL, et al: Magnetic resonance imaging of primary malignant bone tumors. RadioGraphics 7:425, 1987

23. Wetzel LH, et al: A comparison of MR imaging and CT in the evaluation of musculoskeletal masses. RadioGraphics 7:851, 1987

24. Petasnick JP, et al: Soft-tissue masses of the locomotor system: Comparison of MR imaging with CT. Radiology 160:125, 1986

25. Totty WG, et al: Soft-tissue tumors: MR imaging. Radiology 160:135, 1986

26. Harms SE: MRI of the musculoskeletal system. In Scott WW, Magid D, Tieshman EK (eds): CT of the Musculoskeletal System, pp 171–206. New York, Churchill Livingstone, 1987

27. Berquist TH, et al: Miscellaneous conditions and future potential. In Berquist TH, Ehman RL, Richardson ML (eds): Magnetic Resonance of the Musculoskeletal System, pp 185–209. New York, Raven Press, 1987

28. Beltran J, et al: Aneurysmal bone cysts: MR imaging at 1.5 T. Radiology 158:689, 1986

29. Alanen A: Magnetic resonance imaging of hematomas in a 0.02T magnetic field. Acta Radiol (Diagn) (Stockh) 27:589, 1986

30. Hudson TM, et al: Magnetic resonance imaging of bone and soft tissue tumors: Early experience in 31 patients compared with computed tomography. Skeletal Radiol 13:134, 1985

31. Berquist TH, et al: Magnetic Resonance of the Musculoskeletal System, pp 85–107. New York, Raven Press, 1987

32. Sundaram M, et al: Magnetic resonance imaging of lesions of synovial origin. Skeletal Radiol 15:133, 1986

33. Levine E, et al: Malignant nerve-sheath neoplasms in neurofibromatosis: Distinction from benign tumors by using imaging techniques. AJR 149:1059, 1987

34. Atlas SW, et al: MR imaging of intracranial metastatic melanoma. JCAT 11:577, 1987

David W. Stoller

Chapter 4   THE KNEE

The most rapid advances in magnetic resonance (MR) imaging of the musculoskeletal system have been in evaluation of internal knee derangements. In fact, because MR imaging is noninvasive and allows anatomic and pathologic definition of osseous, soft tissue, ligamentous, and cartilaginous structures, it is rapidly replacing arthrography and CT for this purpose. Improvements in dedicated extremity coils, high spatial resolution capabilities, and fast scan techniques have extended application of MR of the knee beyond the routine evaluation of the meniscus. Unlike arthrography (which necessitates the intra-articular injection of contrast material to evaluate the surface of the meniscus), the entire substance and internal structure of the meniscus can be seen on MR images.[1] A routine MR examination with imaging in axial, sagittal, and coronal planes can be performed in less than 10 min of acquisition time. In addition, manipulation of the joint—needed to perform an arthrogram—is not necessary. This is particularly important in patients who have sustained trauma with associated joint effusions and who cannot tolerate physical examination without anesthesia.

The ability to display anatomic features of the knee in direct multiplanar, off-axis, and oblique orientations has enhanced the use of MR in the assessment of trauma, arthritis, infection, and neoplasia.[2,3] The inherently superior soft tissue resolution of MR has facilitated direct visualization and differentiation of cortex, marrow, ligaments, tendons, muscle, synovium, vascular, and cartilage elements, not possible using conventional radiographic techniques.

IMAGING PROTOCOLS FOR THE KNEE

A circumferential extremity coil provides uniform signal-to-noise across the knee, without the posterior to anterior signal drop off observed in imaging with flat surface coils (Fig. 4-1). The routine knee protocol for the

Figure 4-1
Circumferential transmit-and-receive surface coil used in imaging the knee.

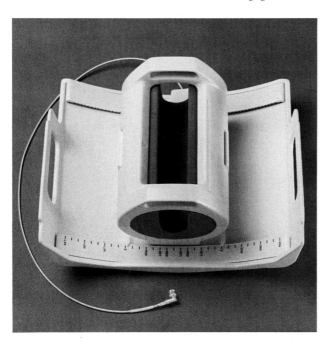

evaluation of internal derangement uses T1-weighted images in the axial, sagittal, and coronal planes. Using a recovery time (TR) of 600 msec and an echo time (TE) of 20 msec, all three orthogonal planes can be imaged in approximately 10 min of acquisition time. High resolution is obtained with a 256 × 256 acquisition matrix and a 16-cm field of view (FOV) at one excitation (NEX). Spatial resolution is recorded at 0.6 mm in both the phase-encoded and the frequency-encoded directions. A 16-cm FOV provides adequate visualization of the quadriceps-patellar mechanism in the sagittal plane; a 12-cm FOV should be used for pediatric patients. The initial axial acquisition is used to evaluate the patellofemoral joint and serves as a localizer for subsequent sagittal and coronal plane images. The sagittal plane is most sensitive for identifying meniscal and cruciate pathology, and the coronal plane is best for displaying collateral ligament anatomy.

Patients are placed in the supine position, with the knee placed in 15° of external rotation (to realign the anterior cruciate ligament parallel to the sagittal imaging plane). The rotation of the knee does not need to be changed for imaging in either the axial or coronal plane. Thin (5 mm) sections with a 1 mm interslice gap are used for studies in the axial plane, 5 mm contiguous sections in the sagittal plane, and 5 mm without an interslice gap in the coronal plane. Three millimeter slices are not necessary to accurately assess meniscal lesions in adults. In pediatric patients, however, a 3-mm slice thickness allows optimum medial to lateral joint coverage in the sagittal plane and allows anterior to posterior coverage in the coronal plane.

In selected cases of acute trauma, arthritis, infection, and neoplasia, T2-weighted images are acquired using either conventional spin echo or fast-scan techniques. Conventional T2-weighted images are generated at a TR of 2000 msec and TE of 20, 60 msec at a 256 × 128 acquisition matrix using 1 NEX. Fast-scan gradient echo (refocused) images with less than a 90° flip angle can be used to give effective T2 or T2* contrast. With this technique studies can be performed in 3 min of imaging time using a TR of 400 msec, a TE of 30 msec, and theta of 30°, at a 256 × 256 acquisition matrix using 2 NEX. With three dimensional Fourier transform (3-DFT) techniques, gradient echo volumetric imaging reduces imaging time and can reduce slice thickness to 0.7 mm. T2-weighting is helpful in highlighting ligamentous edema in either the coronal (collateral ligaments) or the sagittal (cruciate ligaments) imaging plane. In patients with arthritis, sagittal images provide the most information in early synovial reactions and cartilage erosions. Posterior femoral condylar defects, however, are best displayed on coronal images. Neoplastic lesions, both benign and malignant, require both T1- and T2-weighted images in the axial plane. T1-weighted sagittal or coronal images demonstrate the proximal and distal extent of a lesion in one section.

Artifact from pulsation of the popliteal artery, which may interfere with sagittal plane imaging of the cruciate ligaments, can be modified by switching the frequency- and phase-encoded directions.[4] Reversing the frequency-encoded direction in the sagittal plane reduces the apparent thickness of the tibial cortex (chemical shift artifact), allowing optimal visualization of the distal femoral articular cartilage.

High contrast photography of MR images, using narrow window widths, has been used to emphasize or highlight areas of brighter signal intensities within the normally low signal intensity menisci. We have not found this to be routinely necessary when lesions are photographed at proper contrast and intensity levels.

NORMAL MR ANATOMY OF THE KNEE

Axial Images

Axial plane images have an important role in routine knee evaluation. The patellar facets and the articular cartilage, because of their oblique orientation, are most accurately demonstrated in axial images through the patellofemoral joint. Patellofemoral disease (chondromalacia) may be over- or underestimated on sagittal images alone. Axial scans are also used as localizers to determine sagittal and coronal coverage when short TR sequences (TR = 600 msec) are used. Although the axial plane displays meniscal structure, it is not the most sensitive plane for evaluating meniscal degeneration and tears. Sagittal images, which section the meniscus perpendicular to its surface, provide the best demonstration of internal meniscal anatomy and pathology.

The surface of the tibial plateau is visualized on inferior axial sections through the knee joint. The posterior cruciate insertion is displayed on the posterior tibial surface and images with low signal intensity. At the mid joint level, the medial and lateral menisci are demonstrated with low signal intensity (Fig. 4-2). The medial meniscus has a more open "C" shape and a wider posterior horn than does the lateral meniscus. Because of partial voluming, 3-mm sections may be necessary to show both menisci in the same image. On these sections the transverse ligament of the knee is visualized as a band of low signal intensity connecting the anterior horns of the lateral and medial menisci. It can be seen traversing the infrapatellar fat pad that is visualized with high signal intensity. The semimembranosus and the semitendinosus tendons are visualized as circular areas of low signal intensity, located lateral to the medial head of the gastrocnemius muscle and posterior to the medial tibial plateau. The semimembranosus appears larger than the semitendinosus tendon. The sartorius muscle is elliptical in appearance and the gracilis tendon is circular. These muscles are located more medially and posteriorly, in line with the medial collateral ligament that

can be seen crossing the peripheral joint line. Proximal to its insertion on the fibular head, the biceps femoris tendon is visualized anterolateral to the lateral head of the gastrocnemius muscle. The popliteal artery is identified anterior to the popliteal vein, anterior to and between the two heads of the gastrocnemius muscle. In cross section, the low signal intensity lateral or fibular collateral ligament may be surrounded on all sides by high signal intensity fat. The anterior and posterior cruciate insertions can be seen within the intercondylar notch. The infrapatellar fat pad is bordered by the low signal intensity iliotibial band laterally, the medial retinaculum medially, and the thick patellar tendon anteriorly.

The anterior cruciate ligament can be identified superior to the joint line, 15° to 20° off axis, in an anteromedial orientation (Fig. 4-3).[5] The posterior cruciate ligament is circular in cross section. The origin of the anterior cruciate ligament can be seen on the medial aspect of the lateral femoral condyle, and the posterior cruciate ligament can be seen on the lateral aspect of the medial femoral condyle (Fig. 4-4). The plantaris muscle is located anterior to the lateral head of the gastrocnemius muscle. The common peroneal nerve is located lateral to the plantaris muscle, images with low to intermediate signal intensity, and is encased in fat. At the level of the femoral condyles, the tibial nerve is located posterior to the popliteal vein and visualizes with intermediate signal intensity. The larger, lateral patellar facet and the oblique, medial patellar facet are best visualized in the axial plane (Fig. 4-5). Articular cartilage surfaces image with intermediate signal intensity. Both medial and lateral patellar retinacular attachments are seen at the level of the patellofemoral joint and are of low signal intensity.

Sagittal Images

Although visible in axial and coronal plane images, the anterior and posterior cruciate ligaments are best displayed on sagittal images. The lateral or fibular collateral ligament and biceps femoris tendon may also be seen in peripheral sagittal sections. Images in the sagittal plane are key in evaluating meniscal anatomy for both degenerations and tears. The medial collateral ligament is not defined in the sagittal plane, and coronal planar images are needed for its evaluation.

On medial sagittal images, the low signal intensity semimembranosus tendon and intermediate signal muscle are seen posteriorly (Fig. 4-6). The vastus medialis muscle makes up the bulk of the musculature, anterior to the medial femoral condyle. Yellow marrow visualizes with bright signal intensity, whereas adjacent cortical bone images with low signal intensity. Femoral and tibial hyaline articular cartilage visualizes with intermediate signal intensity. The tibial cortex appears thicker than femoral cortical bone because of a chemical shift

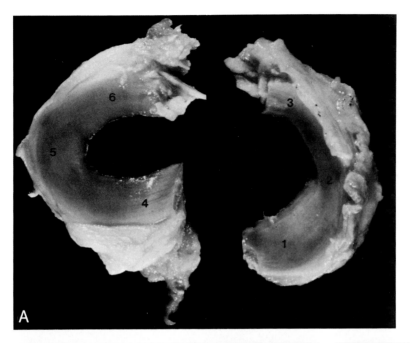

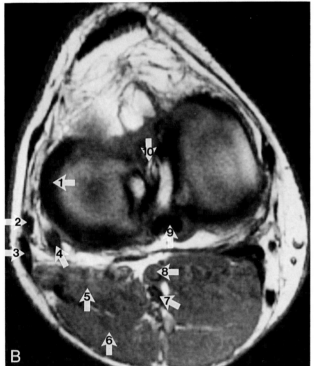

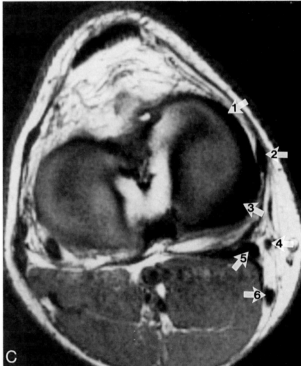

Figure 4-2

Axial anatomy of the menisci. **(A)** Gross anatomy of the lateral meniscus *(left)* and medial meniscus *(right)*. Larger posterior horn of the medial meniscus is evident: posterior horn of medial meniscus *(1)*, body of medial meniscus *(2)*, anterior horn of medial meniscus *(3)*, posterior horn of lateral meniscus *(4)*, body of lateral meniscus *(5)*, anterior horn of lateral meniscus *(6)*. **(B)** Axial image in the plane of the lateral meniscus: lateral meniscus *(1)*, fibular collateral ligament *(2)*, biceps femoris tendon *(3)*, popliteus tendon *(4)*, plantaris muscle *(5)*, lateral head of gastrocnemius muscle *(6)*, popliteal vein *(7)*, popliteal artery *(8)*, posterior cruciate ligament *(9)*, anterior cruciate ligament *(10)*. **(C)** Axial image in the plane of the medial meniscus: anterior horn of medial meniscus *(1)*, medial (tibial) collateral ligament *(2)*, posterior horn of medial meniscus *(3)*, gracilis tendon *(4)*, semimembranosus tendon *(5)*, semitendinosus tendon *(6)*.

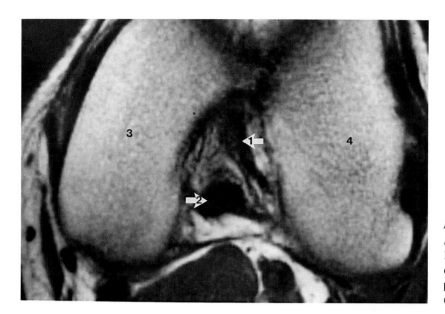

Figure 4-3

Axial anatomy of the cruciate ligaments.
Intercondylar anatomy of the anterior and posterior
cruciate ligaments: anterior cruciate ligament *(1)*,
posterior cruciate ligament *(2)*, medial femoral
condyle *(3)*, lateral femoral condyle *(4)*.

Figure 4-4

Axial anatomy at the origin of the cruciate ligaments: Sartorius muscle *(1)*,
gracilis tendon *(2)*, semitendinosus tendon *(3)*, semimembranosus muscle
(4), medial head of the gastrocnemius muscle *(5)*, popliteal vein *(6)*,
popliteal artery *(7)*, plantaris muscle *(8)*, lateral head of the gastrocnemius
muscle *(9)*, biceps femoris muscle *(10)*, origin of the posterior cruciate
ligament *(11)*, origin of the anterior cruciate ligament *(12)*, iliotibial band
(13).

Figure 4-5

Axial anatomy at the level of the patellofemoral joint: Medial patellar facet
(1), lateral patellar facet *(2)*. Medial retinacular attachments *(straight black
arrows)*, lateral retinacular attachments *(curved black arrows)*, articular
cartilage of medial and lateral patellar facets *(white arrows)*.

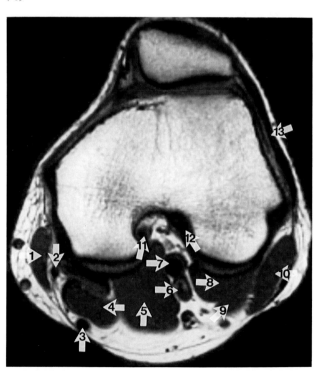

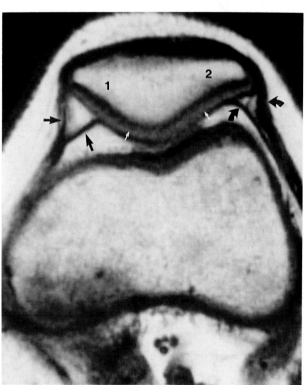

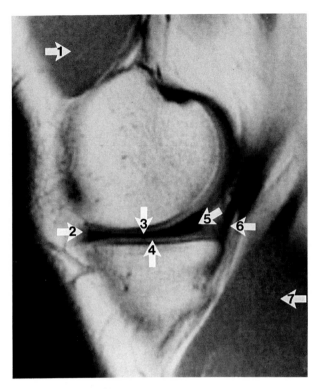

Figure 4-6

Sagittal peripheral medial compartment: Vastus medialis muscle *(1)*, anterior horn of medial meniscus *(2)*, body of medial meniscus *(3)*, tibial hyaline cartilage *(4)*, posterior horn of medial meniscus *(5)*, semimembranosus tendon *(6)*, medial head of the gastrocnemius muscle *(7)*.

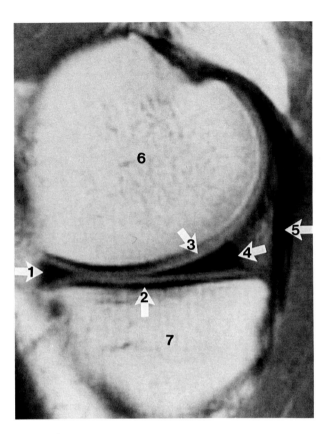

Figure 4-7

Sagittal medial compartment: Anterior horn of medial meniscus *(1)*, cortical bone of tibia *(2)*, femoral articular cartilage *(3)*, posterior horn of medial meniscus *(4)*, semimembranosus tendon *(5)*, medial femoral condyle *(6)*, medial tibial plateau *(7)*.

artifact. The medial meniscus, composed of fibrocartilage, images with uniform low signal intensity. The body of the medial meniscus has a continuous or bow-tie morphology on at least one or two consecutive medial sagittal images. On medial compartment sections closer to the intercondylar notch, the separate anterior and posterior horns of the medial meniscus are visualized (Fig. 4-7). They appear as opposing triangular shapes on a minimum of two to three consecutive sagittal images. The posterior horn of the medial meniscus is larger than the opposing anterior horn. The medial head of the gastrocnemius muscle sweeps posteriorly from its origin along the distal femur. A small band of high signal intensity fat can be seen between the posterior horn of the medial meniscus and the low signal intensity posterior capsule.

When viewing sagittal images in the medial to lateral direction, the posterior cruciate ligament is visualized before the anterior cruciate comes into view. The thick, uniform low signal intensity posterior cruciate ligament arcs from its anterolateral origin on the medial femoral condyle to its insertion on the posterior tibial plateau. With partial knee flexion, the convex curve of the posterior cruciate becomes taut. In the lateral inter-

condylar notch, the anterior cruciate ligament extends from its origin on the posteromedial lateral femoral condyle to its insertion 8 mm posterior to the anterior tibial edge. It is not unusual to see portions of both cruciate ligaments on the same sagittal section (Fig. 4-8). The anterior cruciate ligament is composed of two bands of fibers, anteromedial and posterolateral, which are difficult to separate on the sagittal images. Independent of partial voluming with the lateral femoral condyle, anterior cruciate fibers may image with a minimally higher intensity signal than the posterior cruciate ligament. The anterior cruciate is normally visualized on at least one sagittal section when the knee is properly positioned in 10° to 15° of external rotation. Fiber bundle striations of the anterior cruciate are prominent at femoral and tibial attachment sites.

On midsagittal sections, the quadriceps and patellar tendons (imaged with low signal intensity) are demonstrated in their anterior attachments to the superior and inferior patellar poles, respectively. Hoffa's infrapatellar fat pad is directly posterior to the patellar tendon and images with bright signal intensity. Posterior patellar cartilage displays a smooth convex arc on images through the medial and lateral facets. Without joint fluid, the collapsed suprapatellar bursa is usually not visualized above the superior pole of the patella. On intercondylar sagittal sections, the popliteal vessels are seen in long axis, with the artery anterior and the vein posterior.

The conjoined insertion of the lateral collateral ligament and the biceps femoris tendon on the fibular head can be identified on most lateral sagittal sections. The lateral head of the gastrocnemius muscle is seen posterior to the fibula, and follows an inferior course from the distal lateral femoral condyle behind the popliteus muscle. The popliteus tendon (of low signal intensity) and its sheath (of intermediate signal intensity) are seen in their expected anatomic locations between the capsule and the periphery of the lateral meniscus (Fig. 4-9). Separate synovium-lined fascicles, or struts, of the meniscus allow intra-articular passage of the popliteus tendon. In its middle one third (or body), the C-shaped lateral meniscus also demonstrates a bow-tie shape (Fig.

Figure 4-8
Sagittal intercondylar notch: Suprapatellar bursa with fluid *(1)*, quadriceps tendon *(2)*, patellar tendon *(3)*, popliteal artery *(4)*, femur *(5)*, tibia *(6)*. Anterior cruciate ligament *(white arrows)*, posterior cruciate ligament *(black arrows)*.

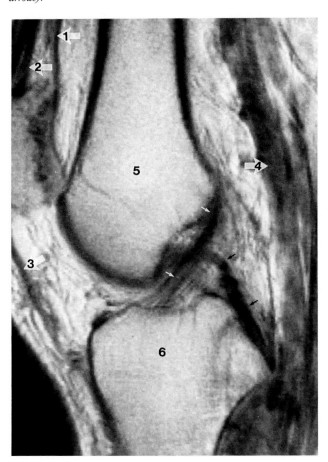

4-10). On more medial sections through the lateral compartment, the separate triangular shapes of the anterior and posterior horns (oriented toward each other and nearly symmetric in size and shape) can be distinguished. The medial collateral ligament is not defined on sagittal images (see coronal plane).

Coronal Images

Coronal planar images are needed to define the collateral ligaments. Posterior coronal images are also best for displaying the posterior femoral condyles, the site of early articular erosions. The cruciate ligaments, although displayed to best advantage in the sagittal plane, can also be identified in coronal images.

The low signal intensity popliteal vessels are identified on posterior coronal images (Fig. 4-11). The fibular collateral ligament is imaged on posterior coronal sections as a low signal intensity cord stretching from its insertion on the fibular head to the lateral epicondyle of the femur (Fig. 4-12). It is separated from the lateral meniscus by the thickness of the popliteus tendon. At the level of the femoral condyles posteriorly, the menisco-femoral ligament of Wrisberg may be visualized as a thin, low spin density band extending from the posterior horn of the lateral meniscus to the lateral surface

Figure 4-9
Sagittal lateral compartment: Anterior horn of lateral meniscus *(1)*, femoral articular cartilage *(2)*, posterior horn of lateral meniscus and popliteus tendon sheath *(3)*, popliteus tendon *(4)*, biceps femoris muscle *(5)*, plantaris muscle *(6)*, Hoffa infrapatellar fat pad *(7)*, physeal scar *(8)*, lateral femoral condyle *(9)*, lateral tibial plateau *(10)*, proximal tibiofibular joint *(11)*, fibula *(12)*.

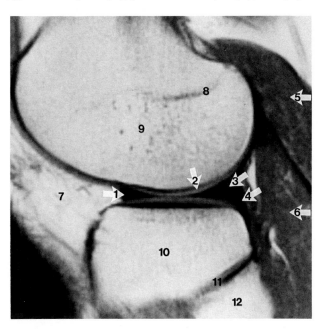

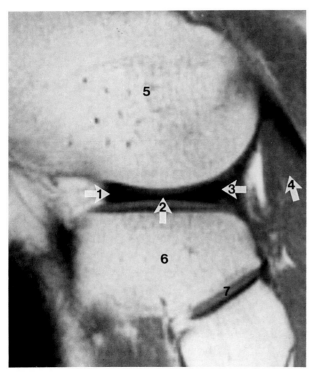

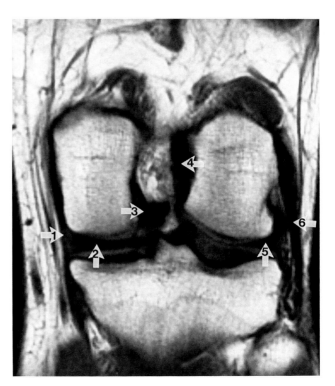

Figure 4-10

Sagittal peripheral lateral compartment: Anterior horn of lateral meniscus *(1)*, body of lateral meniscus *(2)*, posterior horn of lateral meniscus *(3)*, plantaris muscle *(4)*, lateral femoral condyle *(5)*, lateral tibial plateau *(6)*, proximal tibiofibular joint *(7)*.

Figure 4-11

Posterior coronal image: Sartorius muscle *(1)*, semimembranosus *(2)*, medial head of the gastrocnemius muscle *(3)*, popliteal vessels *(4)*, biceps femoris muscle *(5)*, lateral head of the gastrocnemius muscle *(6)*, anterior cruciate *(7)*, posterior cruciate *(8)*, posterior horn of lateral meniscus *(9)*.

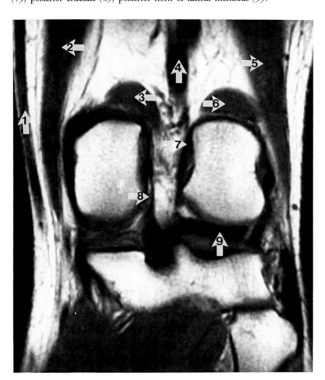

Figure 4-12

Posterior midcoronal image: Medial (tibial) collateral ligament *(1)*, posterior horn of medial meniscus *(2)*, posterior cruciate *(3)*, anterior cruciate *(4)*, body of lateral meniscus *(5)*, lateral (fibular) collateral ligament *(6)*.

of the medial femoral condyle. The anteromedial and posterolateral bands of the anterior cruciate can be discerned on anterior and posterior coronal images, respectively. The posterior cruciate ligament is circular and is of uniform low signal intensity on anterior and midcoronal sections (Fig. 4-13). On posterior coronal images the triangular attachment of the posterior cruciate can be differentiated as it fans out from the lateral aspect of the medial femoral condyle. The medial collateral ligament is identified on midcoronal sections, anterior to sections where femoral condyles appear to fuse together with the distal metaphysis. The tibial or medial collateral ligament visualizes as a band of low signal intensity extending from its medial femoral epicondylar attachment to the medial tibial condyle. It consists of a superficial layer and a deep layer attached to the periphery of the medial meniscus. The femoral and tibial attachments of the uninjured or intact medial collateral ligament image with uniform dark signal intensity, indistinguishable from underlying cortical bone. From the plane of the posterior femoral condyles, the medial collateral ligament is visualized on at least two to three coronal images (when acquired using 5-mm sections without interslice gaps). A line of intermediate signal intensity separates the periphery of the medial meniscus from the deep layer of the medial collateral ligament. This represents either a small bursa or, more probably, vascularized connective tissue. The anterior body and

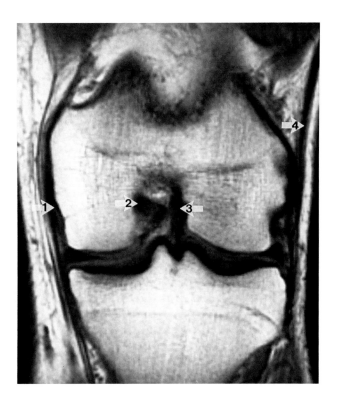

posterior horns of the medial and lateral menisci are visualized as distinct segments and not as opposing triangles as seen on sagittal images. On posterior coronal images the plane of section is parallel to the posterior curve of the C-shaped menisci, and the posterior horn may be displayed as a continuous band of low signal intensity.

Midcoronal sections demonstrate the anterior tibial spine, whereas anterior images are marked by the high signal intensity of Hoffa's infrapatellar fat pad, anterior to the lateral knee compartment (Figs. 4-14 and 4-15). Anteriorly, the iliotibial band blends with the lateral patellar retinaculum, and the vastus medialis is in continuity with its medial retinacular patellar attachment. The low signal intensity fibers of the quadriceps and patellar tendons can be identified on the most anterior sections in the plane of the patella.

Figure 4-13
Midcoronal image: Medial collateral ligament *(1)*, posterior cruciate ligament *(2)*, anterior cruciate ligament *(3)*, iliotibial band *(4)*.

Figure 4-15
Anterior coronal image: Hoffa fat pad *(1)*, physeal scar *(2)*.

Figure 4-14
Midanterior coronal image: Medial collateral ligament *(1)*, body of medial meniscus *(2)*, anterior cruciate ligament *(3)*, anterior horn of lateral meniscus *(4)*, anterior tibial spine *(5)*.

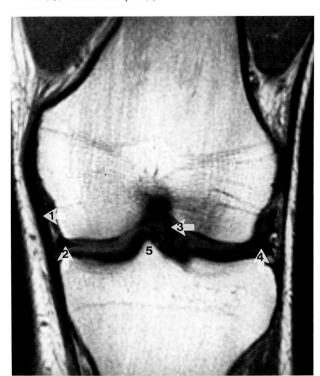

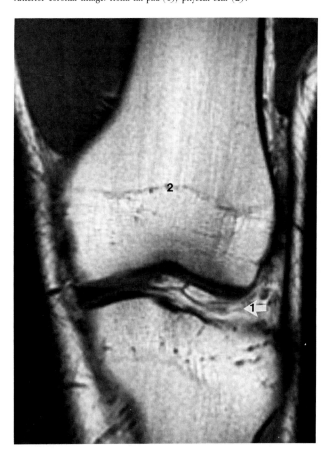

THE MENISCI

Imaging Protocols for the Menisci

T1-weighted or intermediate (proton density)-weighted protocols are most sensitive for the detection of meniscal lesions.[6] Additional images with conventional T2-weighting, using a spin echo sequence, can be used to identify fluid, edema, or hemorrhage in acute ligamentous trauma or fracture. Gradient echo T2* images offer the advantage of effective T2-weighting without compromising the delineation of meniscal degenerations or tears.[7] Gradient recall techniques are also useful for demonstrating articular cartilage, that images with high signal intensity using this sequence. Meniscal examinations should be performed with a dedicated extremity coil, as discussed earlier.

Normal MR Anatomy of the Menisci

The C-shaped fibrocartilaginous menisci or semilunar cartilages are attached to the condylar surface of the tibia and provide added mechanical stability to femorotibial rotations (Fig. 4-16). The intact meniscus images with uniform low signal intensity on both T1- and T2-weighted images. The menisci are triangular in cross section, have an outer convex curve, a medially directed apex, and are arbitrarily divided into thirds—the anterior horn, the body, and the posterior horn. The menisci transmit axial and torsional forces across the joint, cushion mechanical loading, distribute synovial fluid, and provide increased surface area for femoral condylar motion. The lateral meniscus forms a tight C shape and accommodates the popliteus tendon posteriorly. It is separated from the lateral collateral ligament (extracapsular), and has posterior horn attachments to the posterior cruciate ligament and medial femoral condyle through the ligament of Wrisberg. The medial meniscus is wider, with a more open C shape. In addition to intercondylar connections, it is attached to the deep layer of the medial collateral ligament and capsule. The pos-

terior horn of the medial meniscus is wider than the anterior horn or the body. Except for the peripheral perimeniscal capillary plexus, the adult meniscus is relatively avascular.[8] In the pediatric meniscus the geniculate arteries give rise to a more extensive vascular supply.

Meniscal Pathology

Meniscal Degenerations and Tears

Pathogenesis.   Rotation of the femur against a fixed tibia during flexion and extension places the menisci at risk for injury.[9] There is controversy as to whether an unstable meniscus accelerates articular degeneration. Tears involving the medial meniscus usually initiate in the inferior surface of the posterior horn.[6] The lateral meniscus is more prone to transverse or oblique tears. Associated hemorrhage and tearing in peripheral meniscal attachments contribute to the pain perceived in meniscal tears.

Usefulness of MR.   In comparison with arthroscopy, the sensitivity of MR imaging in the detection of meniscal tears has been reported to be between 75% and 100%[2,10,11] In a large series by Mink, et al, the accuracy rate of MR imaging in 600 menisci was 92%, with nine false-negatives and 18 false-positives.[12] Fast three-dimensional MR imaging of the meniscus produced a 95% concurrence between MR and arthroscopy in detection of meniscal tears, and a 100% correlation with meniscal degenerations.[13] The negative predictive value of MR approaches 100% in exclusion of tears in normal MR examinations of the meniscus. Further documentations with both arthrography and arthroscopy are needed to validate clinical efficacy. The variation in detection rates of meniscal lesions when compared to arthroscopy may be due to multiple factors, including: (1) a learning curve on the part of the radiologist in interpreting MR signal intensities, (2) the experience of several different arthroscopists participating in correlative studies, (3) false interpretation of areas of fibrillation or fraying as

Figure 4-16   ▶

Normal anatomy of the meniscus. *(A)* Gross specimen of the lateral meniscus. *Line 1* represents the plane of sagittal section through the body of the lateral meniscus. *Line 2* represents the plane of sagittal section through the anterior and body of the lateral meniscus. *(B)* Corresponding gross sagittal sections (*1* and *2*) through the posterior horns *(curved black arrows)* and anterior and posterior horns *(straight white arrows)* of the lateral meniscus. The periphery or body of the meniscus has a continuous "bow-tie" appearance. The anterior and posterior horns are oriented as opposing triangles of fibrocartilage. *(C–D)* Corresponding sagittal plane images *(1* and *2)* demonstrating low signal intensity body *(curved black arrows)* and anterior and posterior horns *(straight white arrows)* of the lateral meniscus.

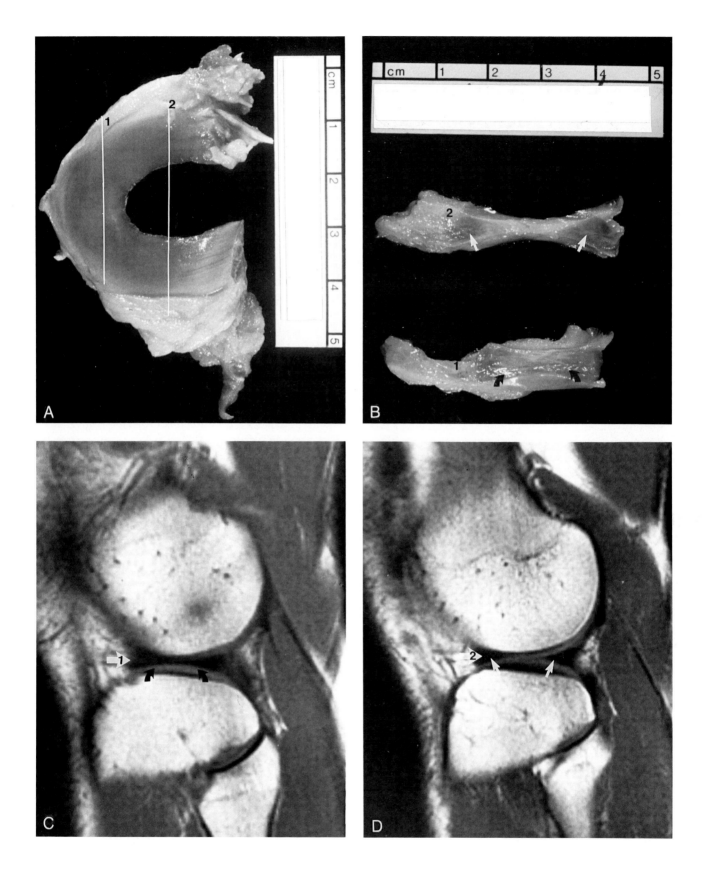

meniscal tears, (4) the inability of arthroscopy to detect degenerative cleavage tears without probing, and (5) the variability in performing examinations with different MR imagers and surface coils at a variety of field strengths.

MR Appearance. Whereas the intact meniscus demonstrates homogeneous low signal intensity regardless of the pulse sequence, degenerations and tears of the meniscus image with increased signal intensity, attributed to imbibed synovial fluid.[6] As synovial fluid diffuses through the meniscus, areas of degeneration and tears trap water molecules onto surface boundary layers, increasing the local spin density. T1 and T2 values are shortened as interaction of synovial fluid with large macromolecules in the meniscus slows the rotation rates of protons.[6] This explains the sensitivity of T1-weighted and intermediate- or proton density-weighted images in visualizing meniscal degenerations and tears. Increased signal intensity in synovial fluid gaps has been confirmed in surgically induced tears in animal models.[14] In MR studies performed after arthrography, increased signal intensity may be observed on T2-weighted images. This change is related to the actions of joint fluid and a hyperosmolar contrast agent that draw fluid into meniscal separations. This creates a motional narrowing effect (free water molecules in motion) allowing more mobile protons to be imaged separately from unbound water molecules.[15] In the absence of a joint effusion, meniscal degenerations and tears may actually decrease in signal intensity on T2-weighted images. On T2* or gradient refocused images, however, degenerations and tears generate increased signal intensities.[7]

In order to understand the significance of increased signal intensity in meniscal abnormalities, a *grading system* has been developed and correlated with a pathologic (histologic) model (Fig. 4-17).[6,10] Areas of

Figure 4-17

Illustration of gross meniscus showing representative grades of meniscal degeneration (grades 1 and 2) and tear (grade 3).

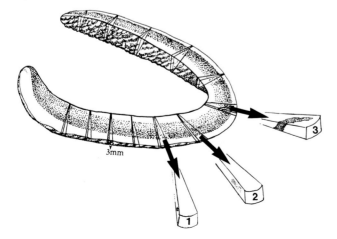

degeneration image with increased signal intensity in a spectrum of patterns or grades that are based on signal distribution relative to an articular surface (exclusive of the peripheral capsular margin of the meniscus that is considered nonarticular).

In MR grade 1 there is focal or globular intrasubstance increased signal intensity that is nonarticular (Fig. 4-18). Histologically, grade 1 signal intensity correlates with foci of early mucinous degeneration and chondrocyte-deficient or hypocellular regions that are pale staining on hematoxylin and eosin (H and E) preparations. (The terms mucinous, myxoid, and hyaline degeneration can be used interchangeably to describe the accumulation or increased production of mucopolysaccharide ground substance in stressed or strained areas of the meniscal fibrocartilage.[16,17] These changes usually occur in response to mechanical loading and degeneration.) Grade 1 signal intensity may be observed in asymptomatic athletes and normal volunteers and is not clinically significant.

In MR grade 2 there is horizontal, linear intrasubstance increased signal intensity that extends from the capsular periphery of the meniscus but does not involve an articular surface (Fig. 4-19). Areas and bands of mucinous degeneration are more extensive in grade 2 than seen in grade 1. Although no distinct cleavage plane or tear is observed in grade 2 menisci, microscopic clefting and collagen fragmentation has been recorded in hypocellular regions of the fibrocartilaginous matrix. The middle perforating collagen bundle, a structure not ordinarily seen on MR images, sends out fibers that horizontally divide the meniscus into superior and inferior halves.[18] It creates a neutral or buffer plane for superior femoral and inferior tibial frictional forces, and is the site for preferential accumulation of mucinous ground substance imaged as grade 2 signal intensity. Although patients with grade 2 menisci may or may not present with symptomatic knee pain, these lesions are prone to fibrocartilaginous tears, especially in the posterior horns of the medial menisci. The presence of mucinous degeneration is thus thought to represent potential structural weakening within collagen fibers. In the immature meniscus, vascular ingrowth along midperforating collagen bundles may contribute to the finding of grade 2 signal in young children; and there may not be areas of degeneration. In the adult, however, vascular penetrations in the meniscus have been resorbed, and the finding of increased signal intensity distinctly correlates with areas of mucinous degeneration.

A meniscus is considered MR grade 3 when the area of increased signal intensity communicates or extends to at least one articular surface (Fig. 4-20). Fibrocartilaginous separation or tears have been found in all menisci with grade 3 signal intensity. In about 5% of grade 3 menisci these disruptions represent what has been referred to in the orthopedic literature as *confined*

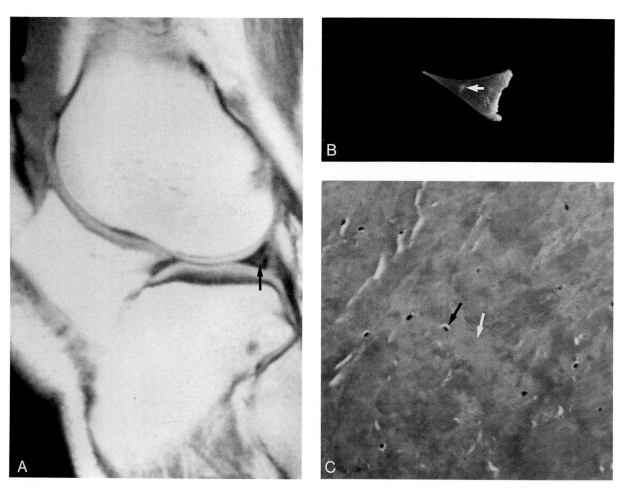

Figure 4-18

Meniscal degeneration. *(A)* Grade 1 signal intensity *(arrow)* in posterior horn of lateral meniscus. T1-weighted sagittal image; TR = 800 msec, TE = 20 msec. *(B)* Focus of degeneration on cut gross section *(arrow)*. *(C)* Corresponding photomicrograph showing hypocellularity with decreased numbers of chondrocytes *(black arrow)* in pale staining areas *(white arrow)* on hematoxylin and eosin stained section.

intrasubstance cleavage tears (Fig. 4-21).[19] Diagnosis of these closed meniscal tears may require surgical probing during arthroscopy and might be missed altogether on arthrographic examination. These disruptions also explain in part the 6% false-positive interpretations of grade 3 signal when correlated with arthroscopy.[10] A similar rate of false-negative correlations with arthroscopy may relate to spurious interpretation of areas of fraying and fibrillation as meniscal tears. Even without joint locking, the mechanical instability created by confined horizontal cleavage tears may be responsible for the clinical presentation of acute knee pain. In addition to observing increased signal intensity within tears, the morphology (size and shape) of the meniscus should be assessed when evaluating meniscal lesions (Figs. 4-22 and 4-23).

A displaced longitudinal tear of the medial meniscus, called a *bucket-handle tear*, is so named because the separated central fragment resembles the handle of a bucket.[6] The remaining larger peripheral section of the medial meniscus is the bucket. A bucket-handle tear effectively reduces the width of the meniscus, and peripheral sagittal images fail to demonstrate a normal bow-tie configuration in the body of the medial meniscus (Fig. 4-24). The remaining anterior and posterior horns are often hypoplastic or truncated with internal signal intensity. When the posterior horn of the medial meniscus is intact, it is wider and taller than the anterior horn. The displaced meniscal fragment can frequently be identified within the intercondylar notch on coronal images (Fig. 4-25). In complex bucket-handle tears, axial images show the anatomic relationship of the tear to the remaining meniscus in a single section. This information is valuable for directing an arthroscopic approach for repair or resection.

Regenerative chondrocytes and synovial metaplasia have been documented along the tear-meniscal interface, resulting from an attempt at meniscal repair.[6]

Text continues on p. 114

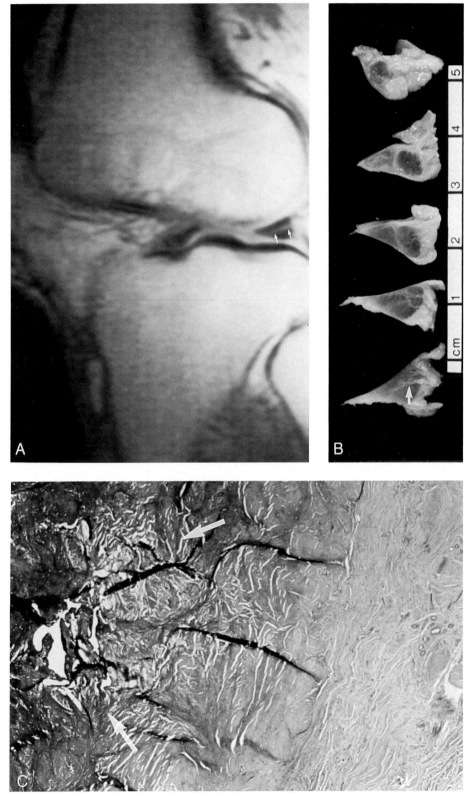

Figure 4-19

Meniscal degeneration. *(A)* Grade 2 signal intensity in the posterior horn of the lateral meniscus *(arrows)*. T1-weighted sagittal image; TR = 800 msec, TE = 20 msec. *(B)* Corresponding gross section demonstrating linear mucinous degeneration *(arrow)*. *(C)* Histologic correlation identifying focus of mucinous degeneration within meniscal fibrocartilage *(arrows)*.

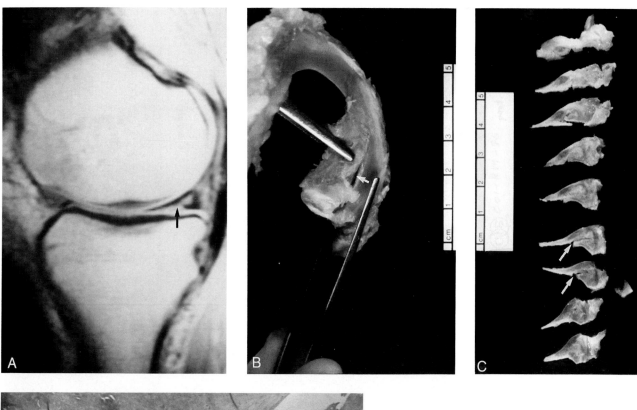

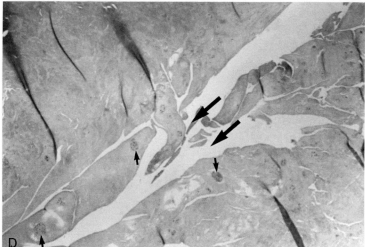

Figure 4-20

Meniscal tear. *(A)* Grade 3 signal intensity extending to inferior articular surface in posterior horn of medial meniscus flap tear *(arrow)*. TR = 800 msec, TE = 20 msec. *(B)* Corresponding inferior surface tear revealed with probing of gross medial meniscus specimen *(arrow)*. *(C)* Cut gross sagittal sections identifying orientation of inferior surface flap tear *(arrows)*. *(D)* Photomicrograph of grade 3 meniscal tear showing complete fibrocartilaginous separation *(large arrows)* with regenerative chondrocytes observed along the free edge of the torn meniscus *(small arrows)*.

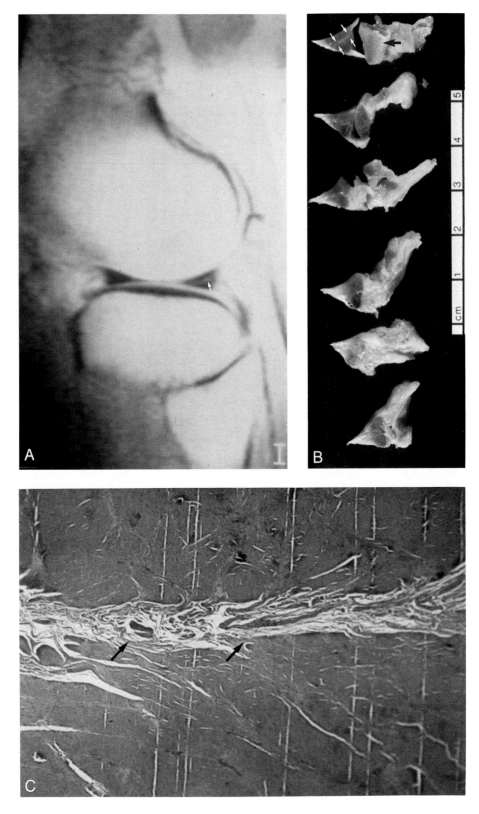

Figure 4-21

Closed meniscal tear. **(A)** Horizontal intrasubstance cleavage tear is visualized as grade 3 signal intensity *(white arrow)*. T1-weighted sagittal image; TR = 800 msec, TE = 20 msec. **(B)** Sagittal gross section identifying degeneration approaching the inferior surface of the meniscus without a visible surface tear *(white arrows)*. Popliteus tendon is indicated *(black arrow)*. **(C)** Corresponding photomicrograph demonstrating confined fibrocartilaginous separation *(arrows)*.

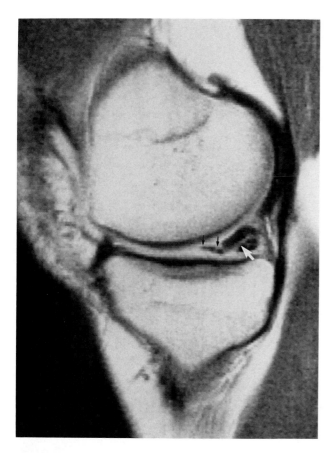

Figure 4-22
Flap tear (grade 3) of posterior horn of medial meniscus *(white arrow)* with truncated meniscal apex *(black arrows)*. TR = 1500 msec, TE = 40 msec.

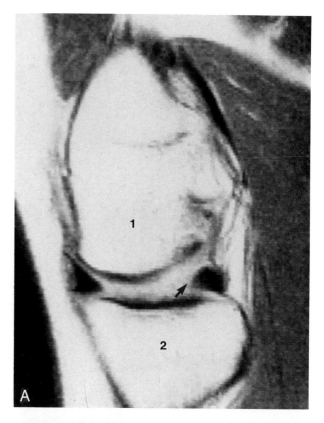

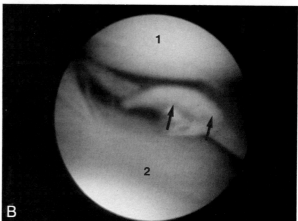

Figure 4-23
Torn medial meniscus with abnormal morphology. *(A)* Blunted and foreshortened apex of the posterior horn of the medial meniscus *(arrow)*: femur *(1)*, tibia *(2)*. T1-weighted sagittal image; TR = 600 msec, TE = 20 msec. *(B)* Arthroscopic view demonstrates complete flap tear *(arrows)* to the truncated medial meniscus: femur *(1)*, tibia *(2)*.

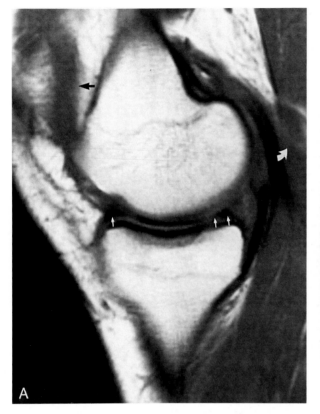

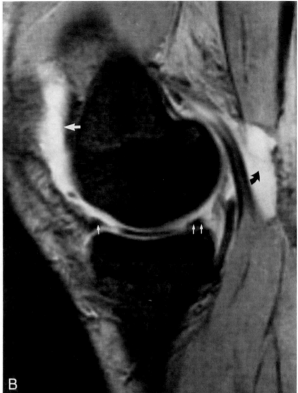

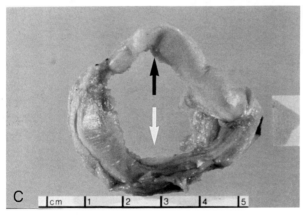

Figure 4-24

Bucket-handle tear. Bucket-handle tear with foreshortened anterior *(single white arrow)* and posterior *(double white arrows)* horns. Suprapatellar fluid *(large straight arrow)* and popliteal cyst *(curved arrow)* image with low signal intensity on T1-weighted images *(A)* and with high signal intensity on T2* gradient echo sagittal image *(B)*. *(A)* TR = 600 msec, TE = 20 msec; *(B)* TR = 400 msec, TE = 30 msec; flip angle = 30°. *(C)* Gross specimen demonstrates displaced longitudinal bucket-handle tear *(black arrow)* from the medial meniscus *(white arrow)*.

Synovial metaplasia in degenerative tears is thought to contribute to the development of acute and chronic pain. Peripheral perimeniscal capillary ingrowth has been observed perforating areas of degeneration and fibrocartilaginous separation, explaining the preferential healing in this location (Fig. 4-26).

Fresh traumatic tears have less predictable orientations than degenerative horizontal cleavage or flap tears, and have smaller areas of associated mucinous degenerations as sites for structural weakening (Fig. 4-27).[20] Grade 3 signal intensity is most frequent in the posterior horn of the medial meniscus, a finding supported by observations of increased stress and strain generated on the undersurface of the meniscus with femorotibial rotations. MR makes a significant contribu-

tion in imaging this frequently injured site. The accuracy of arthroscopy in identifying inferior surface tears of the posteromedial meniscus is reported to be as low as 45% to 69%.[21,22] Furthermore, arthrography and arthroscopy are insensitive to grades 1 and 2 degenerations as precursors to a visibly detected tear. MR allows detection of multiple meniscal tears that may be overlooked on an arthrogram study (Fig. 4-28).

Pitfalls in the Interpretation of Meniscal Tears. Knowledge of some of the more common pitfalls encountered in MR imaging of the meniscus will help to maintain high specificity and accuracy of diagnostic interpretations of meniscal tears.[23]

In a small percentage of cases (less than 5% in our

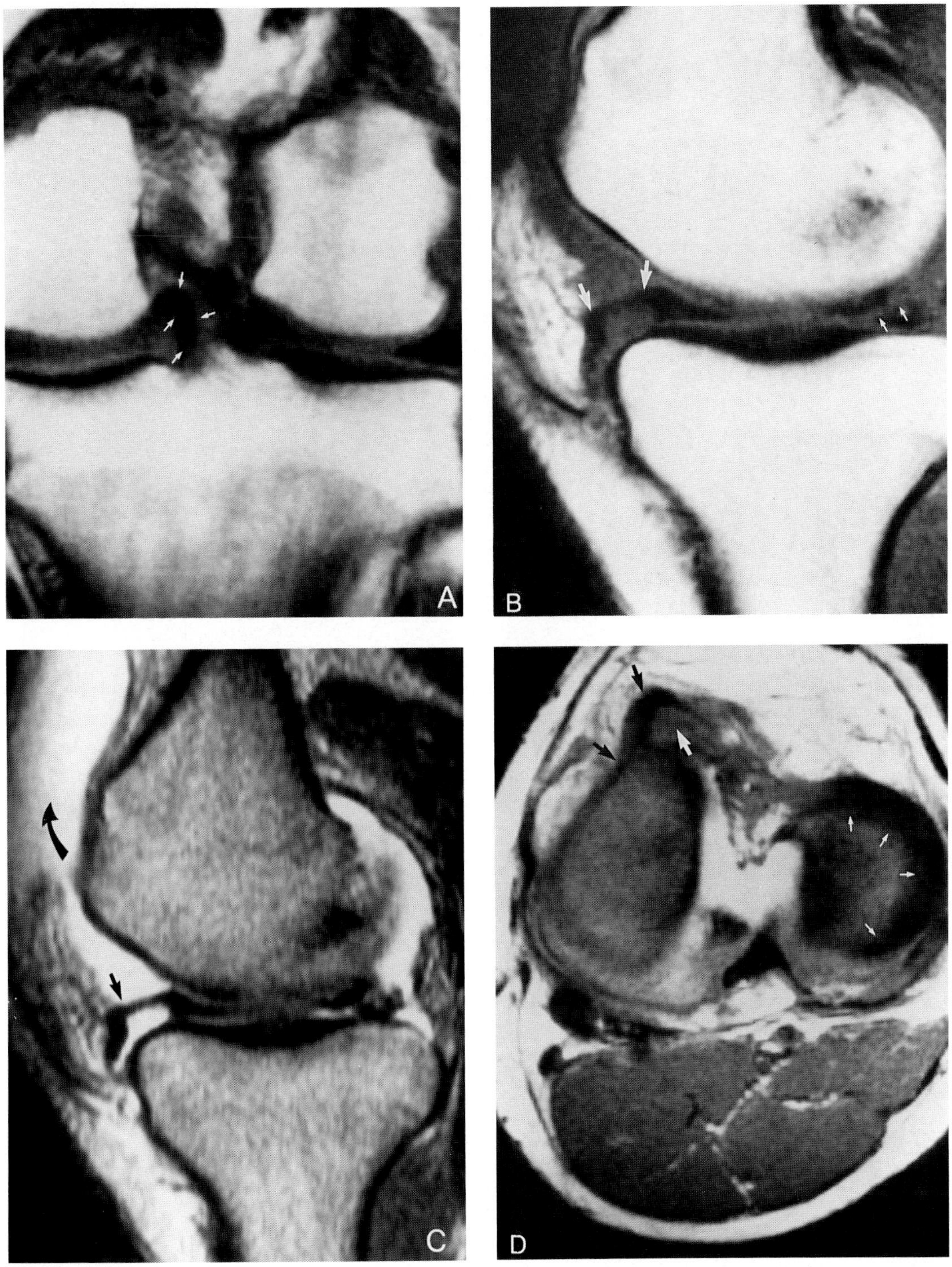

Figure 4-25

Displaced bucket-handle tear. *(A)* Intercondylar meniscal fragment identified on coronal image *(arrows)*. T1-weighted image; TR = 600 msec, TE = 20 msec. *(B)* Flipped anterior horn *(large arrows)*, medial meniscal tissue, and posterior horn tear *(small arrows)* are identified on a T1-weighted sagittal image. TR = 600 msec, TE = 20 msec. *(C)* Corresponding T2-weighted sagittal image demonstrating arthrographiclike effect with high signal intensity fluid *(curved arrow)* outlining low signal intensity meniscus *(straight arrow)*. TR = 2000 msec, TE = 60 msec. *(D)* Corresponding axial image demonstrating displaced bucket handle tear *(black arrow)* with associated low signal intensity fluid *(large white arrow)*. Intact lateral meniscus *(small white arrows)* is identified. TR = 600 msec, TE = 20 msec.

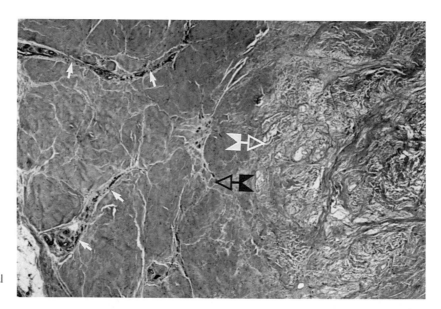

Figure 4-26

Perimeniscal capillary ingrowth *(solid arrows)* directed toward area of mucinous degeneration *(white flagged arrow)*. Normal adjacent meniscal tissue is demonstrated *(black flagged arrow)*.

Figure 4-27

Traumatic meniscal tear in a 12 year old. Complex tear of the posterior horn of the lateral meniscus communicating with both superior and inferior articular surfaces *(small white arrows)*. Physeal scar *(black arrows)* and associated joint effusion *(open arrow)* are indicated.

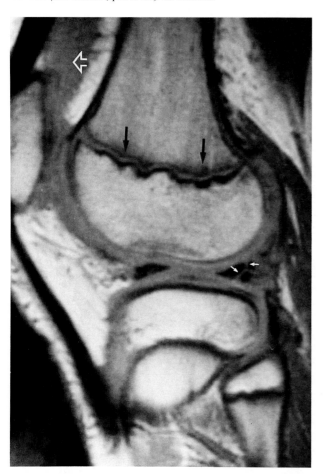

experience), it may be difficult to distinguish articular surface extension of signal intensity. In this circumstance, evaluation of the morphology of the meniscus as well as the degree of increased signal intensity and thickness of generated signal may facilitate an accurate interpretation. Weakening or decreased signal intensity of a grade 3 lesion as it approaches an articular surface, for example, favors a diagnosis of an intrasubstance cleavage tear that, at arthroscopy, might require surgical probing for detection. In the presence of a joint effusion, grade 3 signal, which becomes more conspicuous on T2-weighting, indicates a disrupted meniscal surface that facilitates the influx of free water molecules (T2 prolongation; Fig. 4-29).

Fibrillation or *fraying* of the concave free edge of the meniscus (facing the intercondylar notch) is visualized as increased signal intensity restricted to the apex of the meniscus and does not represent meniscal tearing (Fig. 4-30). However, a *truncated* or foreshortened meniscus represents abnormal morphology in a meniscal tear. A *macerated meniscus* will imbibe synovial fluid throughout its substance and images with a diffuse increase in signal intensity (multiple grade 3 signals; Fig. 4-31).

The *transverse ligament* of the knee, which connects the anterior horns of the medial and lateral menisci, can simulate an oblique tear adjacent to the anterior horn of the lateral meniscus (Fig. 4-32). In up to 30% of MR examinations, the fat that surrounds the low signal intensity ligament mimics grade 3 signal intensity (Fig. 4-33). Axial images have been most successful in demonstrating the entire course of the transverse ligament as a low signal intensity band through Hoffa's fat pad (Fig. 4-34). On serial sagittal images, the round

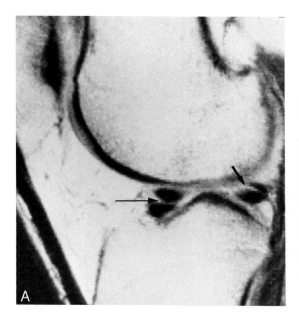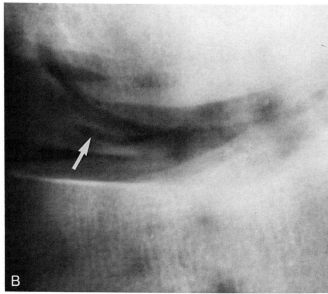

Figure 4-28

Meniscal tear. **(A)** Horizontal tears in the anterior *(long arrow)* and posterior *(short arrow)* horns of the lateral meniscus. T1-weighted sagittal image; TR = 1000 msec, TE = 40 msec. **(B)** Corresponding arthrogram confirming anterior horn tear *(arrow)*. Posterior horn tear was missed on the arthrogram.

Figure 4-29

Posterior horn medial meniscus tear *(small arrows)* with associated joint effusion *(open arrow)* on T1-weighted **(A)** and T2-weighted **(B)** images. Tear demonstrates increased signal intensity on T2-weighted image. **(A)** TR = 800 msec, TE = 20 msec; **(B)** TR = 2000 msec, TE = 80 msec.

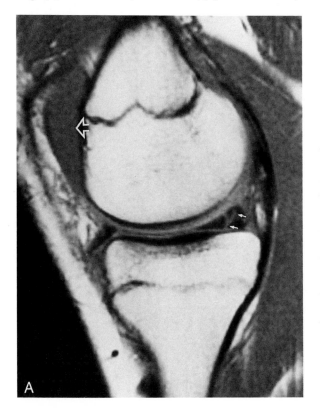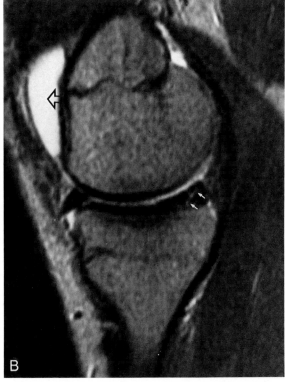

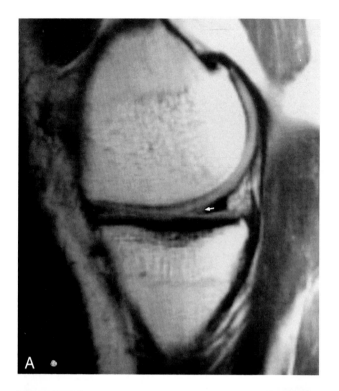

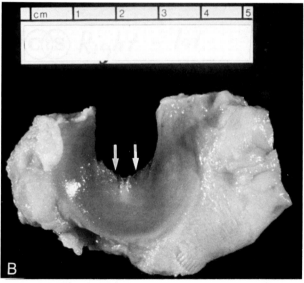

Figure 4-30

Fibrillation. **(A)** Increased signal intensity restricted to the apex of the meniscus represents degenerative fibrillation or fraying *(arrow)*. **(B)** Gross meniscus with fibrillation along concave free edge *(arrows)*.

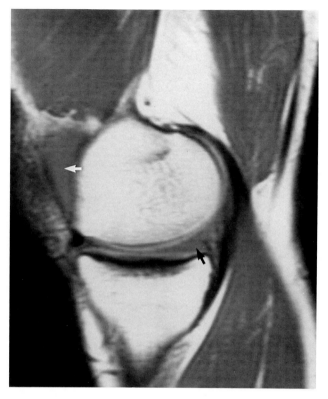

Figure 4-31

Increased signal intensity from imbibed synovial fluid in the macerated posterior horn of the medial meniscus *(black arrow)*. Adjacent joint effusion *(white arrow)* is indicated. T1-weighted sagittal image; TR = 600 msec, TE = 20 msec.

transverse ligament may be traced from the anterior horns of the lateral to medial meniscus in 15% of cases. Isolated tears of the anterior horn of the lateral meniscus are unusual, but can easily be differentiated from the transverse ligament pseudotear. Rarely would prominent branch vessels off the *lateral inferior geniculate artery* simulate a second pseudotear in this location.

In the posterior horn of the lateral meniscus the

popliteus tendon sheath can be mistaken for a grade 3 signal and be falsely interpreted as a tear (Fig. 4-35). The popliteus tendon sheath is intermediate in signal intensity on T1- and T2-weighted images and courses in an oblique anterosuperior to posteroinferior direction, anterior to the low signal intensity popliteus tendon (Fig. 4-36). In the presence of a joint effusion, fluid in the popliteus sheath visualizes with bright signal intensity on T2-weighted images (Fig. 4-37). In addition, the fascicles (superior and inferior) of the posterior horn of the lateral meniscus are best displayed on T2-weighted images in the presence of a small effusion. A fascicle tear should not be equated with the normal superior and inferior *meniscocapsular defects,* which allow passage of the popliteus tendon (Fig. 4-38). The thickness of the popliteus tendon sheath is variable and may image as a thin line or as a thick band. A true peripheral lateral meniscus tear will image with a different obliquity than that described for the popliteus sheath (Fig. 4-39).

Complex meniscal tears may present with unique MR imaging characteristics. In a patient without visualization of the posterior horn of the lateral meniscus,

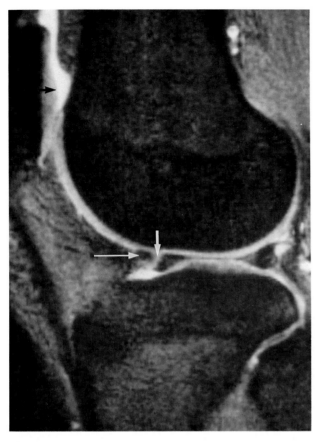

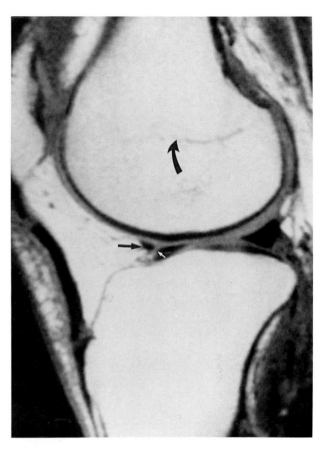

Figure 4-32

Transverse ligament of the knee *(long white arrow)* separated from the anterior horn of the lateral meniscus by high signal intensity fluid *(small white arrow)*. Bright signal intensity suprapatellar effusion is demonstrated *(small black arrow)*. T2* weighted image; TR = 400 msec, TE = 30 msec; flip angle = 30°.

Figure 4-33

Transverse ligament of the knee. Oblique pseudotear created by fat *(white arrow)* associated with the low signal intensity transverse ligament of the knee *(straight black arrow)*. Physeal scar is identified in the distal femur *(curved arrow)*. T1-weighted sagittal image; TR = 600 msec, TE = 20 msec.

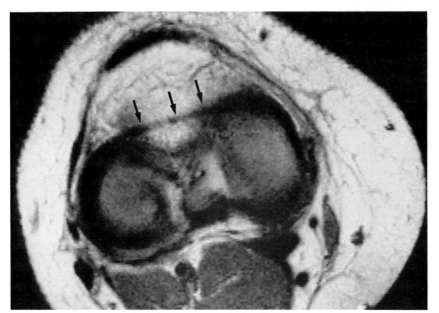

Figure 4-34

The low signal intensity transverse ligament of the knee is shown connecting the anterior horns of the medial and lateral menisci *(arrows)*. The ligament is surrounded by high signal intensity fat in Hoffa's infrapatellar fat pad. T1-weighted axial image; TR = 1000 msec, TE = 40 msec.

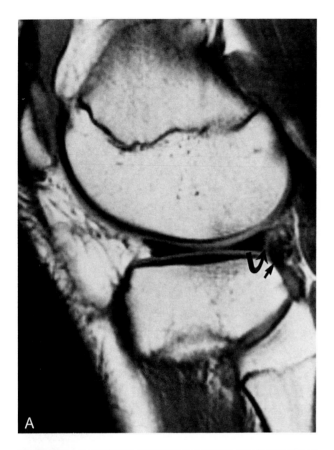

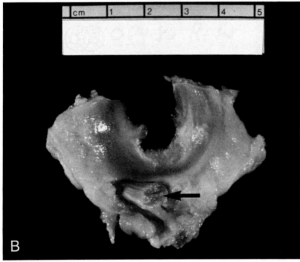

Figure 4-35

Popliteus tendon and sheath. **(A)** Intermediate signal intensity popliteus tendon sheath *(curved arrow)* and low signal intensity popliteus tendon *(straight arrow)* demonstrated on T1-weighted sagittal image. TR = 600 msec, TE = 20 msec. **(B)** Corresponding gross specimen showing the course of the popliteus tendon *(arrow)* along the posterior horn of the lateral meniscus.

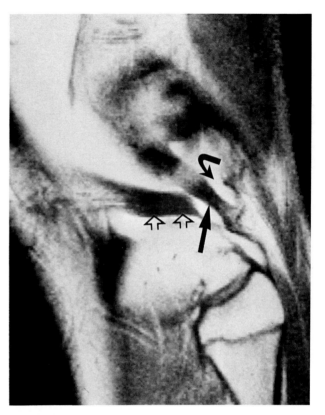

Figure 4-36

Peripheral sagittal image identifying the oblique course of the popliteus tendon *(straight arrow)* to its superior attachment along the lateral femoral condyle. Adjacent body of the lateral meniscus *(open arrows)* and high signal intensity synovial effusion *(curved arrow)* are shown. T2-weighted image; TR = 1500 msec, TE = 80 msec.

the posterior horn was identified to be flipped anteriorly, occupying the space adjacent to the anterior horn, and creating pseudohypertrophy of the anterior horn (Fig. 4-40).

Miscellaneous Conditions of the Meniscus

Postoperative Menisci. MR may also be useful in evaluating patients with pain or mechanical symptoms after partial or total meniscectomy (Fig. 4-41).[24] The same criteria used for assessing meniscal degenerations and tears in native menisci apply to partial-meniscectomy remnants. The signal intensity in a meniscal or fibrous remnant may image with a grayer signal than normally seen with low spin density fibrocartilage. Small postoperative meniscal fragments adjacent to the site of a meniscectomy have been identified on MR examination; however, the clinical significance of this finding relative to a patient's symptoms requires further investigation. Although the morphology of postmeniscectomy menisci is variable, we have documented several cases

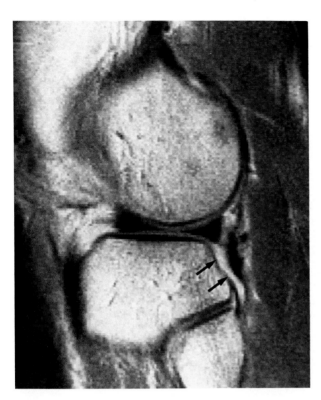

Figure 4-37
High signal intensity fluid shown distending the popliteus tendon sheath
(arrows) on T2-weighted sagittal image. TR = 1500 msec, TE = 80 msec.

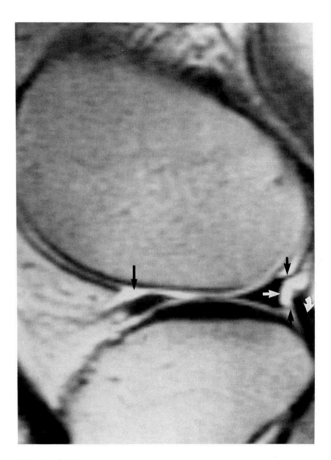

Figure 4-38
T2-weighted sagittal image demonstrating high signal intensity joint fluid
reflected over the lateral meniscus *(large black arrow)* and contained within
the popliteus sheath *(straight white arrow)*. Lateral meniscal struts *(small
black arrows)* and popliteus tendon *(curved white arrow)* are visualized.
TR = 2000 msec, TE = 60 msec.

of grade 3 signal intensity in such menisci, confirmed as
tears at arthroscopy. In two of four cases of primary
meniscal repair, grade 3 signal intensity was observed
and tears confirmed at arthroscopy. Further MR documentation of primary meniscal repairs is needed to understand the significance of signal intensity at the suture
line. A track made previously by an arthroscope leaves a
visible low signal intensity track in Hoffa's infrapatellar
fat pad.

Discoid Menisci. A discoid meniscus is a dysplastic
meniscus that has lost its normal "C" or semilunar shape
and has a broad disclike configuration.[25–27] Lateral discoid menisci are more common than medial discoid
menisci, and the enlargement varies from mild hypertrophy to a bulky slab of fibrocartilage. It has been postulated that an abnormal posterior horn attachment,
involving the inferior fascicle, contributes to the
development of discoid growth. Discoid menisci are
susceptible to tears and cysts, and in the young patient
present with symptoms of a torn cartilage.

Plain films of discoid menisci may demonstrate
widening of the involved compartment, and arthrography demonstrates an elongated meniscus (Fig. 4-42).

On MR, a discoid meniscus images with a continuous or
bow-tie appearance on three or more successive sagittal
images (Fig. 4-43).[2] Visualization of anterior and posterior horns is limited to one or two sagittal sections near
the intercondylar notch. On both coronal and sagittal
images, the increased inferior–superior dimensions can
be appreciated. The central tapering, seen in the normal
meniscus on sagittal images, is lost in discoid fibrocartilage. In a series of six patients with discoid menisci,
grade 3 signal intensity was observed in three cases. In
the presence of an effusion, the enlarged meniscus is
outlined with high signal intensity fluid on T2-weighted
images.

Meniscal Cysts. Meniscal cysts are collections of
mucinous or synovial fluid traceable to the joint line
(Fig. 4-44). They may develop in response to trauma or
degeneration and are associated with meniscectomy.[28,29]
Meniscal cysts are more common laterally and often
present at the peripheral margin of the meniscus. A horizontal meniscal tear is frequently identified in line with

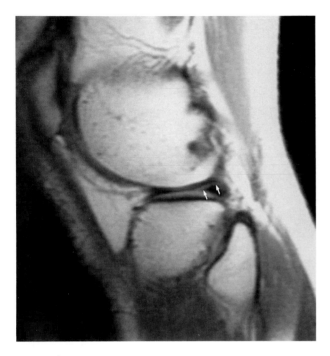

Figure 4-39
Peripheral tear of the lateral meniscus *(arrows)* with obliquity opposite to the orientation of the popliteus tendon sheath. T1-weighted sagittal image; TR = 600 msec, TE = 20 msec.

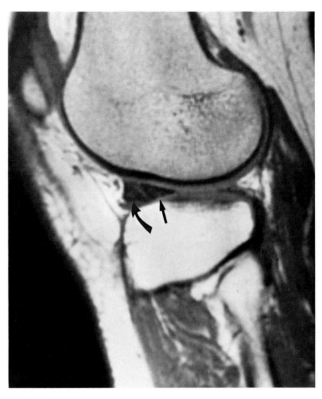

Figure 4-40
Pseudohypertrophy of the meniscal horn. A complex tear of the lateral meniscus demonstrates a flipped posterior horn *(curved arrow)* lying in tandem with the anterior horn fibrocartilage *(straight arrow)*. T1-weighted sagittal image; TR = 600 msec, TE = 20 msec.

the meniscal cyst, suggesting decompression of synovial fluid. Meniscal cysts image with uniform low signal intensity on T1-weighted images and with high signal intensity on T2-weighted images. Loculations of a complex meniscal cyst have also been visualized on MR examination (Fig. 4-45).

Meniscocapsular Separations. Peripheral meniscocapsular separations or tears usually involve the less mobile medial meniscus.[23] The posterior horn of the medial meniscus, fixed to the tibia by meniscotibial or coronary ligaments, is especially likely to tear at its capsular attachment. On sagittal MR images the tibial plateau cartilage should be covered by the posterior horn of the medial meniscus without an exposed articular surface. Uncovered tibial articular cartilage, or fluid interposed between the peripheral edge of the meniscus and capsule, is suggestive of peripheral detachment (Fig.

4-46). Associated grade 3 signal intensity is often visualized within the posterior horn (Fig. 4-47). Complete peripheral detachment of the posterior horn is visualized as a free floating meniscus, especially if it is associated with a medial collateral ligament tear. Peripheral detachments involving the meniscocapsular or meniscosynovial junction have a propensity to improve clinically, perhaps because of their proximity to vascular tissue and synovium.

Calcifications. In chondrocalcinosis, meniscal calcifications are frequently identified using conventional radiographic techniques. We have performed MR studies on one patient with *calcium pyrophosphate disease* (CPPD) and, using high contrast settings for photography, were able to differentiate focal, low signal intensity calcifications from the low spin density menisci.

Text continues on p. 128

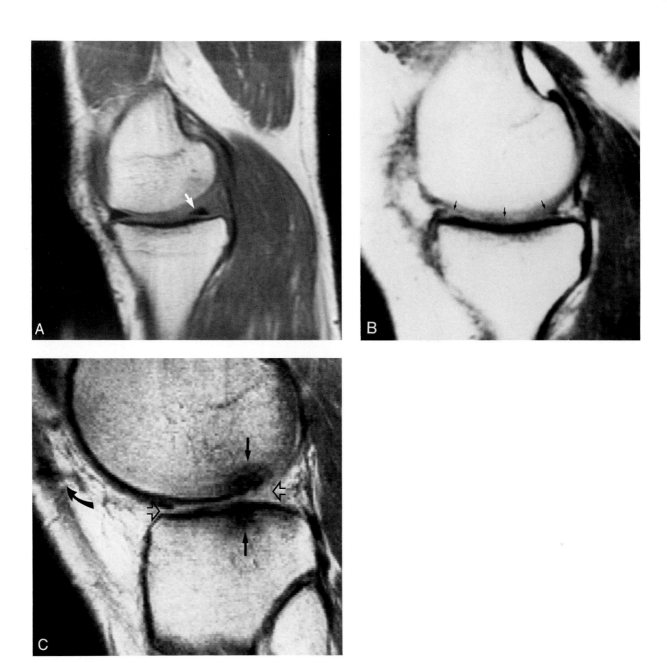

Figure 4-41

Meniscectomy. *(A)* Partial medial meniscectomy with diminished size of the posterior horn of the medial meniscus *(arrow)*. T1-weighted sagittal image; TR = 600 msec, TE = 20 msec *(B)* Total medial meniscectomy *(arrows)* with loss of joint space. T1-weighted sagittal image; TR = 800 msec, TE = 20 msec. *(C)* Total lateral meniscectomy *(open arrows)* with secondary degenerative subchondral sclerosis visualized as low signal intensity *(closed arrows)*. Arthroscopy track is identified anteriorly as low signal intensity *(curved arrow)*. T1-weighted sagittal image; TR = 1000 msec, TE = 40 msec.

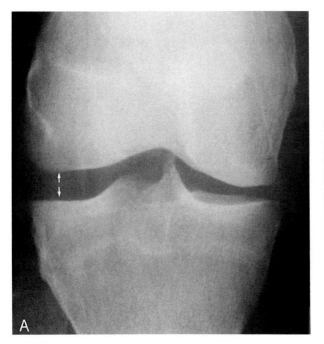

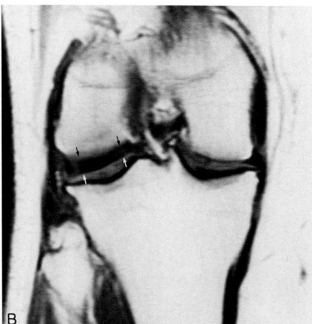

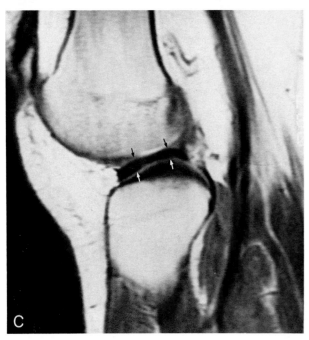

Figure 4-42

Discoid lateral meniscus. *(A)* AP radiograph with widened lateral joint compartment *(arrows)*. Corresponding coronal *(B)* and sagittal *(C)* images demonstrating the thick slab of lateral meniscal fibrocartilage imaging as a continuous low signal intensity band *(arrows)*. TR = 600 msec, TE = 20 msec.

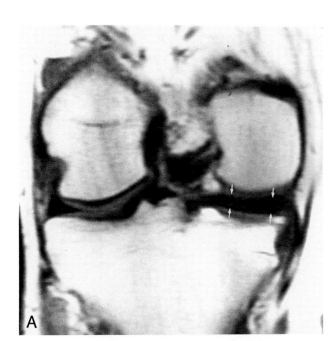

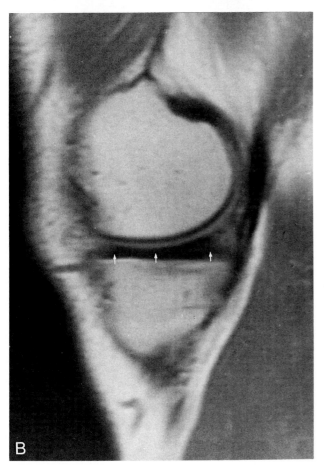

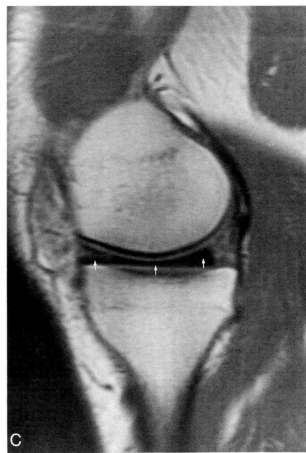

Figure 4-43

Discoid medial meniscus. *(A)* Coronal image demonstrating dysplastic and hypertrophied band of medial meniscal tissue *(arrows)*. A discoid medial meniscus is a rare finding. Continuous low signal intensity "bow-tie" appearance *(arrows)* seen on multiple sagittal images from the periphery *(B)* toward the intercondylar notch *(C)*. TR = 600 msec, TE = 20 msec.

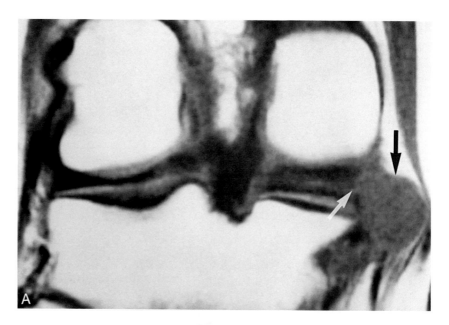

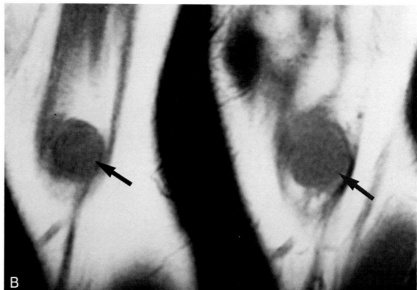

Figure 4-44

Meniscal cyst. Medial meniscal cyst shown projecting medial to the joint line *(black arrow)* on coronal *(A)* and peripheral sagittal *(B)* T1-weighted images. Communication with a meniscal tear is identified on coronal image *(white arrow)*. TR = 1000 msec, TE = 20 msec.

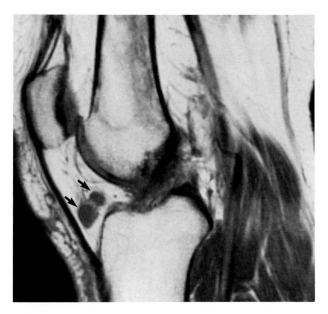

Figure 4-45

Bilobed meniscal cyst *(arrows)* seen dissecting through Hoffa's fat pad. Synovial fluid contents are of low signal intensity on this T1-weighted sagittal image. TR = 600 msec, TE = 20 msec.

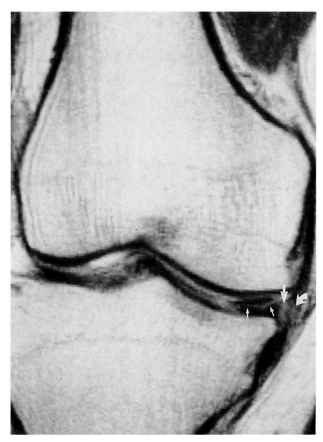

Figure 4-47

Grade 3 signal intensity in medial meniscal tear *(small straight arrows)*, associated meniscocapsular separation *(large straight arrow)*. Medial collateral ligament disruption is visualized *(curved arrow)*. Intermediate weighted coronal image; TR = 1500 msec, TE = 40 msec.

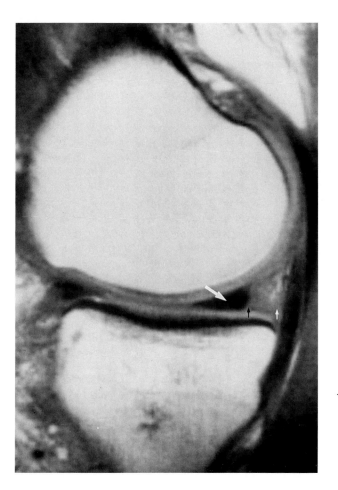

◄ **Figure 4-46**

Meniscocapsular separation with exposed tibial cartilage. The periphery of the meniscus *((black arrow)* should cover the periphery of the hyaline cartilage surface *(small white arrows)*. Posterior horn medial meniscus is identified *(large white arrow)*. T1-weighted sagittal image; TR = 600 msec, TE = 20 msec.

THE CRUCIATE LIGAMENTS

Anterior Cruciate Ligament

The cruciate ligaments are extrasynovial and intracapsular. The anterior cruciate ligament (ACL) extends from its tibial attachment, anterior to the intercondyloid eminence, to the medial aspect of the lateral femoral condyle. The ACL is composed of two fiber bundles, an anteromedial band and a posterolateral band.[30,31] It is 4 cm long and 1 cm wide and functions to limit hyperextension and tibiofemoral rotation. Anterior translation of the tibia is also controlled by ACL support. The ACL is composed of multiple fascicles that spiral along its long axis; it is taut in full knee extension and relaxed at about 45° of flexion. Anterior cruciate failure can occur with external rotation and abduction with hyperextension, with direct forward displacement of the tibia, and with internal tibial rotation with the knee in full extension.[9] The larger anteromedial band of the ACL is always taut and must be disrupted before a positive anterior drawer sign, indicating forward tibial displacement, is elicited. Tears of the ACL occur most frequently in its midsubstance, and avulsions usually occur from its femoral attachment. Isolated tears of the ACL are unusual, and hemorrhagic joint effusions and tears of the meniscus and medial collateral ligament are associated with ACL injuries.[31,32] Clinically, anterior tibial translation or subluxation greater than 5 mm is associated with an attenuated or torn anterior cruciate. On arthrography, the ACL can be only indirectly visualized by observing air and contrast along its reflected synovial surface.

For MR examination of the anterior cruciate, the knee should be in 15° of external rotation to orient the ligament with the sagittal imaging plane (Fig. 4-48). In cases where visualization is suboptimal, direct oblique imaging of the ACL is possible using the axial plane as a localizer (Fig. 4-49). We use all three planes (axial, sagittal, and coronal) to evaluate the ACL, although sagittal images are most informative (Fig. 4-50). T2-weighted or gradient echo images may be necessary to differentiate edema and hemorrhage in partial or complete ligamentous tears (Fig. 4-51). Although partial voluming effects may be minimized with 3-mm sections, we have not found them to be more sensitive than 5-mm contiguous slices in identifying ligamentous disruptions. In the presence of a joint effusion, T2-weighting may be necessary for assessment of the ACL.

On coronal and sagittal images, the normal ACL images as a band of low signal intensity with separate fiber striations visible near attachment points. Independent of partial voluming, the ACL may visualize with a minimally greater signal than that observed in the homogeneously dark posterior cruciate ligament.

In complete tears of the ACL there is discontinuity in the low signal intensity band, with or without loss of

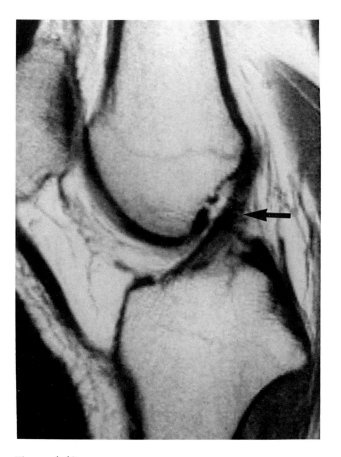

Figure 4-48

Intact low signal intensity anterior cruciate ligament *(arrow)* is identified on T1-weighted sagittal image. TR = 600 msec, TE = 20 msec.

its normally taut parallel margins (Fig. 4-52).[5,33] Partial or complete ligamentous disruptions may be associated with blurring of the cruciates's fascicles, from edema or hemorrhage (Fig. 4-53). In acute tears or strains, fluid or edema will image with high signal intensity on T2-weighted images. On sagittal images, partial voluming of the ACL with the lateral femoral condyle may be mistaken for a tear. However, in partial voluming no increase in signal intensity is observed on T2-weighting. Hemorrhagic joint effusions associated with tears of the anterior cruciate ligament may incite a synovitic reaction, associated with irregularity of the infrapatellar fat pad (Fig. 4-54).[34]

Accurate assessment of partial ligamentous tears is more difficult than detection of complete disruptions. Posterior bowing of the ACL or buckling of the posterior cruciate ligament may be associated with increased laxity or with a chronic tear of the ACL (Fig. 4-55). Absence of the ACL on both sagittal and coronal images is diagnostic of ACL disruption. Forward displacement of the tibia visualized on MR is the equivalent of a positive anterior drawer test on physical examination seen in the injured or deficient anterior cruciate (Fig. 4-56).

Text continues on p. 133

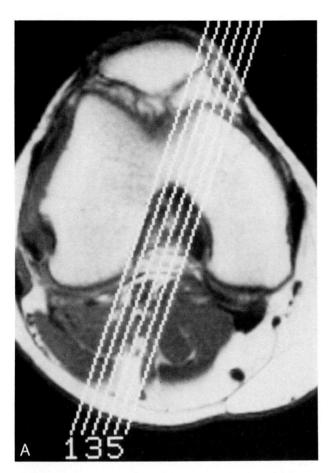

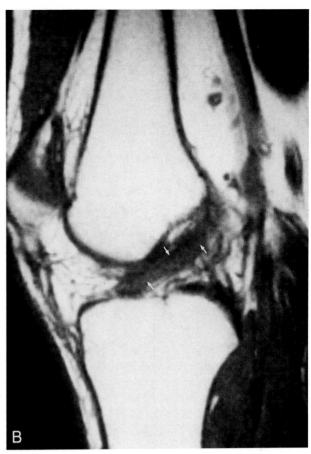

Figure 4-49

Anterior cruciate oblique imaging. Axial plane image through the intercondylar notch **(A),** used as a localizer for direct oblique–sagittal 3-mm images through the anterior cruciate ligament *(arrows; **B**).* TR = 600 msec, TE = 20 msec.

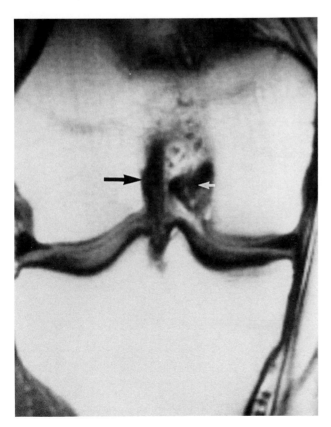

Figure 4-50

Anatomy of anterior cruciate *(black arrow)* and posterior cruciate *(white arrow)* ligaments on T1-weighted coronal image. The anterior cruciate images as a band, whereas the posterior cruciate ligament is circular in cross section. TR = 600 msec, TE = 20 msec.

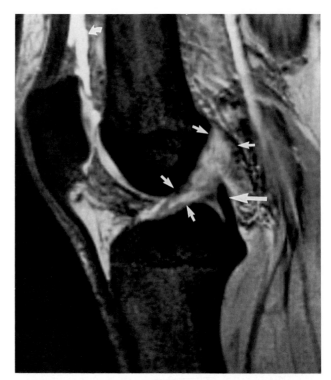

Figure 4-51

High signal intensity edema imaged in torn anterior cruciate ligament *(small straight arrows)* on T2* gradient echo image. Normal low signal intensity posterior cruciate ligament shown in contrast *(large straight arrow)*. Bright signal intensity suprapatellar effusion is demonstrated *(curved arrow)*. TR = 400 msec, TE = 30 msec; flip angle = 30°.

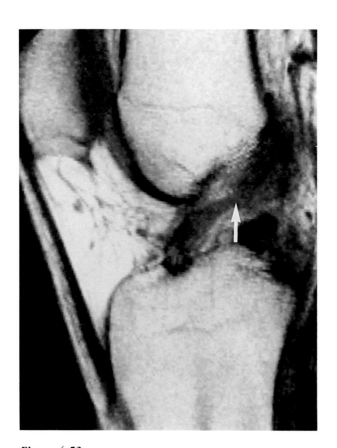

Figure 4-52

Midsubstance tear of the anterior cruciate ligament *(arrow)* with loss of continuity of its normally parallel margins. TR = 1000 msec, TE = 40 msec.

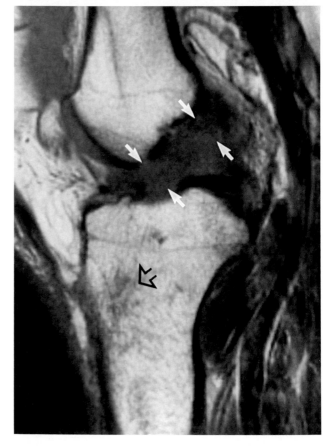

Figure 4-53

Torn and edematous anterior cruciate ligament *(white arrows)* with blurring of ligamentous fibers. Low signal intensity marrow edema is visualized in bone contusion *(open arrow)*. T1-weighted sagittal image; TR = 800 msec, TE = 20 msec.

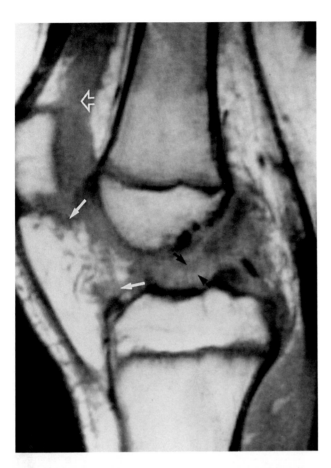

Figure 4-54

Disrupted anterior cruciate ligament *(black arrows)* associated with hemorrhagic effusion *(open arrow)* and synovitis, inferred by the presence of an irregular infrapatellar fat pad *(solid white arrows)*. TR = 800 msec, TE = 20 msec.

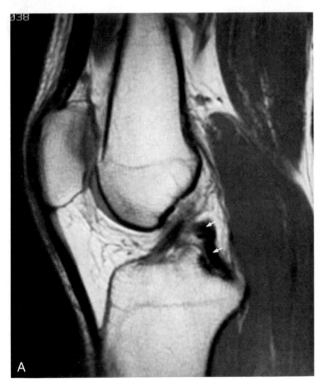

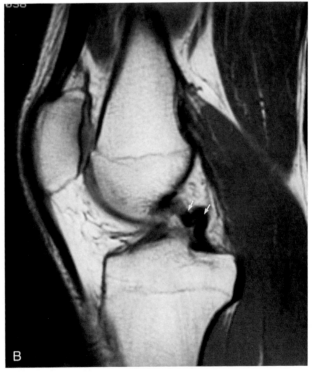

Figure 4-55

Buckled posterior cruciate ligament. *(A–B)* Increase laxity of anterior cruciate ligament associated with buckling of the posterior cruciate ligament *(arrows)*. Secondary forward translation of the tibia relative to the femur. TR = 800 msec, TE = 20 msec.

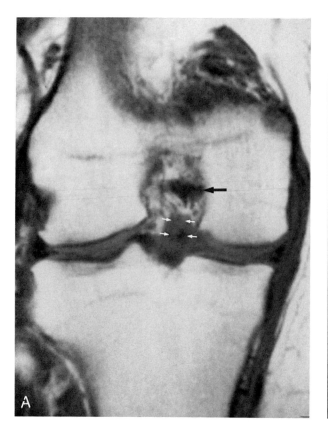

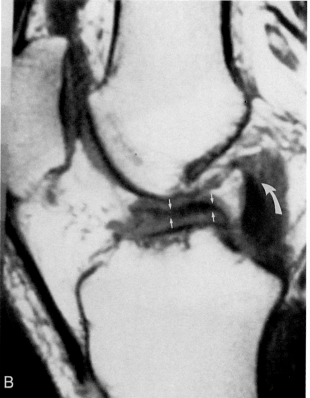

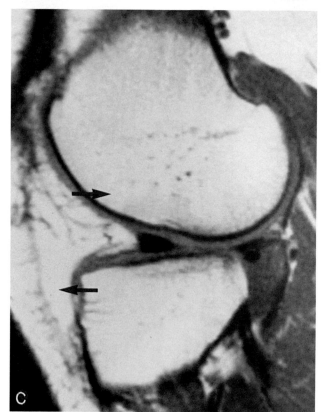

Figure 4-56

Anterior drawer sign. **(A)** Complete tear of the anterior cruciate ligament with tibial remnant *(small white arrows)* imaged on T1-weighted coronal image. Intact posterior cruciate ligament is indicated *(black arrow)*. TR = 600 msec, TE = 20 msec. **(B)** Disrupted anterior cruciate *(small white arrows)* seen in association with buckling of the posterior cruciate ligament *(curved white arrow)*. T1-weighted sagittal image; TR = 600 msec, TE = 20 msec. **(C)** "Auto"-anterior drawer sign with forward displacement of the tibia on the femur *(arrows)*. T1-weighted sagittal image; TR = 600 msec, TE = 20 msec.

The type of treatment for an ACL injury is often dependent on whether or not there is an associated meniscal injury. Primary repair of the ACL is most successful when avulsion has occurred at either its femoral or tibial attachment (Fig. 4-57). Reconstruction or excision is often necessary in substance tears. ACL reconstruction can be performed using the semitendinous, gracilis or patellar tendons.[35–37] Synthetic (prosthetic) replacements of the ACL (with Dacron, Teflon, and most recently, Gortex) have provided long-term function and stability not possible with fascial and tendon procedures (Fig. 4-58). MR has been used successfully to evaluate ACL reconstruction. Reconstruction procedures using tunneling in the intercondylar notch and anterior tibia, as well as points of ligamentous fixation (provided there is minimal metallic artifact) can be evaluated with MR.

On T2-weighted images, torn Gortex prosthetic ligaments visualize with increased signal intensity in areas of fluid accumulation around separated fascicles.

Posterior Cruciate Ligament

The posterior cruciate ligament (PCL) arises from the lateral aspect of the medial femoral condyle, crosses the anterior cruciate ligament, and attaches to the posterior intercondyloid fossa of the tibia.[38,39] Posterior to the PCL, the ligament of Wrisberg connects with the posterior horn of the lateral meniscus and inserts on the medial femoral condyle (Fig. 4-59). The ligament of Humphrey passes anteriorly to the PCL. The PCL controls posterior displacement of the tibia on the femur and stabilizes against excessive varus and valgus angulation.[9]

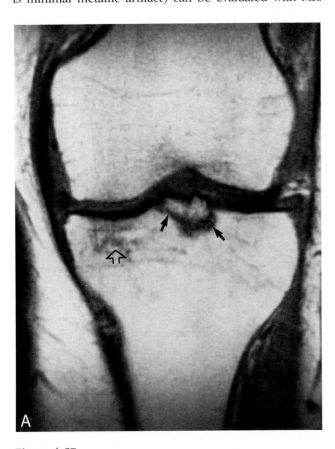

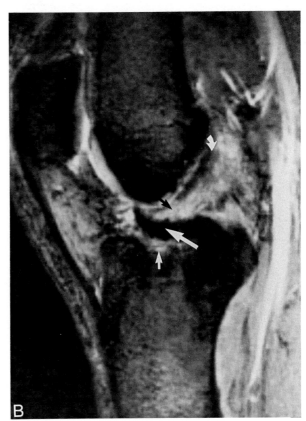

Figure 4-57

Anterior cruciate ligament avulsion. **(A)** Avulsion of the anterior tibial plateau (tibial spine) *(solid arrows)* from the pull of the anterior cruciate ligament. Associated low signal intensity edema is visualized in a medial tibial plateau compression fracture *(open arrow)*. T1-weighted coronal image; TR = 600 msec, TE = 20 msec. **(B)** Corresponding T2* gradient echo image demonstrating high signal intensity hemorrhage in the tibial portion of the anterior cruciate ligament *(black arrow)*. Normal anterior cruciate ligament fibers are shown as low signal intensity *(curved arrow)*. Low signal intensity fracture avulsion *(large white arrow)* and undermining high signal intensity fluid are identified *(small white arrow)*.

The PCL is composed of anterolateral and posteromedial bands that tighten on flexion and extension, respectively.

Tears of the PCL are most common in its midsubstance, whereas avulsions occur at its tibial insertion.[5,33] Rupture can be caused by excessive rotation, by hyperextension, by dislocation, or by direct trauma while the knee is flexed. Injuries to the PCL are usually associated with tears of either the ACL, meniscus, or collateral ligaments. A posterior drawer sign (posterior tibial displacement) can be seen in up to 60% of cases, provided the acutely injured patient can cooperate.

In the sagittal plane the PCL is visualized as a uniform dark band usually displayed on a single sagittal image (Fig. 4-60). The anatomy of the PCL is not as sensitive to positioning as that of the ACL, and in partial knee flexion, the PCL is taut on MR images. An abnormally high arc or buckling in the PCL, however, may indicate a tear of the ACL with forward tibial displacement (see Figs. 4-55 and 4-56). Any increase in signal, on either T1- or T2-weighted images, within this normally low signal intensity ligament should be interpreted as abnor-

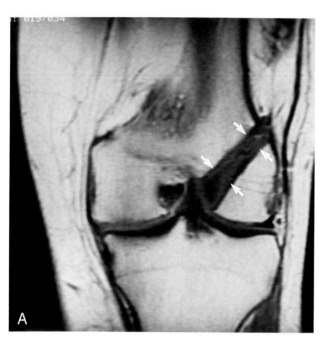

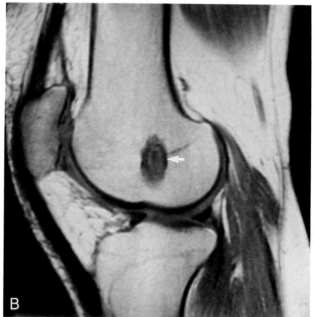

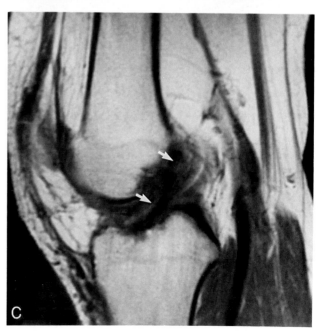

Figure 4-58

Gortex anterior cruciate ligament. Gortex anterior cruciate ligament *(white arrows)* images through osseous tunnel on T1-weighted coronal *(A)* and sagittal *(B–C)* images. Intact synthetic fibers image with low signal intensity *(C)*. TR = 800 msec, TE = 20 msec.

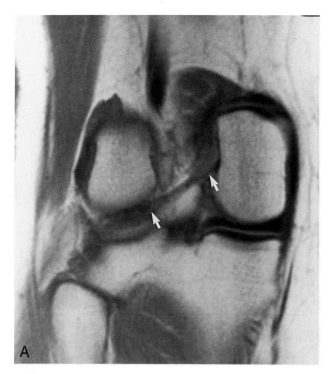
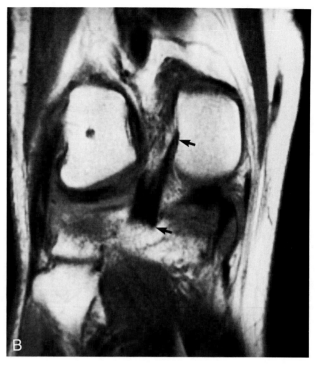

Figure 4-59

Ligament of Wrisberg. **(A)** Coronal image of low signal intensity ligament of Wrisberg *(white arrows)* extending from the posterior horn of the lateral meniscus to the medial femoral condyle. **(B)** The coronal anatomy of the posterior cruciate *(black arrows)* is visualized just anterior to the ligament of Wrisberg's (menisco-femoral ligament) insertion on the medial femoral condyle.

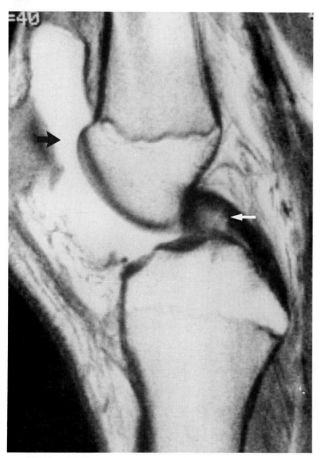

Figure 4-60

Intact low signal intensity posterior cruciate ligament *(white arrow)*. Adjacent high signal intensity joint effusion is indicated *(black arrow)*. T2-weighted sagittal image; TR = 2000 msec, TE = 40 msec.

mal (Fig. 4-61). Hemorrhage and edema, seen in acute injuries, are bright on T2-weighted images and cause less distortion or mass effect than with tears of the ACL (Fig. 4-62). Complete disruption of the PCL images with a loss or "gap" in ligament continuity (Fig. 4-63). Partial tears may be more difficult to assess. Chronic tears with fibrous scarring do not show increased signal intensity on T2-weighted images, and image with intermediate signal intensity on T1-weighted images. Coronal images, with the PCL on cross-sectional display, are also helpful in identifying increased signal intensity. An avulsion tear off the tibial plateau may be associated with high signal intensity in a bone fragment containing marrow (Fig. 4-64).[40] The presence of a large joint effusion does not interfere with visualization of the PCL.

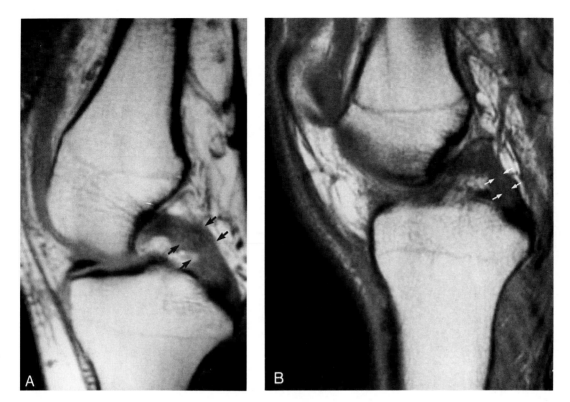

Figure 4-61

Posterior cruciate ligament tear. **(A–B)** Low signal intensity edema and hemorrhage in torn posterior cruciate ligament *(arrows)* demonstrated in two separate patients. T1-weighted sagittal images; TR = 600 msec, TE = 20 msec.

Figure 4-62

Posterior cruciate ligament tear with edema and hemorrhage visualized as high signal intensity *(curved arrow)* on T2* gradient echo image. Interface between cartilage *(small white arrows)* and fluid *(large white arrow)* is defined. Sagittal image; TR = 400 msec, TE = 30 msec; flip angle = 30°.

Figure 4-63

Complete transection of the posterior cruciate ligament with hemorrhage *(open arrow)* and loss of ligamentous continuity *(closed arrows)*. T1-weighted sagittal image; TR = 800 msec, TE = 20 msec.

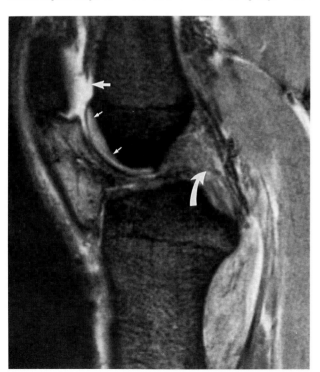

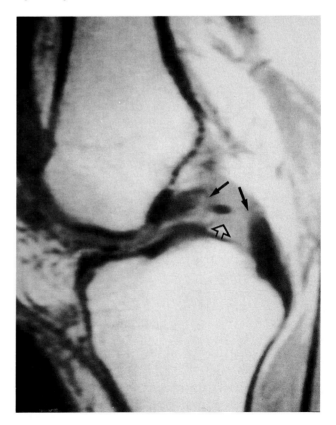

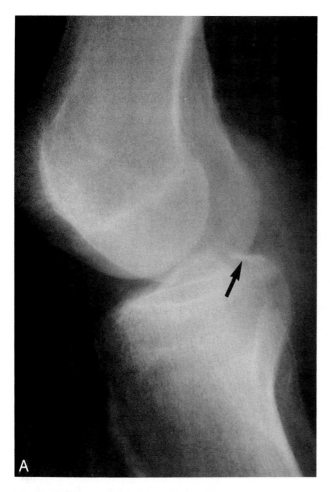
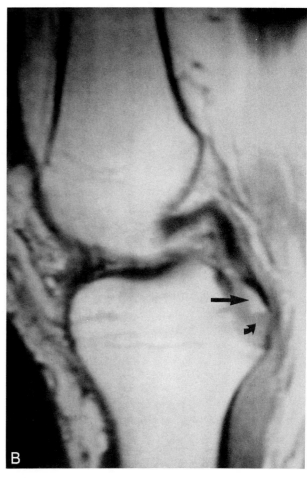

Figure 4-64

Posterior cruciate avulsion. **(A)** Lateral radiograph identifying avulsed bony fragment off posterior tibial plateau *(arrow)*. **(B)** Corresponding T1-weighted sagittal image demonstrating avulsed bone, containing high signal intensity yellow marrow from the attachment site of the posterior cruciate ligament *(straight arrow)*. Intermediate signal intensity is generated from associated edema and hemorrhage *(curved arrow)*. TR = 800 msec, TE = 20 msec.

THE COLLATERAL LIGAMENTS

Medial Collateral Ligament

The medial or tibial collateral ligament (MCL) is 8 to 10 cm long and extends from its posteromedial attachment, 4 to 5 cm below the tibial plateau, to the medial epicondyle of the femur (Fig. 4-65). The MCL is composed of two layers—a deep band, that attaches to the capsule and medial meniscus peripherally, and a more superficial band. When the knee is extended, the tibial collateral ligament fibers are taut and limit hyperextension. When the knee is flexed, the MCL provides primary valgus stability. Commonly, the MCL is injured when a valgus force is applied to the flexed knee. Partial ruptures or sprains frequently involve fibers attaching to the medial femoral condyle. In complete MCL ruptures there may be associated tears of the medial and posterior cap-

sule, of the anterior cruciate, and of the medial meniscus.[9] A fracture caused by the impact of the lateral femoral condyle on the lateral tibial plateau during valgus injury is not uncommon.

Arthrography is limited in its ability to detect MCL injuries, especially after 48 hours when extravasation of contrast material can no longer be seen. MR evaluation of these injuries is best accomplished with coronal images, that demonstrate the low signal intensity MCL and its attachment points where it merges with low signal intensity cortical bone. Occasionally, separation of the deep and superficial layers can be distinguished on T2-weighted images (Fig. 4-66). A thin band of intermediate signal intensity, thought to be fat or an intraligamentous bursa, is often seen between the MCL and its peripheral meniscal attachment and does not represent a meniscocapsular separation (Fig. 4-67)[41] Signal intensity above or below the level of the meniscus, however, is abnormal.

On MR examination, partial tears or strains of the MCL are seen with increased distance between the subcutaneous tissue and cortical bone (Fig. 4-68). T2-weighted images demonstrate edema and or hemorrhage around low signal intensity ligamentous fibers. There is loss of continuity of ligament fibers in tears compared with ligamentous strains. Complete tears are associated with extensive joint effusions (hemarthrosis) and extravasation of joint fluid that tracks along the MCL. Focal hemorrhage can be visualized at the femoral epicondylar attachment in complete ligamentous avulsions. Subacute hemorrhage visualizes with increased signal intensity on T1- and T2-weighted images. Conventional T2-weighted and gradient echo T2* images have been useful in documenting interval healing with reattachment of the torn MCL ligament (Fig. 4-69). Tearing of the MCL with capsular disruption may be associated with a peripheral meniscal tear and widening of the medial joint space (Fig. 4-70). Adjacent subcutaneous edema is

seen as low signal intensity on T1-weighted images and high signal intensity on T2-weighted images. In response to a chronic tear, the medial collateral ligament is thickened, but without increase in signal intensity.

In the acute setting, nondisplaced compression fractures of the lateral tibial plateau, seen in conjunction with MCL injuries, are visualized with low signal intensity on T1-weighted images and with high signal intensity on T2-weighted images.[42] These fractures or bone contusions can be identified on MR scans even though initial radiographs are normal.

Lateral Collateral Ligament

The lateral or fibular collateral ligament (LCL) is extracapsular and free from meniscal attachment in its course to the conjoined insertion with the biceps femoris tendon on the fibular head from the lateral femoral epicondyle.[43] The intracapsular popliteus tendon passes medial

Figure 4-65
Intact low signal intensity superficial band of the medial (tibial) collateral ligament *(arrows)* on anterior T1-weighted coronal image. A more posterior coronal section would show attachment with the deep band of the medial collateral ligament and periphery of the medial meniscus at the meniscocapsular insertion. TR = 1000 msec, TE = 40 msec.

Figure 4-66
Linear high signal intensity fluid *(arrow)* is visualized delineating the deep and superficial layers of the medial collateral ligament. T2* gradient echo image; TR = 400 msec, TE = 30 msec; flip angle = 30°.

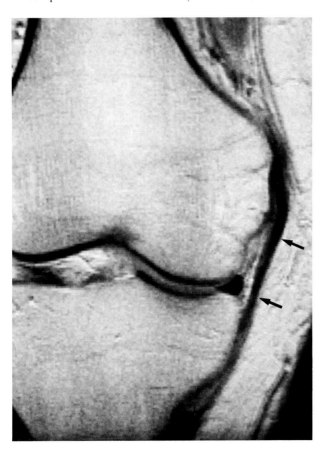

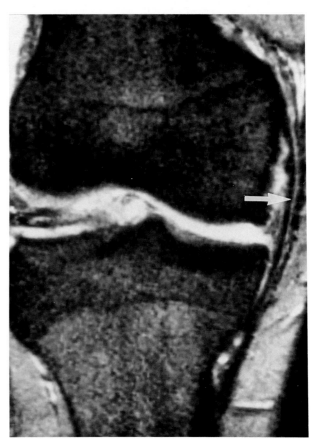

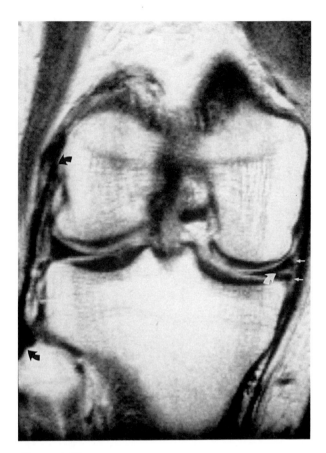

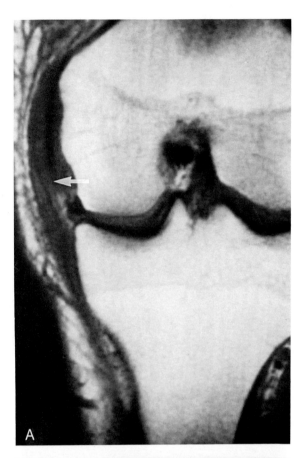

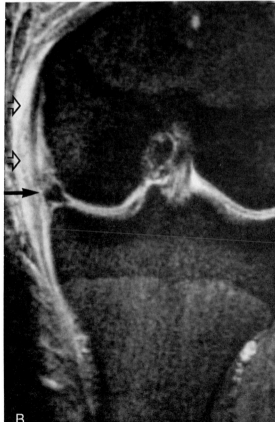

Figure 4-67

Normal intermediate signal intensity connection between the medial collateral ligament and the periphery of the medial meniscus *(straight white arrows)*. Linear grade 2 degeneration is also demonstrated *(curved white arrow)*. The intact fibular (lateral) collateral ligament is imaged on the same coronal section *(curved black arrows)*. Intermediate weighted image; TR = 1500 msec, TE = 40 msec.

Figure 4-68

Medial collateral ligament tear. *(A)* Torn medial collateral ligament *(arrow)* shown as thickened band of low signal intensity with increased separation between the subcutaneous tissue and cortical bone. T1-weighted coronal image; TR = 600 msec, TE = 20 msec. *(B)* Corresponding T2* gradient echo coronal image delineates disrupted medial collateral ligament and meniscocapsular separation *(solid arrow)*. Surrounding edema shown with high signal intensity *(open arrows)*. TR = 400 msec, TE = 30 msec; flip angle = 30°.

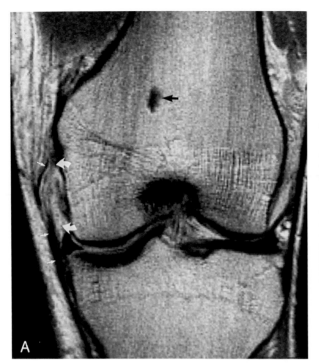

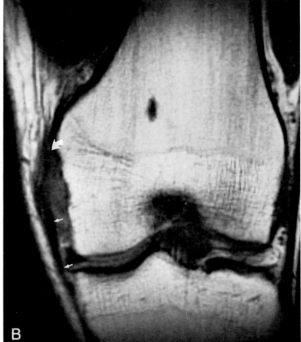

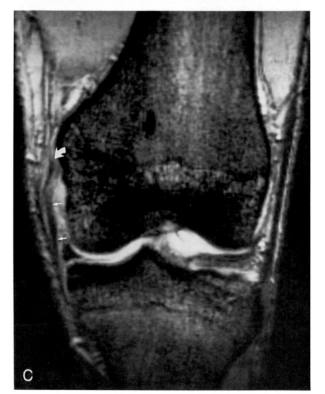

Figure 4-69

Medial collateral ligament avulsion. *(A)* Subacute avulsion of the medial collateral ligament from its femoral epicondylar cortical attachment *(small white arrows)*. Focal hemorrhage *(curved arrows)* images with high signal intensity. Incidental bone island identified as low signal intensity focus *(black arrow)*. Intermediate weighted coronal image; TR = 2000 msec, TE = 40 msec. After 6 months of brace treatment the medial collateral ligament *(small white arrows)* is shown in continuity with its thickened proximal portion *(curved arrow)*. *(B–C)* Delineation of femoral cortical attachment improves as weighting progresses from T1-weighted image *(B)* to T2* gradient echo sequence *(C)*. *(B)* TR = 600 msec, TE = 20 msec; *(C)* TR = 400 msec, TE = 30 msec; flip angle = 30°.

to the LCL. With the leg in internal rotation, an applied varus force can cause injury to the LCL and capsule. Injury or disruption of the LCL is significantly less frequent than injury to the MCL. Cruciate and lateral meniscus tears may be associated with lateral compartment ligamentous tears. Conventional radiographs may reveal a widened joint space, fracture of the fibular head, and Segond fracture (avulsion of the tibial insertion of the lateral capsular ligament).

The LCL is best seen on posterior coronal images and is visualized as a band of low signal intensity (Fig. 4-71). Occasionally, peripheral sagittal images demonstrate LCL anatomy at the level of the fibular head (Fig. 4-72). Edema and hemorrhage, although less frequent in this location, are seen as ligamentous thickening with increased signal intensity on T2-weighted images. The degree of increased signal in LCL injuries is less noticeable than that demonstrated in medial collateral ligament disruptions. This may be related to the normal capsular separation of the lateral collateral ligament that excludes the accumulation of extravasated joint fluid. In complete disruptions, the LCL images with a wavy contour and loss of ligamentous continuity (Fig. 4-73). Edema and hemorrhage in LCL tears may also be confirmed on peripheral sagittal images (Fig. 4-74).

Medial tibial plateau compression fractures can be detected on MR scans and are associated with significant varus injuries.[42] Tears of the iliotibial band may also be associated with LCL disruptions. The iliotibial band provides lateral compartment support and images as a thin band of low signal intensity, parallel to the femur, with anterolateral tibial insertion on Gerdy's tubercle.

Figure 4-71

Intact low signal intensity lateral collateral ligament on posterior coronal image *(large arrows)*. The ligament is visualized separate from the lateral meniscus *(small arrows)*. T1-weighted image; TR = 600 msec, TE = 20 msec.

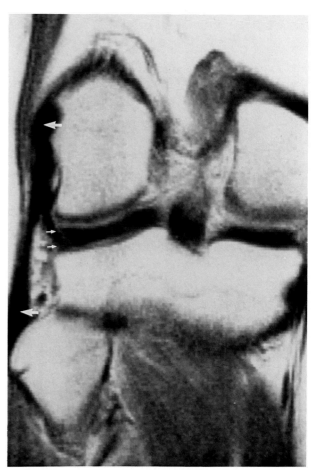

Figure 4-70

Medial collateral ligament tear *(black arrows)* with meniscocapsular separation and valgus instability. Widening of the medial joint compartment *(white arrows)* is identified. Intermediate weighted coronal image; TR = 1500 msec, TE = 40 msec.

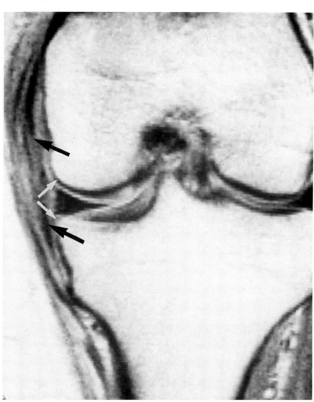

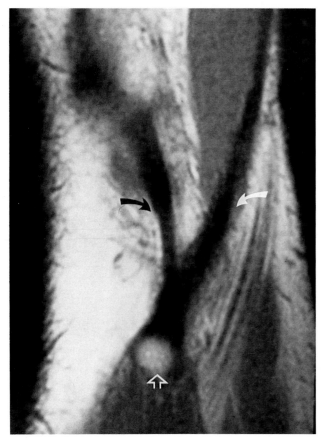

Figure 4-72

The conjoined insertion on the fibular head *(open arrow)* of the separate lateral collateral ligament *(curved black arrow)* and biceps femoris tendon *(curved white arrow)* are imaged on a peripheral sagittal image. T1-weighted image; TR = 800 msec, TE = 20 msec.

Figure 4-73

Complete tear of the lateral collateral ligament near its distal fibular attachment *(arrow)*. The disrupted ligament has a wavy contour. T1-weighted coronal image; TR = 800 msec, TE = 20 msec.

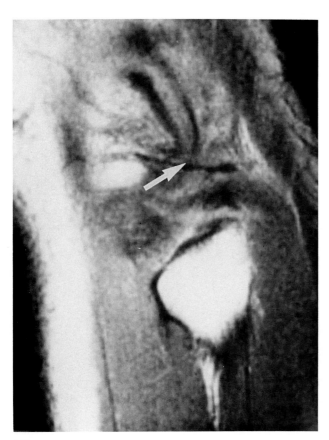

Figure 4-74

Complete disruption of the fibular (lateral) collateral ligament at the level of the joint line *(arrow)* on a T1-weighted sagittal image. TR = 800 msec, TE = 20 msec.

THE PATELLOFEMORAL JOINT AND EXTENSOR MECHANISM

Axial images are required to characterize the patellofemoral articulation accurately. The lateral and medial patellar facets are oblique and cannot be characterized precisely on sagittal or coronal images. Patellar cartilage and retinacular attachments are defined in axial sections through the patellofemoral joint. The quadriceps muscles and tendon can be visualized on sagittal or axial images. The patellar tendon is imaged en face in the coronal plane, in profile in the sagittal plane, and in cross section on axial planar images.

Chondromalacia Patellae

Chondromalacia patellae is characterized by patellofemoral joint pain, accentuated in knee flexion, with associated crepitus.[44–46] Softening of the articular cartilage, with associated degenerative changes, is responsible for the spectrum of changes seen. Chondromalacia most often affects adolescents and young adults, and may be primary and idiopathic or may occur subsequent to patellar trauma.[47] There is also an adult form of the disease in which there are osteoarthritic changes in adolescence, but no symptoms until middle age. The point of contact between the convex medial patellar facet and

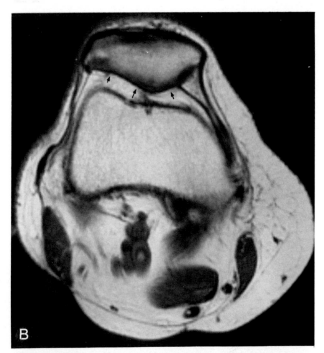

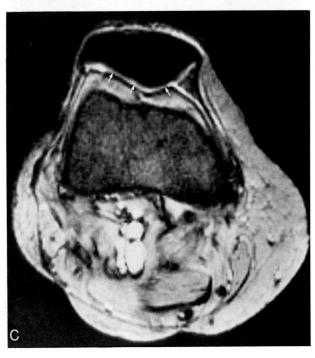

Figure 4-75
Early chondromalacia patellae. Attenuated hyaline cartilage *(arrows)* of the patellar facets as imaged on T1-weighted sagittal *(A)* and axial *(B)* images and T2* weighted axial images *(C)*. Thinned articular cartilage is displayed with high signal intensity on gradient echo sequence *(C)*. *(A–B)* TR = 600 msec, TE = 20 msec; *(C)* TR = 400 msec, TE = 30 msec; flip angle = 30°.

the medial femoral condyle represents the earliest site of cartilage fissuring and softening in chondromalacia. Patella alta, an increased valgus angle, and femoral condylar hypoplasia may predispose to cartilage changes involving both the medial and lateral patellar facets. Softening of the subchondral bone may be associated with softening, edema, and fissuring of the overlying articular cartilage. Symptoms of chondromalacia may mimic meniscal pathology.

On axial MR images, early cartilage attenuation or erosions can be appreciated in either the medial or lateral facets (Fig. 4-75).[48] Frequently, the opposing femoral cartilage also demonstrates thinning on sagittal images. Sagittal images, which are less sensitive to cartilage erosions, may show a straightening or loss of the normal convex curve seen in patellar hyaline cartilage when viewed in profile. T2-weighted or gradient echo sequences are useful for demonstrating inhomogeneity of the signal obtained from patellar cartilage in areas of focal edema. Subchondral low signal intensity, representing sclerosis, may be associated with irregular surface erosions (Fig. 4-76). Low signal intensity patellar cysts are sometimes seen in early stages of patellar softening, preceding cartilage erosions (Fig. 4-77).

In one study, arthroscopic grades of chondromalacia patellae were correlated with findings on MR imaging.[49] Arthroscopic grade 1 (patellar softening) and grade 2 (blisterlike swelling) were imaged with areas of decreased signal on T1- and T2-weighted images. Arthroscopic grade 3 surface irregularity and attenuation correlated with irregularity and thinning of the facet articular cartilage on MR. The finding of ulceration and exposure of subchondral bone in arthroscopic grade 4 was represented by frank articular cartilage defects, exposed subchondral bone, and undermining fluid.

Joint effusions, imaging with low signal intensity on T1-weighted images and bright signal intensity on T2-weighted images, are commonly associated with patellofemoral chondromalacia. Treatment by shaving of the patellar surface cartilage can be identified on MR evaluation as an artificially straight articular surface with microscopic metallic artifacts (Fig. 4-78).

Figure 4-76

Lateral facet chondromalacia. **(A)** Lateral patellar facet cartilage degeneration *(small arrows)* with subchondral irregularity and low signal intensity sclerosis *(open arrow)* as imaged in a professional ballet dancer. **(B)** Asymptomatic knee shown for comparison with thicker articular cartilage surface *(arrows)*. TR = 600 msec, TE = 20 msec.

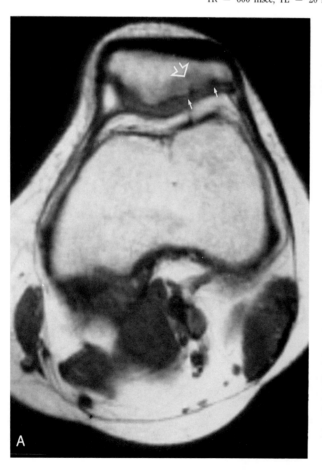
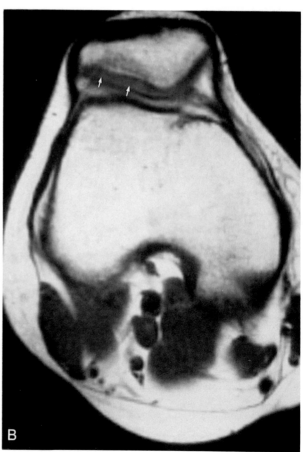

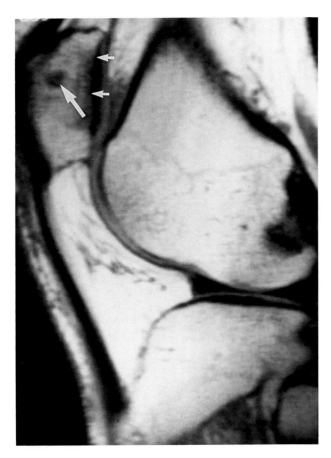

Figure 4-77
Chondromalacia patellae visualized with subchrondral (low signal intensity) sclerosis *(small arrows)* and degenerative patellar cyst *(large white arrow)*. T1-weighted sagittal image; TR = 800 msec, TE = 20 msec.

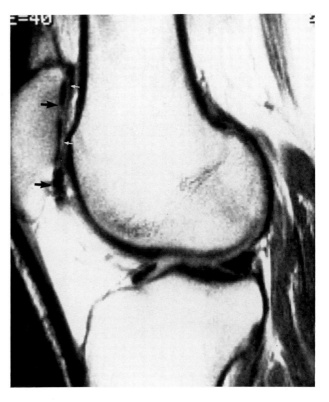

Figure 4-78
Low signal patellar cortex *(black arrows)* with thin rim of shaved hyaline articular cartilage *(white arrows)* shown as intermediate signal intensity. Intermediate-weighted sagittal image; TR = 1500 msec, TE = 40 msec.

Patellar Subluxation and Dislocation

Patellar subluxation sometimes presents with symptoms of joint locking and may be mistaken for a torn meniscus.[50] The repetitive trauma caused by lateral displacements of the patella accelerates articular surface degeneration (Fig. 4-79). Torn medial retinacular attachments can be identified on axial images subsequent to patellar dislocation and traumatic subluxations. Patella alta, lateral femoral condyle hypoplasia, genu valgum or recurvatum, and abnormal (lateral) insertion of the patellar tendon can precipitate displacements. We have used MR imaging to identify a dysplastic patella with no medial facet or central ridge as the cause for lateral subluxation (Fig. 4-80). This was classified as a Wiberg type 5 or Jagerhut patella.[51]

Retinacular Attachments

The medial and lateral retinacula are fascial extensions of the vastus medialis and lateralis muscle groups, respectively.[4] The retinacula reinforce and guide normal patellar tracking. On anterior coronal images, the retinacular attachments can be visualized as low signal intensity structures converging on the medial and lateral patellar facets. The single band of the lateral retinaculum and the Y-shaped bands of the medial retinaculum, however, are best seen on axial images through the patellofemoral joint (see Fig. 4-5).

The *medial retinaculum* is more frequently torn than the lateral, especially after patellar dislocation (Fig. 4-81). Axial MR images may demonstrate a free floating retinaculum, without patellar attachment, or a masslike effect in compressed torn retinacular fibers or chondral fragments. Associated edema and hemorrhage produce increased signal intensity on T2-weighted images.

A tight lateral retinaculum *(excessive lateral pressure syndrome)* tilts the patella in a lateral direction without subluxation. To minimize the development of lateral facet degenerative disease, a retinacular release may be performed. The site of retinacular division following release can be evaluated with MR studies.

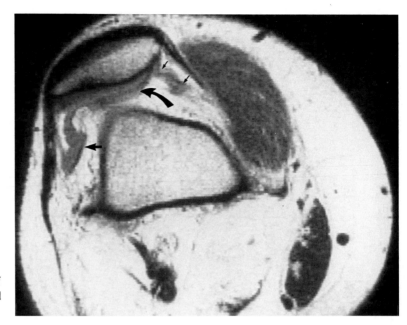

Figure 4-79

Lateral patellar subluxation *(curved arrow)* with associated effusion *(large straight arrow)* and tear of the inner limb of the medial retinaculum *(small straight arrows)*. T1-weighted axial image; TR = 600 msec, TE = 20 msec.

Figure 4-80

Lateral subluxation *(open arrow)* of a dysplastic patella with medial facet missing *(white arrows)*—referred to as a Jagerhut patella. Lax lateral retinaculum is identified *(black arrows)*. T1-weighted axial image; TR = 600 msec, TE = 20 msec.

Patellar Tendon Abnormalities

Patellar tendon tears, resulting in loss of extension and a high riding patella, can occur with avulsion injuries from the tibial tubercle or inferior pole of the patella.[52] Bony fragments that image with the signal intensity of marrow, may be identified on sagittal MR images. Increased tendon laxity with a wavy contour can be visualized in acute or chronic tears (Fig. 4-82). A thickened patellar tendon may be seen after arthroscopy or trauma.

The *patellar tendon to patella ratio* is considered abnormal when the lengths of the patella and patella tendon are unequal.[52] Patella alta (high position of the patella) and patella baja (low position of the patella) can be determined on direct sagittal images that show the entire length of the patellar tendon and the superior to inferior dimensions of the patella. Patella alta[53] has been associated with subluxation, chondromalacia, Sinding–Larsen–Johansson syndrome, cerebral palsy, and quadriceps atrophy (Fig. 4-83). Patella baja is seen with polio, achondroplasia, and juvenile rheumatoid arthritis (Fig. 4-84).

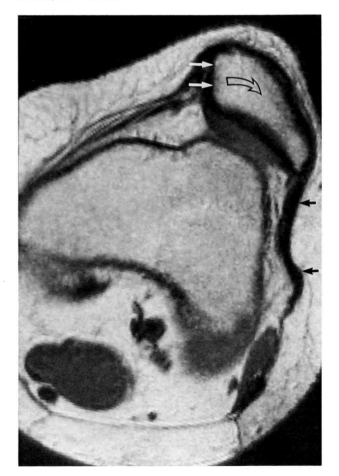

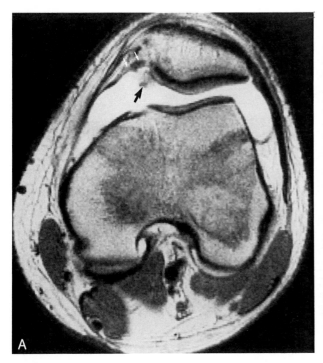

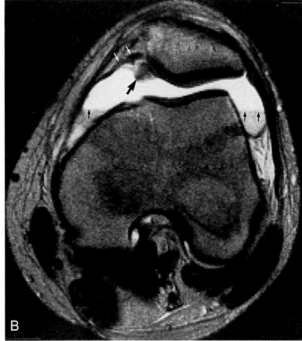

Figure 4-81

Retinacular tear. Medial retinacular tear *(white arrows)* with chondral fragment *(large black arrow)* on intermediate *(A)* and T2-weighted *(B)* axial images. Hemorrhagic serum-sediment fluid level is demonstrated on T2-weighted image *(small black arrows)*. TR = 2000 msec, TE = 20, 60 msec.

Figure 4-82

Tear of the patellar tendon imaged with increased laxity and redundant contour *(arrows)*. T1-weighted sagittal image; TR = 800 msec, TE = 20 msec.

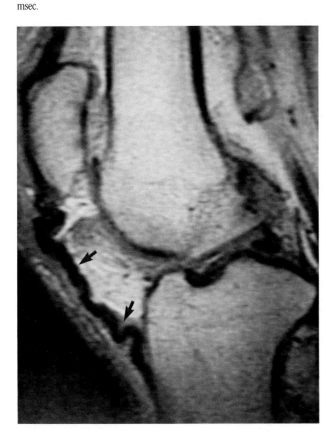

Patella Bursa

Prepatellar bursitis is visualized as a localized soft tissue mass anterior to the patella. It images with low signal intensity on T1-weighted images and with high signal intensity on T2-weighted images (Fig. 4-85). Infrapatellar bursitis is identified posterior to the patellar tendon and inferior to Hoffa's fat pad.[4]

Extensor Muscle Tears

The quadriceps muscle group is composed of the rectus femoris and vastus intermedius muscles (which insert on the base of the patella) and the vastus lateralis and medius muscles (which insert on the lateral and medial patella, respectively). Quadriceps tears or ruptures occur in the young athlete either with forced muscle contraction or direct trauma (see Fig. 5-28). Myositis ossificans may be a sequela to injury, especially when the vastus medialis is involved.

For MR evaluation of extensor muscle tears, an initial set of coronal or sagittal images is used to display the longitudinal extent of muscle involvement. Axial images are used to identify both the precise muscle group involved and adjacent anatomic relations. Axial images

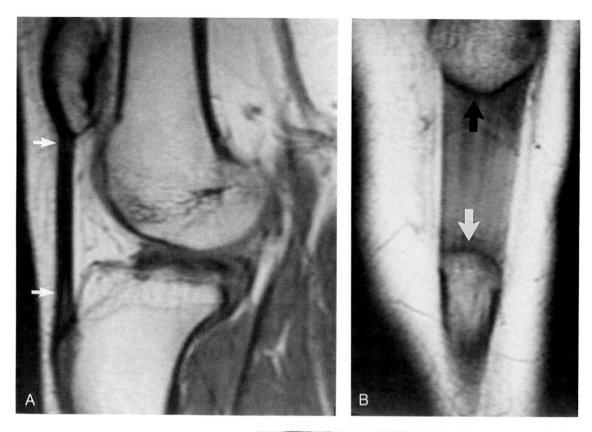

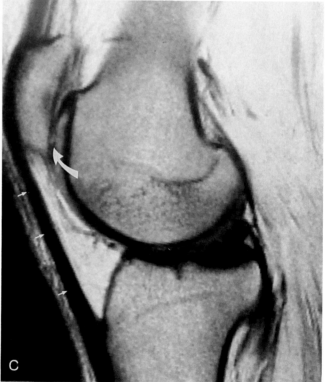

Figure 4-83

Patella alta. *(A)* High riding patella with elongated patellar tendon *(arrows)* in a patient with atrophy of the quadriceps muscle. T1-weighted sagittal image; TR = 600 msec, TE = 20 msec. *(B)* Corresponding coronal image demonstrating stretched patellar tendon en face. Patellar *(black arrow)* and tibial tubercle *(white arrow)* attachments identified. TR = 600 msec, TE = 20 msec. *(C)* Patella alta in a separate patient showing lengthened patella tendon *(small straight arrows)* in a patient with patella subluxation *(curved arrow).*

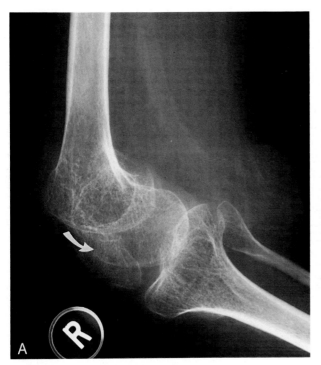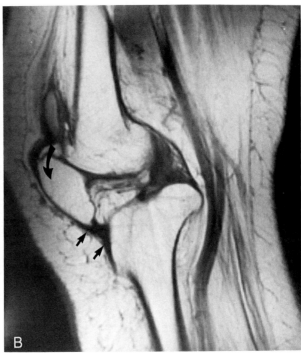

Figure 4-84

Patella baja. Low position of the patella *(curved arrow)* with shortened patellar tendon *(straight arrows)* visualized on lateral radiograph *(A)* and on T1-weighted sagittal image *(B)* in a patient with polio.

Figure 4-85

Low signal intensity prepatellar bursitis with thickening of soft tissue anterior to the patella *(arrows)*. T1-weighted axial image; TR = 600 msec, TE = 20 msec.

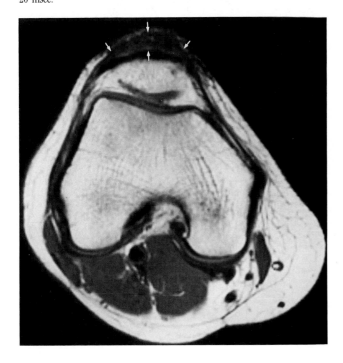

are also useful in differentiating between complete muscle tears with diastases or partial tears with associated atrophy. MR imaging is sensitive to both acute and chronic hemorrhage in extensor muscle tears. Edema and areas of fraying in the affected muscle image with intermediate signal intensity on T1-weighted images. Edema and hemorrhage demonstrate increased signal intensity on T2-weighted images. Muscle atrophy and fatty infiltration are visualized as regions of increased signal intensity on T1-weighted images. A retracted proximal or distal muscle bundle can be identified as a soft tissue mass with higher signal intensity than the native muscle. Any increase in signal intensity within the quadriceps tendon is abnormal, and ranges from intrasubstance signal in degeneration or tendinitis to high signal intensity hemorrhage or edema in complete avulsions or ruptures of the tendon.

GENERAL PATHOLOGIC CONDITIONS AFFECTING THE KNEE

Arthritis

Assessment of the extent, progression, and therapeutic response in adult arthritic disorders and in juvenile chronic arthritis is enhanced by MR imaging of articular cartilage.[34] Even in patients with negative conventional radiographs, joint effusions, synovial reactions, popliteal cysts, and osteonecrosis can be demonstrated and evaluated with MR studies.

Cartilage

Cartilage of the patellar, femoral, and tibial articular surfaces is best visualized on T1-weighted images.[34] Because of its hydropic composition, normal hyaline cartilage images with intermediate signal intensity, compared to the low signal intensity of cortex and fibrocartilaginous menisci (Fig. 4-86). On conventional T2-weighted images, hyaline cartilage maintains an intermediate signal intensity. With gradient echo, chemical shift, and fast low angle shot (FLASH) techniques, however, hyaline cartilage images with high signal intensity; thus, it is possible to detect early stages of hyaline cartilage degeneration (Fig. 4-87).[7] A decrease in the signal intensity of cartilage has been attributed to a loss of water-binding proteoglycan molecules. With gradient echo T2* images, articular cartilage defects as small as 3 mm have been identified in trauma, arthritis, osteochondritis, and osteonecrosis (Fig. 4-88). These defects were not detected with conventional T1- or T2-weighted spin echo images. Chemical shift artifact in the frequency-encoded direction may underestimate the apparent thickness of the curvilinear hyaline cartilage on the femoral condylar surface. The thinner articular surface of the tibia is a less predictable indicator of disorders affecting

Figure 4-86

Thick intermediate signal intensity hyaline articular cartilage *(solid arrows)* in a child. Epiphyseal yellow marrow images with bright signal intensity *(open arrow)*. T1-weighted coronal image; TR = 600 msec, TE = 20 msec.

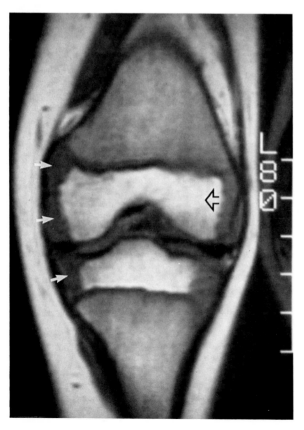

Figure 4-87

Articular cartilage images with bright signal intensity with T2* gradient echo contrast *(small arrows)*. Grade 2 degeneration in the posterior horn of the medial meniscus is shown *(large arrow)*. Sagittal image; TR = 400 msec, TE = 30 msec; flip angle = 30°.

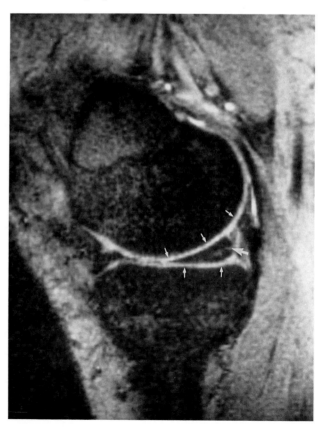

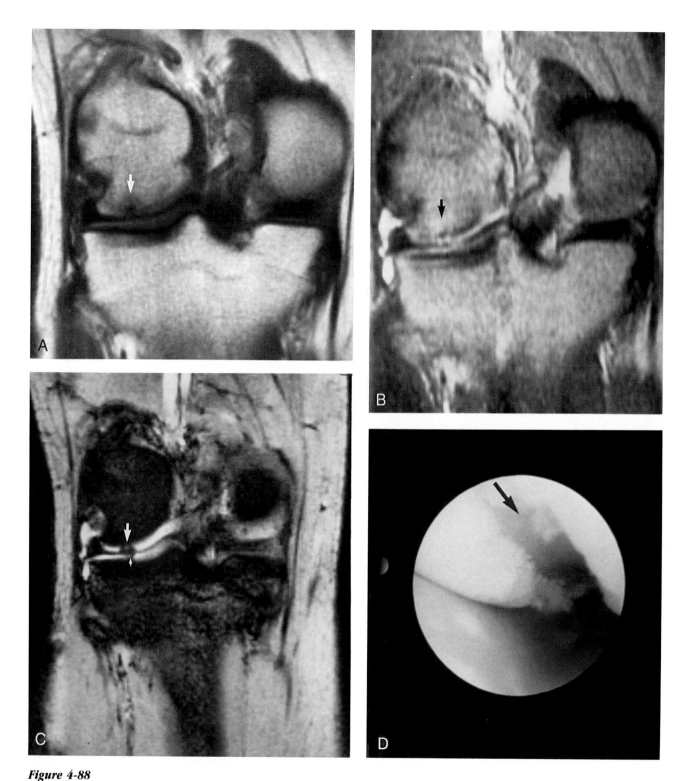

Figure 4-88

Osteochondral injury in a javelin thrower. *(A)* T1-weighted coronal image demonstrating low signal intensity traumatic osteochondral defect involving the posterior lateral femoral condyle *(arrow)*. TR = 600 msec, TE = 20 msec. *(B)* Corresponding conventional T2-weighted image displaying increased signal intensity within osteochondral defect *(arrow)*. TR = 2000 msec, TE = 60 msec. *(C)* T2* gradient echo image in the same patient showing hyaline articular cartilage defects in the femoral condyle *(large arrow)* and opposing tibial plateau *(small arrow)* not appreciated on the previous T1- or T2-weighted images. TR = 400 msec, TE = 30 msec; flip angle = 30°. *(D)* Subsequent arthroscopy identifying an articular cartilage defect in the lateral femoral condyle *(arrow)*.

articular congruity. With T1- and conventional T2-weighted sequences, joint effusions reduce the definition of articular cartilage surfaces. With gradient echo T2* contrast there is better delineation of the cartilage-fluid interface, because effusions generate higher signal intensity than adjacent cartilage surfaces. Inversion recovery sequences set at the null point of water (water is imaged as black) have also shown potential for more accurate assessment of cartilage thicknesses in effusions associated with arthritis and trauma.

The thicker articular cartilage in children allows an increased sensitivity in detecting focal erosions and cartilage thinning. In infants, the articular cartilage is visualized prior to the appearance of the distal femoral and proximal tibial ossific nuclei and images with a higher signal intensity than adjacent red marrow (Fig. 4-89). Before there is any radiographic evidence of joint narrowing, focal erosions and uniform attenuation of articular cartilage have been observed in MR studies of patients with juvenile rheumatoid arthritis, hemophilia, and degenerative joint disease. Loss of subchondral signal intensity in sclerosis has been observed, in association with initial cartilage loss. Intraosseous cysts and hemorrhage may develop at sites of denuded hyaline cartilage and image with increased signal intensity on T2-weighted images.

Synovium and the Irregular Infrapatellar Fat Pad Sign

Synovial reaction and proliferations are imaged as changes in the contour of synovial reflections. Irregularity, with loss of the smooth posterior concave free border of the infrapatellar fat pad, can be observed with a variety of synovial reactions, and is referred to as the *irregular infrapatellar fat pad sign* (Fig. 4-90).[34] Although the synovium cannot be imaged directly in early synovitis, a corrugated surface along Hoffa's fat pad is evident in the initial stages of synovial irritation. This irregular fat pad sign has been seen in patients with hemophilia, rheumatoid arthritis, pigmented villonodular synovitis, Lyme arthritis, and in cases of hemorrhagic effusions (from arthritis or trauma), with reactive synovium. *Synovial hypertrophy* and *pannus* generally image with low to intermediate signal intensity on T1- and T2-weighted sequences. Fluid associated with synovial masses generates increased signal intensity on T2-weighted images.

Juvenile Chronic Arthritis

In *juvenile rheumatoid (chronic) arthritis* (JRA), MR studies have characterized early synovitis with an irregular infrapatellar fat pad in the initial states of clinical presentation (Fig. 4-91).[54] Articular cartilage erosions

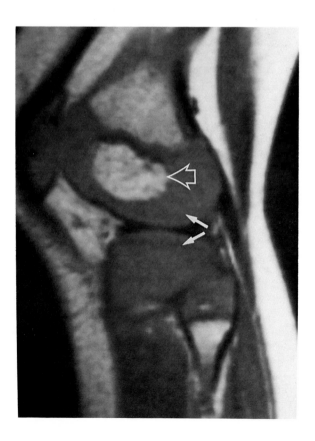

Figure 4-89

Normal thick hyaline articular cartilage of intermediate signal intensity *(solid white arrows)* on T1-weighted sagittal image. Femoral ossific nucleus seen with high signal intensity marrow fat *(open arrow)*. Tibial ossific nucleus is not yet developed. TR = 600 msec, TE = 20 msec.

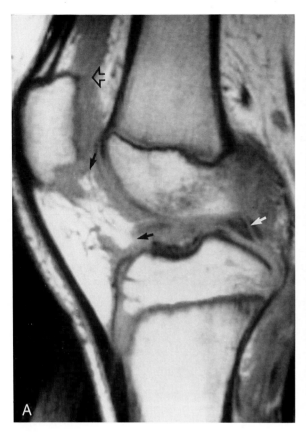 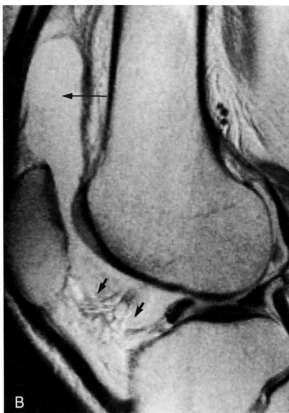

Figure 4-90

Infrapatellar fat pad sign. *(A)* Hemorrhagic effusion *(open arrow)* resulting in synovial irritation imaging with an irregular infrapatellar fat pad *(solid black arrows)*. Torn posterior horn of lateral meniscus is indicated *(white arrow)*. When there is no arthritis, a nonhemorrhagic effusion will not give a positive infrapatellar fat pad sign. T1-weighted sagittal image; TR = 800 msec, TE = 20 msec. *(B)* Glanzman's thrombasthenia with hemorrhagic effusion *(long black arrow)* and irregular infrapatellar fat pad *(short black arrows)*. Intermediate weighted sagittal image; TR = 1500 msec, TE = 40 msec.

and synovial hypertrophy can be identified before joint space narrowing is evident on plain film radiography. Posterior popliteal cysts of the gastrocnemius and semimembranosus bursa are commonly associated with JRA, and image with low signal intensity on T1-weighted images and with uniform high signal intensity on T2-weighted images (Fig. 4-92). Thickening of the synovium of the suprapatellar bursa can be visualized with low signal intensity on T1- and T2-weighted images (Fig. 4-93). With MR scans, subarticular cysts, subchondral sclerosis, and osteonecrosis can be detected on both femoral and tibial surfaces in more advanced disease, findings that are frequently not evident on conventional radiographs (Figs. 4-94 and 4-95). Hypoplastic menisci with small anterior, body and posterior horns have also been observed on MR studies in JRA patients. This finding might be related to an alteration in the fluid composition of synovial fluid, impairing normal fibrocartilage development.

Rheumatoid Arthritis

In adult patients with *rheumatoid arthritis,* bicompartmental and tricompartmental disease is displayed on MR images through the medial and lateral femorotibial compartments and patellofemoral joint (Fig. 4-96).[34] Marginal and subchondral erosions with diffuse loss of hyaline articular cartilage are evident on both femoral and tibial surfaces. Large-joint effusions with popliteal cysts are commonly seen and demonstrate uniform high signal intensity on T2-weighted images. Less frequently, signs of degenerative arthritis with osteophytosis and subchondral sclerosis are visualized on MR scans as low signal intensity. An irregular fat pad may be seen in the more active stages of the disease. Hypertrophied synovial masses remain low in signal intensity with T1- and T2-weighted contrast. Osteonecrosis and infarcts have been observed with MR evaluation in rheumatoid patients before corresponding radiographic changes were demonstrated.

Text continues on p. 160

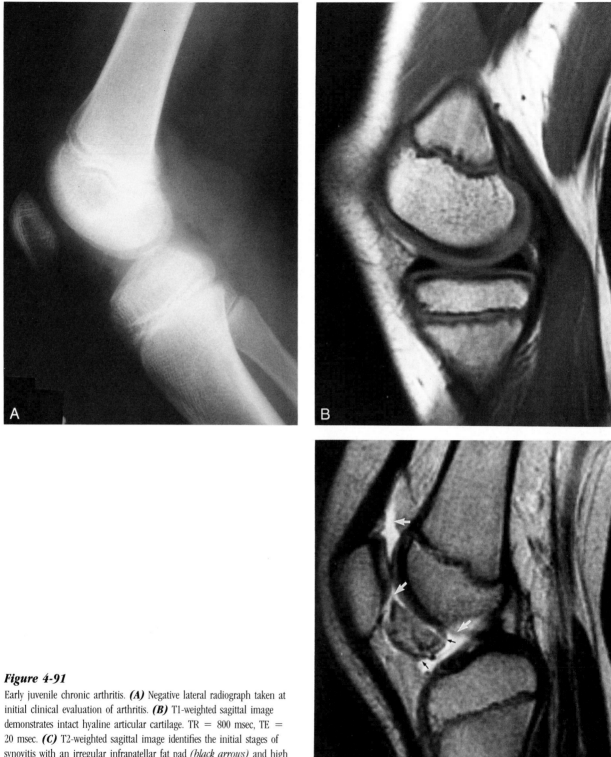

Figure 4-91

Early juvenile chronic arthritis. *(A)* Negative lateral radiograph taken at initial clinical evaluation of arthritis. *(B)* T1-weighted sagittal image demonstrates intact hyaline articular cartilage. TR = 800 msec, TE = 20 msec. *(C)* T2-weighted sagittal image identifies the initial stages of synovitis with an irregular infrapatellar fat pad *(black arrows)* and high signal intensity effusion *(white arrows)*. TR = 2000 msec; TE = 60 msec.

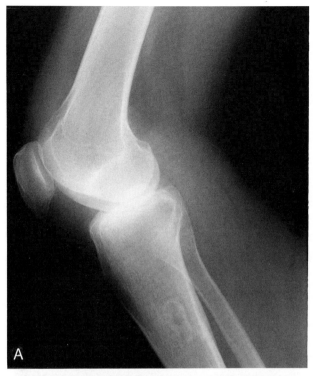

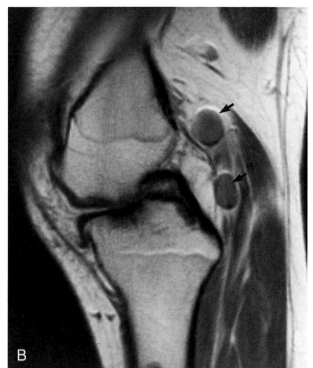

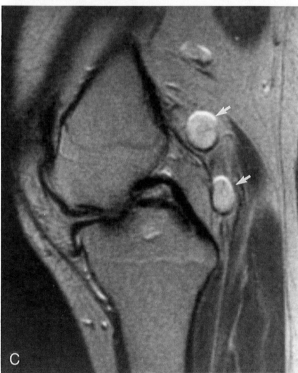

Figure 4-92

Popliteal cysts. Popliteal cysts *(arrows)* of the gastrocnemius-semimembranosus bursa, not detected on lateral radiograph *(A)*, are demonstrated as low and high signal intensity on T1-weighted *(B)* and T2-weighted *(C)* sagittal images, respectively. *(B)* TR = 800 msec, TE = 20 msec; *(C)* TR = 2000 msec, TE = 60 msec.

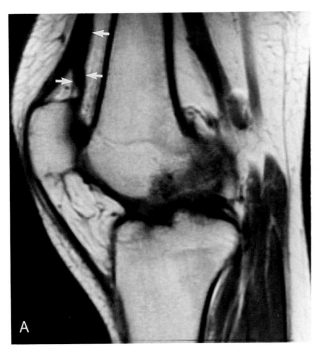
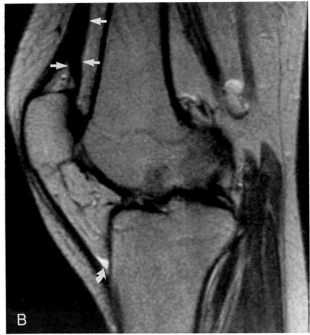

Figure 4-93

Juvenile rheumatoid (chronic) arthritis (JRA) Suprapatellar synovial hypertrophy *(white arrows)* images with low signal intensity on T1-weighted *(A)* and T2-weighted *(B)* sagittal images. In contrast, focus of fluid is visualized as bright signal intensity *(curved arrow)*. *(A)* TR = 800 msec, TE = 20 msec; *(B)* TR = 2000 msec, TE = 60 msec.

Figure 4-94

Juvenile rheumatoid (chronic) arthritis. Advanced JRA with marked joint space narrowing *(black arrows)* as seen on AP radiograph *(A)* and T1-weighted coronal image *(B)*. Articular cartilage erosion *(white arrow)* and subchondral sclerosis *(curved arrow)* are best appreciated on MR. TR = 800 msec, TE = 20 msec.

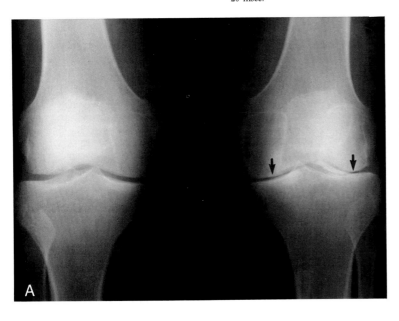
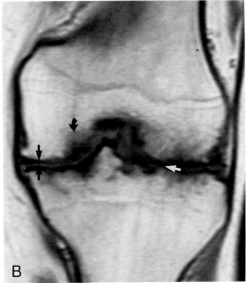

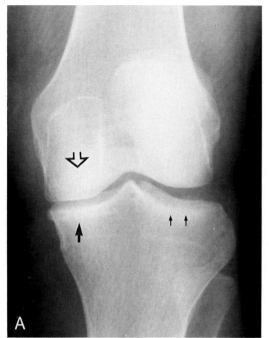

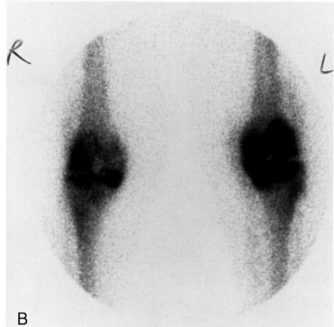

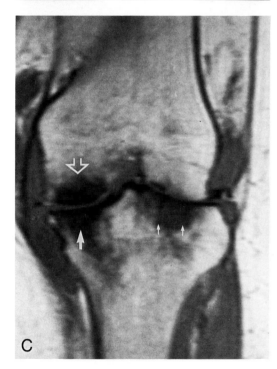

Figure 4-95

Juvenile rheumatoid (chronic) arthritis with steroid-induced osteonecrosis **(A)** AP radiograph with subchondral sclerosis in the medial femoral *(open arrow)* and tibial *(large solid arrow)* condyles and in the lateral tibial plateau *(small solid arrows)*. **(B)** Corresponding 99mTc-MDP scintigraphy showing increased uptake of bone tracer in the left femur and tibia. **(C)** T1-weighted coronal image demonstrating three separate foci of low signal intensity necrotic bone in the medial femoral condyle *(open arrow)* and medial *(large solid arrow)* and lateral *(small solid arrows)* tibial plateaus. All three sites of osteonecrosis were confirmed at biopsy.

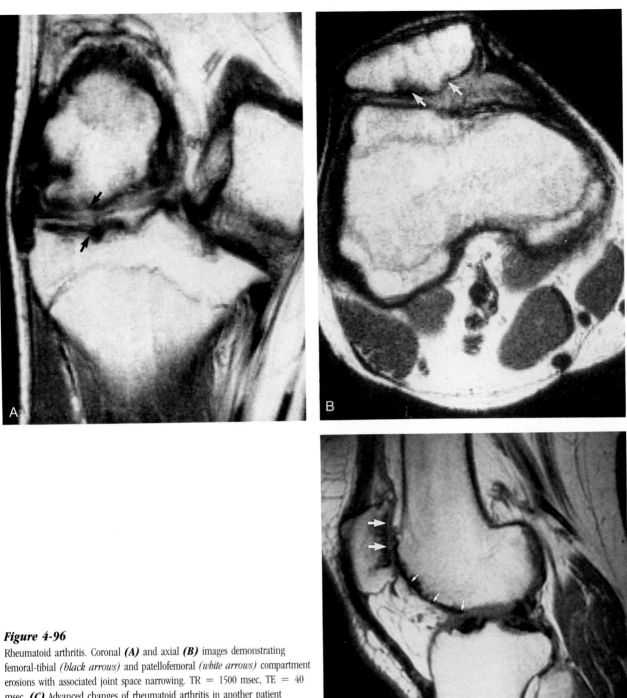

Figure 4-96

Rheumatoid arthritis. Coronal *(A)* and axial *(B)* images demonstrating femoral-tibial *(black arrows)* and patellofemoral *(white arrows)* compartment erosions with associated joint space narrowing. TR = 1500 msec, TE = 40 msec. *(C)* Advanced changes of rheumatoid arthritis in another patient showing severe patellofemoral arthritis *(large arrows)* with subchondral low signal intensity sclerosis and erosive changes. Denuded femoral articular cartilage is indicated *(small arrows)*.

Figure 4-97

Pigmented villonodular synovitis (PVNS). Unremarkable AP *(A)* and lateral *(B)* radiographs of the distal femur and proximal tibia. *(C)* Coronal image identifying low signal intensity hyperplastic synovium on the lateral aspect of the knee *(arrows)*. Intermediate-weighted image; TR = 1500 msec, TE = 40 msec. *(D)* Synovial mass of fibrous tissue and hemosiderin *(white arrows)* remains low in signal intensity while adjacent effusion is shown as bright signal intensity *(black arrow)*. T2-weighted sagittal image; TR = 2500 msec, TE = 40 msec. *(E)* Low signal intensity hemosiderin is visualized deposited in a thickened synovial reflection along the concave surface of the infrapatellar fat pad *(arrows)*. T2-weighted sagittal image; TR = 2500 msec, TE = 40 msec. Intermediate- *(F)* and T2-weighted *(G)* axial images demonstrating no change in signal intensity within posterior hemosiderin-laden synovial mass *(open arrow)*. Suprapatellar effusion *(closed arrow)* increases in signal intensity on T2-weighted image.

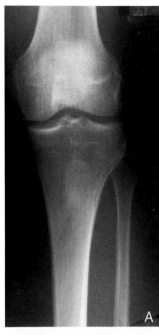

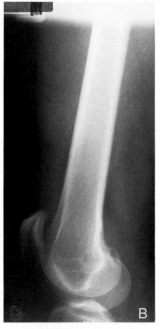

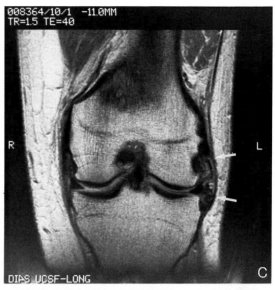

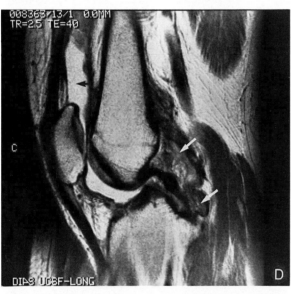

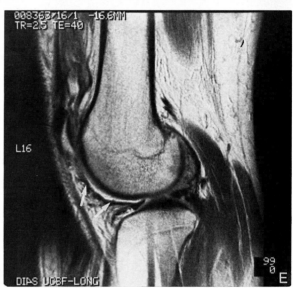

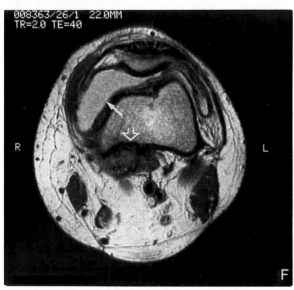

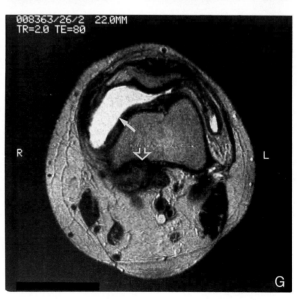

Pigmented Villonodular Synovitis

Pigmented villonodular synovitis (PVNS) is a monoarticular synovial proliferative disorder. It usually presents as a nonpainful soft tissue mass, and the knee is a frequent site of involvement, especially in the diffuse form of the disease. Hemosiderin-laden macrophages are frequently deposited in hyperplastic synovial masses, and there may be associated sclerotic bone lesions.

In a series of ten cases of PVNS of the knee, pathologic changes were correctly identified on MR studies, with surgical confirmation in all cases.[55,56] The hemosiderin-infiltrated synovial masses imaged with low signal intensity of T1- and T2-weighted images because of the paramagnetic effect of iron (Fig. 4-97). Adjacent synovial fluid, however, visualized with increased signal intensity on T2-weighted images. In two cases, hemosiderin deposits were observed in a thickened synovial reflection, superior to Hoffa's infrapatellar fat pad. In one case, lateral femoral condylar erosions, adjacent to a mass of synovial and fibrous tissue, were also visualized (Fig. 4-98). A more localized nodular form of PVNS, presenting as a well-circumscribed mass within the infrapatellar fat pad, has also been reported.

Hemophilia

In MR studies of patients with hemophilic arthropathy, hemosiderin and fibrous tissue—formed from repeated episodes of joint hemorrhage—image with low signal intensity on T1- and T2-weighted images (Fig. 4-99).[57,58] Irregular fat pads and markedly thickened, hemosiderin-laden synovial reflections (of low signal intensity) were present in each of five separate cases we have studied (Fig. 4-100).[34] Although conventional radiographs were normal, articular cartilage irregularities and erosions were detected on MR scans.

Subchondral and intraosseous cysts or hemorrhage can be identified on coronal and sagittal MR images (Fig. 4-101). Fluid-filled cysts generate high signal intensity on T2-weighted images. Areas of fibrous tissue remain low in signal intensity on T1- and T2-weighted images, and low signal intensity synovial effusions can be differentiated from adjacent hemosiderin and fibrous

Figure 4-98
Pigmented villonodular synovitis (PVNS). **(A)** PVNS *(black arrow)* mass seen in posterolateral femoral condyle on T1-weighted sagittal image. TR = 500 msec, TE = 40 msec. **(B)** Femoral condylar erosion *(white arrows)* is demonstrated in axial CT.

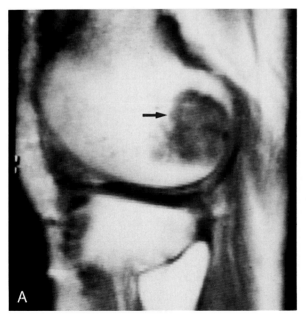
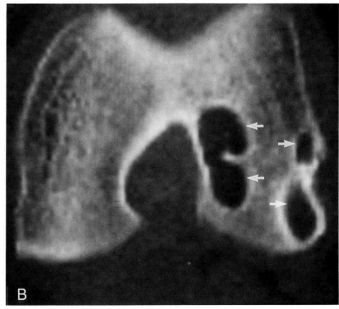

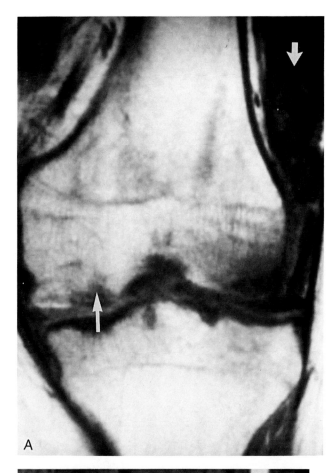

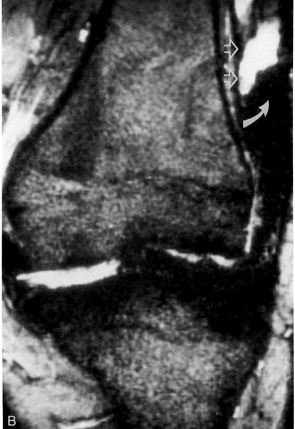

depositions on T2-weighted sequences. In a study of the knees of ten hemophiliacs, articular and subchondral abnormalities were found in 80% (Fig. 4-102).

Lyme Arthritis

Lyme disease and resultant arthritis are transmitted by the *Ixodes* tick, and are characterized by the delayed appearance of an oligo- or polyarticular inflammatory arthritis.[59] The knee is most commonly affected, with development of inflammatory synovial effusions, synovial hypertrophy, infrapatellar fat pad edema, and (in severe chronic cases) cartilage erosions. In one patient, studied 3 months after a documented tick bite, MR studies revealed an extensive joint effusion and an irregular corrugated infrapatellar fat pad (Fig. 4-103).[34] After MR imaging was performed, contrast material was injected into the joint to confirm the scalloped synovium, characteristic of the synovitis initially identified on MR. No cartilage erosions were documented.

Osteoarthritis

The MR findings in *degenerative arthrosis* represent a spectrum varying from osteophytic spurring (which images with the bright signal intensity of marrow), to compartment collapse, denuded articular cartilage, torn and degenerative meniscal fibrocartilage, and diminished marrow signal intensity in areas of subchondral sclerosis (Fig. 4-104).[3,24,60] The ability to assess hyaline cartilage surfaces accurately gives MR an advantage over plain film radiography in preoperative planning for joint arthroplasty procedures. Chondral fragments, of intermediate signal intensity, and loose bodies, with the high signal intensity of marrow fat, may be associated with more advanced degenerative disease (Fig. 4-105).

In *synovial chondromatosis,* multiple synovium-based chondral fragments are visualized with low to intermediate signal intensity (Fig. 4-106). In primary chondromatosis these metaplastic fragments are usually similar to one another in size. In secondary chrondromatosis they are visualized in a variety of sizes.

Text continues on p. 167

Figure 4-99

Hemophilia. *(A)* T1-weighted coronal image demonstrating erosive changes *(long arrow)* and surrounding low signal intensity areas along the lateral femur *(short arrow).* TR = 600 msec, TE = 20 msec. *(B)* T2* gradient echo image differentiating high signal intensity fluid or hemorrhage *(open arrows)* from chronic hemosiderin deposition *(curved arrow).* TR = 400 msec, TE = 30 msec; flip angle = 30°.

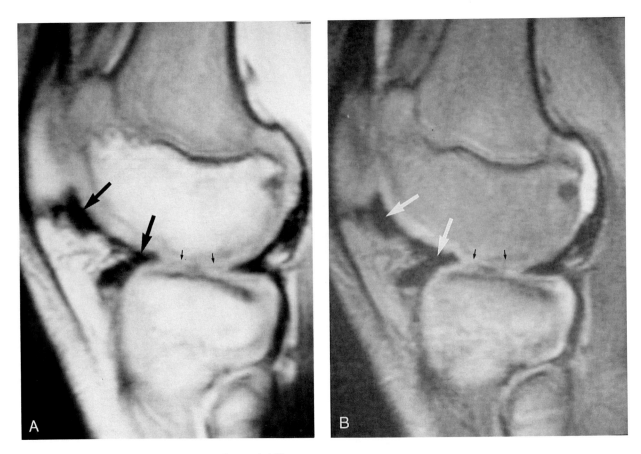

Figure 4-100

Knee in hemophiliac patient showing early cartilage erosions *(small arrows)* and thickened hemosiderin-laden synovium imaging with low signal intensity *(large arrows)* on T1-weighted *(A)* and T2-weighted *(B)* images. Irregularity of Hoffa's infrapatellar fat pad indicates synovial irritation. *(A)* TR = 800 msec, TE = 20 msec; *(B)* TR = 2000 msec, TE = 60 msec.

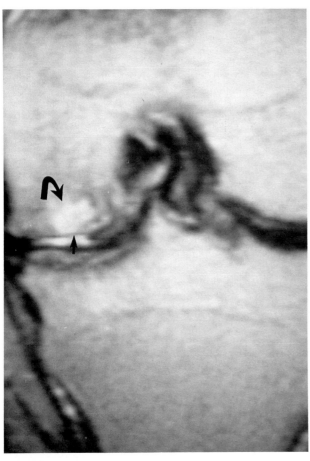

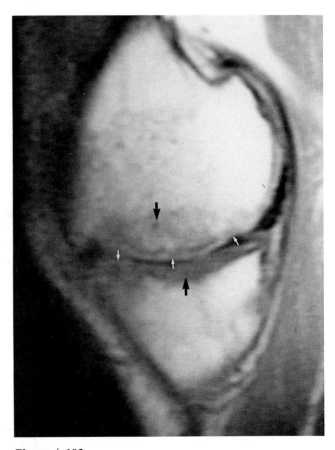

Figure 4-101

High signal intensity intraosseous cyst *(curved arrow),* formed through defect in femoral articular cartilage *(straight arrow)* in hemophiliac patient. T2-weighted coronal image; TR = 2000 msec, TE = 60 msec.

Figure 4-102

Adult hemophiliac with low signal intensity subchrondral sclerosis *(black arrows)* and denuded articular cartilage *(white arrows).* T1-weighted sagittal image; TR = 800 msec, TE = 20 msec.

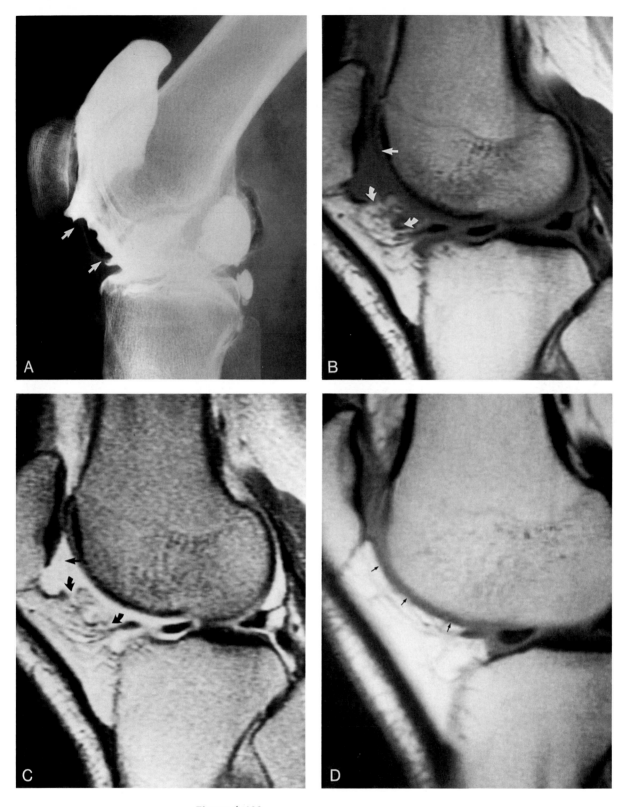

Figure 4-103

Lyme arthritis. **(A)** Lateral view arthrogram demonstrating scalloped appearance of contrast *(arrows)* indicating synovitis. T1-weighted **(B)** and T2-weighted **(C)** sagittal images identify irregular infrapatellar fat pad *(curved arrows)* with interdigitation of synovial effusion *(straight arrow)*. Joint effusion is bright on T2-weighted image **(C)**. **(B)** TR = 800' msec, TE = 20 msec; **(C)** TR = 2000 msec, TE = 60 msec. **(D)** Asymptomatic knee in the same patient displaying normal concave contour to the free edge of Hoffa's infrapatellar fat pad *(arrows)*. Intermediate-weighted sagittal image; TR = 2000 msec, TE = 20 msec.

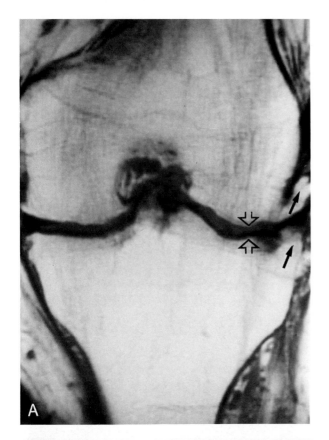

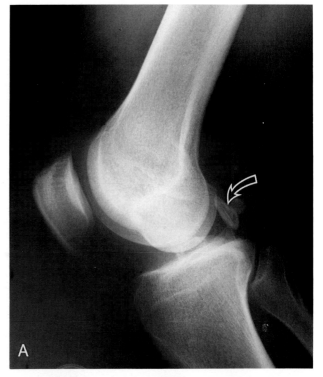

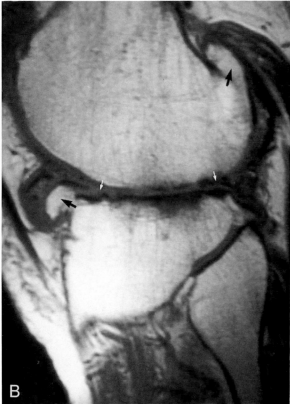

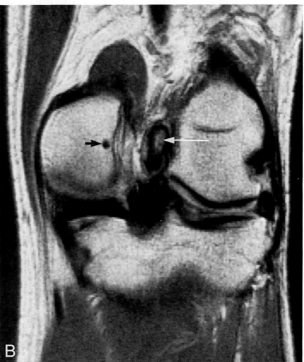

Figure 4-104

Coronal **(A)** and sagittal **(B)** images of degenerative osteoarthritis identifying marrow containing osteophytes *(black arrows)*, joint space narrowing *(open arrows)*, eroded hyaline articular cartilage *(white arrows)*, and macerated menisci. T1-weighted images; TR = 600 msec, TE = 20 msec.

Figure 4-105

Intraarticular loose body. **(A)** Intraarticular loose body is identified posteriorly on plain film lateral radiograph *(open arrow)*. **(B)** On T1-weighted coronal image it is seen in the intercondylar notch *(white arrow)*. The free fragment is imaged with central marrow signal intensity (high) and peripheral cortical signal intensity (low). Incidental bone island is shown as focus of low signal intensity in compact bone *(black arrow)*. TR = 1000 msec, TE = 40 msec.

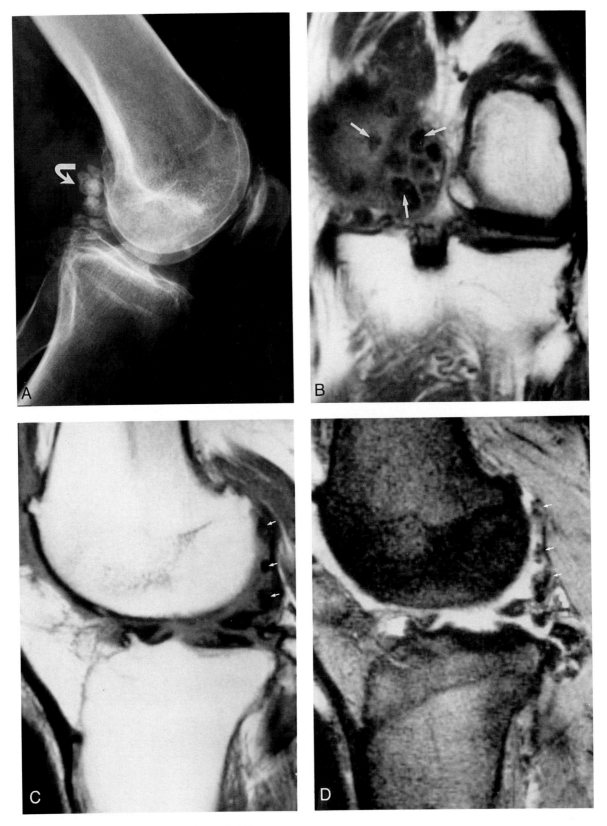

Figure 4-106

Synovial chondromatosis. **(A)** Multiple calcified loose bodies shown on lateral radiograph *(curved arrow)*. **(B)** Osteochondral loose bodies *(arrows)* collecting in posteromedial joint capsule. T1-weighted coronal image; TR = 600 msec, TE = 20 msec. T1-weighted **(C)** and T2* gradient echo **(D)** sagittal images identifying synovium-based osteochrondral fragments *(arrows)*. Surrounding joint effusion is visualized with bright signal intensity on T2* weighted contrast.

Osteonecrosis and Related Disorders

Spontaneous osteonecrosis of the knee typically affects an older patient group, predominantly female, and presents with acute medial joint pain.[24,61,62] Most often, spontaneous osteonecrosis involves the weight-bearing surface of the medial femoral condyle (Fig. 4-107), although cases have been described in which the medial and lateral tibial plateaus and the lateral femoral condyle were involved (Fig. 4-108).[63] In tibial involvement, the weight-bearing surface may or may not be affected. Meniscal tears are often associated with this condition.

Conventional radiographic evaluation is not sensitive to identification of the osteonecrotic focus prior to the development of sclerosis and osseous collapse. With MR imaging in osteonecrosis, however, a low signal intensity focus can be detected on T1- and T2-weighted images in patients with no radiographic findings. We have also observed a more diffuse pattern of low signal intensity in early stages of the disease, and with time,

better demarcation of the lesion. The overlying articular cartilage and status of the meniscus can also be evaluated on T1-weighted images or on T2* gradient echo images. We have documented osteonecrosis in both the medial and lateral tibial plateaus on MR. In a patient with juvenile rheumatoid arthritis, osteonecrosis of the tibial plateau was observed on MR and confirmed at biopsy (see Fig. 4-95).

Osteochondritis dissecans differs from spontaneous osteonecrosis of the knee in that it primarily affects young male patients and involves the nonweight-bearing surface of the medial femoral condyle (Fig. 4-109).[64–66] (We have seen, however, one case of osteochondritis involving the inferior portion of the medial patellar facet.) A history of knee trauma presents in up to 50% of patients. On MR scans, the focus of osteochondritis images with low signal intensity on T1- and T2-weighted images even prior to detection on conventional radiographs (Fig. 4-110). Overlying defects in the hyaline articular cartilage are best appreciated on T2*

Figure 4-107

Spontaneous osteonecrosis of the medial femoral condyle imaged with low signal intensity *(open arrow)* on T1-weighted coronal *(A)* and sagittal *(B)* images. Macerated and torn posterior horn of medial meniscus is identified *(white arrows)*. TR = 800 msec, TE = 20 msec.

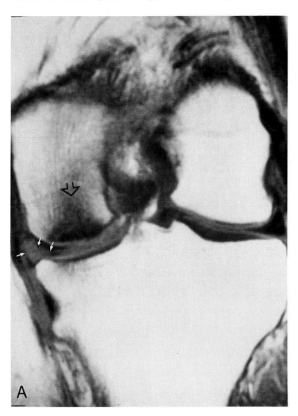 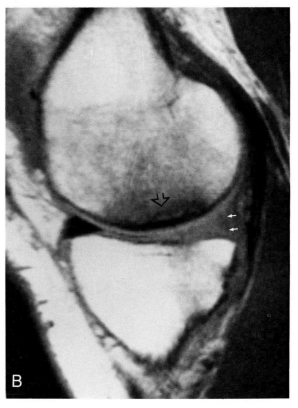

gradient echo images, where cartilage contrast is of high signal intensity (see Fig. 4-88). MR is particularly valuable in demonstrating associated free and loose osseous and chondral fragments.

Osgood–Schlatter disease represents an osteochondrosis of the developing tibial tuberosity and is thought to be secondary to trauma occurring during adolescent growth.[67] Radiographic changes include soft tissue edema anterior to the tibial tuberosity and avulsion and fragmentation of the tibial tubercle ossification center. MR findings include irregularity of the distal patellar tendon and infrapatellar fat pad. In one patient with Osgood-Schlatter disease, multiple small ossicles (anterior to the tibial tuberosity) were imaged with the high signal intensity of marrow fat (Fig. 4-111). In another case, MR findings included patellar tendon thickening and focal low signal intensity in underlying subchondral bone.[4]

Bone infarcts are usually metaphyseal in location but have also been imaged in more epiphyseal and diaphyseal locations.[68] The MR appearance of a bone infarct is characteristic, with a serpiginous low signal intensity border of reactive bone and a central compartment of high signal intensity equivalent to yellow marrow (Fig. 4-112). On T2-weighted images, a chemical shift artifact may be seen as a linear segment of high signal intensity paralleling the outline of the infarct. Bone infarcts can be differentiated from enchondromas on MR, the latter lacking a serpiginous border and having a central region of low signal intensity on T1-weighted images that increases with progressive T2-weighting. Calcified bone infarcts, however, will image with central low signal intensity on T1- and T2-weighted images (Fig. 4-113). Bone infarcts may be seen in association with steroid therapy, as part of a chemotherapy protocol, for example (Fig. 4-114).

Joint Effusions

Joint effusions image with low signal intensity on T1-weighted images and with bright signal intensity on corresponding T2-weighted images (Fig. 4-115).[69] With the

Text continues on p. 172

Figure 4-108

Osteonecrosis of the medial tibial plateau. **(A)** Sclerotic focus in medial tibial plateau *(arrows)* seen on AP radiograph. **(B)** Well-defined region of subchondral low signal intensity in the medial tibial plateau *(black arrows)* with thinning of overlying hyaline articular cartilage *(white arrows)*. T1-weighted coronal image; TR = 800 msec, TE = 20 msec.

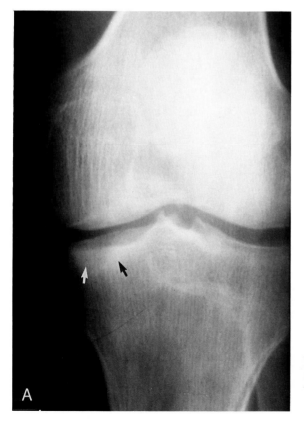
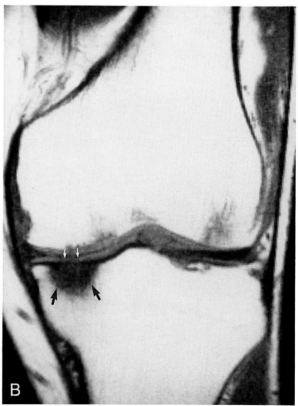

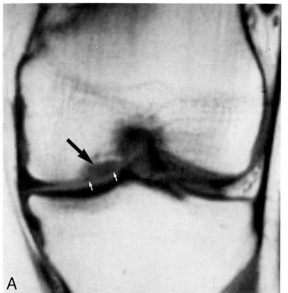

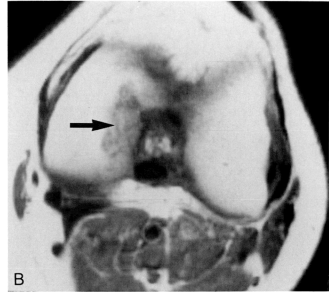

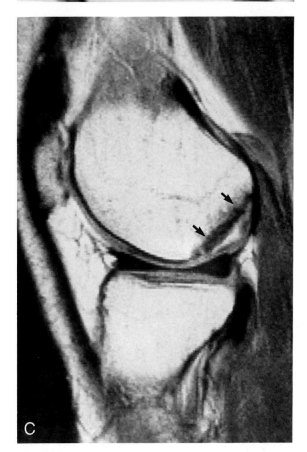

Figure 4-109

Osteochondritis dissecans *(black arrow)* involving the lateral aspect of the medial femoral condyle on T1-weighted coronal *(A)* and axial *(B)* images. Overlying hyaline articular cartilage is bowed *(white arrows)*. TR = 600 msec, TE = 20 msec. *(C)* Osteochondritis dissecans in another patient, identifying the low signal intensity focus of devitalized bone in the non-weight-bearing portion of the medial femoral condyle *(arrows)*. T1-weighted sagittal image; TR = 1000 msec, TE = 40 msec.

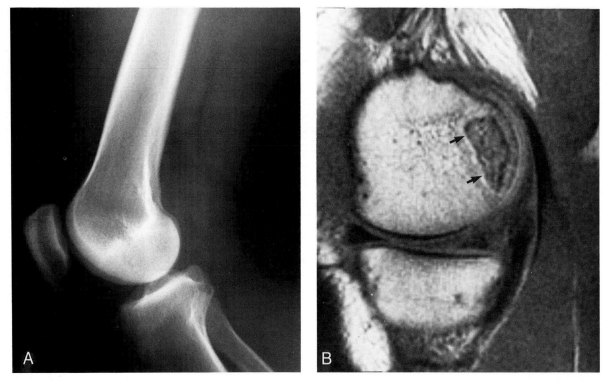

Figure 4-110

Osteochondritis dissecans. **(A)** Negative lateral radiograph. **(B)** Osteochondritis dissecans focus imaged as low signal intensity in the posterior medial femoral condyle *(arrows)*. T1-weighted sagittal image; TR = 600 msec, TE = 20 msec.

Figure 4-111

Unresolved or chronic Osgood-Schlatter's disease with avulsion and irregularity of the tibial tuberosity ossicle *(straight arrow)* on lateral radiograph **(A)** and T1-weighted sagittal image **(B).** Unrelated osteochondral fragment posteriorly is identified *(curved arrow)*. TR = 600 msec, TE = 20 msec.

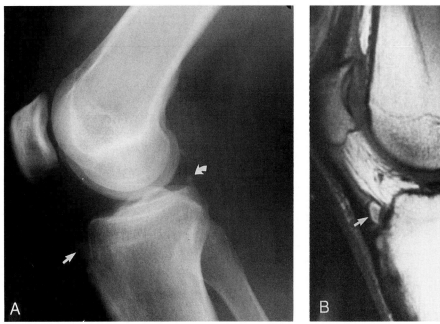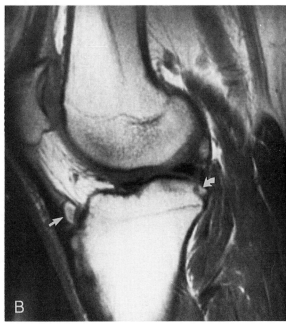

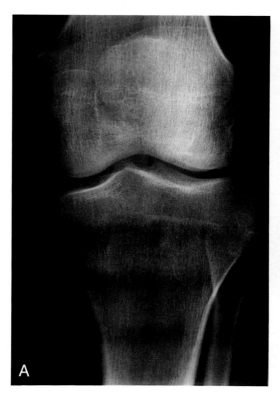

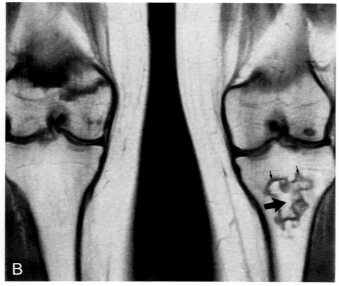

Figure 4-112

Bone infarct not appreciated on AP radiograph *(A)* is delineated on coronal image *(B)* with characteristic serpiginous low signal intensity peripheral sclerosis *(small arrow)* and high signal intensity central portion *(large arrow)*. T1-weighted image; TR = 1000 msec; TE = 40 msec.

Figure 4-114

Multiple bone infarcts in a leukemic patient on steroids.

Figure 4-113

Calcified bone infarct is visualized with multiple central punctate areas of low signal intensity *(large arrow)*. Adjacent noncalcified bone infarct shown with central portion isointense with yellow marrow *(small arrow)*. T1-weighted axial image; TR = 800 msec, TE = 20 msec.

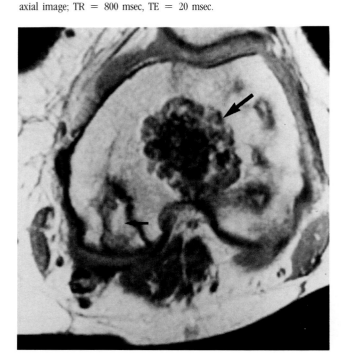

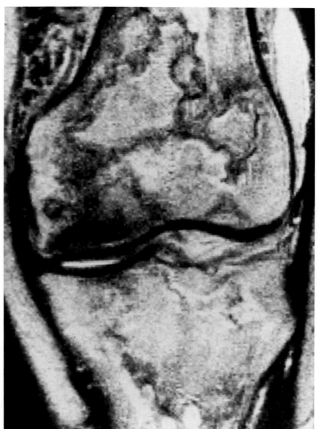

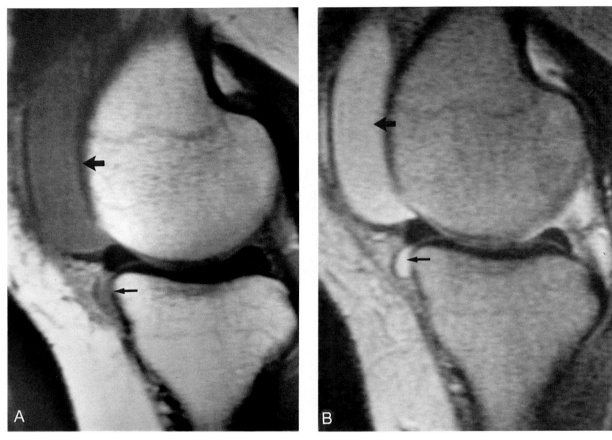

Figure 4-115

Suprapatellar effusion. Joint effusion—low signal intensity on T1-weighted sagittal image ***(A)*** and high signal intensity on T2-weighted sagittal image ***(B)***—distends suprapatellar bursa *(large arrow)* and anterior capsule *(small arrow)* without obscuring visualization of the lateral meniscus. ***(A)*** TR = 800 msec, TE = 20 msec; ***(B)*** TR = 2000 msec, TE = 60 msec.

knee in 15° of external rotation, the effusion may be more prominent in the lateral compartment of the joint capsule, simulating an artificial bloutement. With the patient in the supine position, the posterior capsule is preferentially distended and will collect fluid before there is suprapatellar bursal distention. Layers of fat–fluid, fluid–fluid, and air–fluid levels (postaspiration) can be demonstrated in suprapatellar fluid collections. When MR is performed after arthrography, contrast material coating articular cartilage and extending into the suprapatellar recess can be observed. Fluid, initially trapped between meniscal surfaces, is seen on T2-weighted images as a bright signal intensity interface, and does not obscure diagnostic interpretation of meniscal fibrocartilage. Inflammatory and noninflammatory effusions are indistinguishable in their MR appearance. Our experience indicates that T1-weighted sequences are adequate for detecting small effusions, and there is

no need for longer TR settings. Coronal images are complementary, and the "saddle bag" distribution of fluid in the medial and lateral gutters extending into the suprapatellar bursa can be seen (Fig. 4-116).

Popliteal Cysts

Classically, *popliteal* or *Baker's cysts* of the gastrocnemiosemimembranosus bursa arise between the medial head of the gastrocnemius muscle and the more lateral semimembranosus muscle (Fig. 4-117).[70,71] These cysts image with low signal intensity on T1-weighted images and with uniform increased signal intensity on T2-weighted images. Septations may be visualized, dividing the cyst into compartments. However, this is more frequently seen in atypical cyst locations. A narrow neck

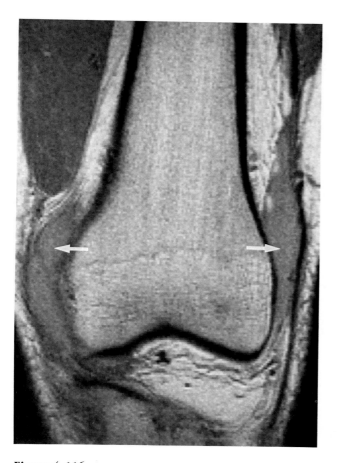

Figure 4-116

The "saddle bag" distribution of joint effusion in medial and lateral gutters of the suprapatellar bursae *(arrows)*. Intermediate-weighted coronal image; TR = 1500 msec, TE = 40 msec.

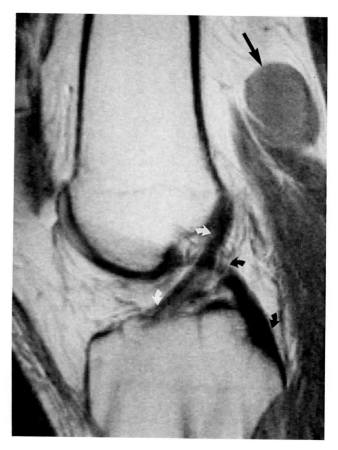

Figure 4-117

Characteristic location of popliteal cyst medial to the medial head of the gastrocnemius muscle *(straight black arrow)*. Cyst contents image with intermediate signal intensity on intermediate-weighted sagittal image. Normal anterior *(curved white arrows)* and posterior *(curved black arrows)* cruciate ligament anatomy is also demonstrated. TR = 1500 msec, TE = 40 msec.

connecting the cyst to the joint is usually identified on axial images. MR is valuable in identifying associated intraarticular pathology, commonly meniscal tears (Fig. 4-118). Hemorrhagic joint effusions may be visualized with a fluid–fluid level in the cyst. In two patients we have studied, multiple loose bodies collecting in a posterior popliteal cyst were identified (Fig. 4-119). Because of the presence of subacute blood, dissecting or ruptured popliteal cysts with hemorrhage image with high signal intensity on T1- and T2-weighted images (Fig. 4-120).

Atypical locations for popliteal cysts include the tibiofibular joint and the bursa between the lateral head of the gastrocnemius and biceps femoris. They may also present as soft tissue masses proximal or distal to the popliteal fossa (Fig. 4-121). In very young children, popliteal cysts may occur in the absence of concurrent intraarticular pathology.[72] Popliteal cysts are frequent in patients with JRA or adult rheumatoid arthritis. With MR

evaluation, a cyst can be differentiated from a *popliteal artery aneurysm* (Fig. 4-122) or a *venous malformation* (Fig. 4-123), which may present with a similar clinical picture. MR offers the advantage of evaluating both popliteal and intraarticular pathology, areas of limited diagnostic efficacy with ultrasound or conventional radiography.

Plicae

Synovial plicae are embryonic remnants of the septal division of the knee joint into three compartments.[73] They may be found as a normal variant in 20% to 60% of adult knees. The suprapatellar, mediopatellar, and infrapatellar are the common plicae. The mediopatellar and infrapatellar plicae are best visualized on axial images (Fig. 4-124), whereas the suprapatellar plica is best visualized on sagittal images traversing the suprapatellar bursa (Figure 4-125). Plica tissue images with low signal

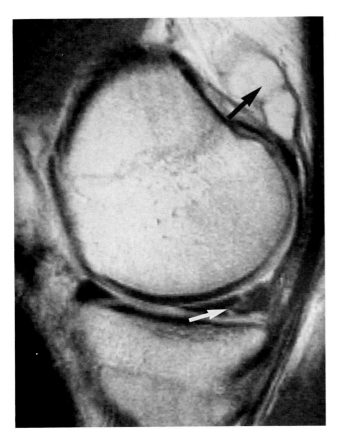

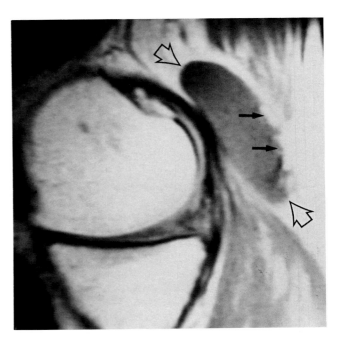

Figure 4-119

Baker cyst *(open arrows)* containing multiple high signal intensity loose bodies imaging with marrow fat signal intensity *(closed arrows)*. T1-weighted sagittal image; TR = 800 msec, TE = 20 msec.

Figure 4-118

T2-weighted sagittal image identifying increased signal intensity synovial fluid in popliteal cyst *(black arrow)* and vertical tear in the posterior horn of the medial meniscus *(white arrow)*. TR = 2000 msec, TE = 40 msec.

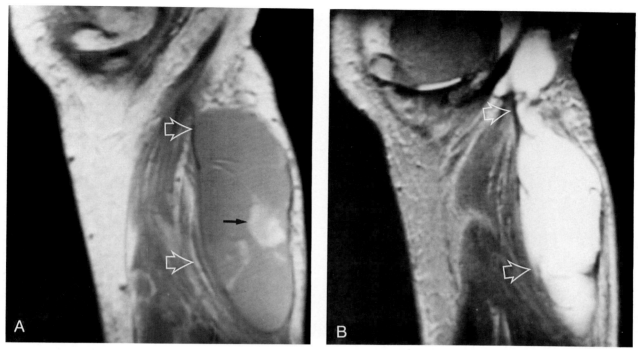

Figure 4-120
Hemorrhagic popliteal cyst. **(A)** Dissecting popliteal cyst *(open arrows)* with area of high signal intensity subacute hemorrhage *(closed arrow)* identified on T1-weighted sagittal image. TR = 1000 msec, TE = 20 msec. **(B)** High signal intensity cyst *(open arrows)* traceable to the joint line on T2-weighted sagittal image. TR = 2000 msec, TE = 60 msec.

intensity on T1- and T2-weighted images.[74] The infrapatellar plica, the most common, may be confused with the anterior cruciate ligament on arthrography.

In one patient presenting with a suprapatellar soft tissue mass, MR study revealed a persistent plica that divided the suprapatellar bursa into two separate compartments and which contained hemorrhagic synovial fluid and debris (Fig. 4-126). An inflamed mediopatellar plica becomes thickened and may interfere with normal quadriceps function (Fig. 4-127). Erosion or abrasion of femoral condylar or patellar articular cartilage can occur as the plica loses its flexibility and gliding motion. On axial MR images, a symptomatic mediopatellar plica may be seen as a thickened band of low signal intensity with underlying irregularity of the medial patellar facet cartilage surface.

Fractures

Fractures about the knee can involve the femoral condyle, the tibial plateau surface, or the patella.[42] Tibial plateau fractures are the most frequent, with predominant lateral plateau involvement (Fig. 4-128).[75] The most common mechanism of injury is impaction of the anterior portion of the lateral femoral condyle in a valgus mechanism of injury. Axial loading, or pure compression force, produces an *impaction* or *compression fracture of the plateau,* whereas a pure valgus force results in a *split condylar fracture.* A valgus compressive force is responsible for the frequent occurrence of *lateral tibial condylar plateau fractures* with tears of the medial meniscus, anterior cruciate, and medial collateral ligaments.

Text continues on p. 183

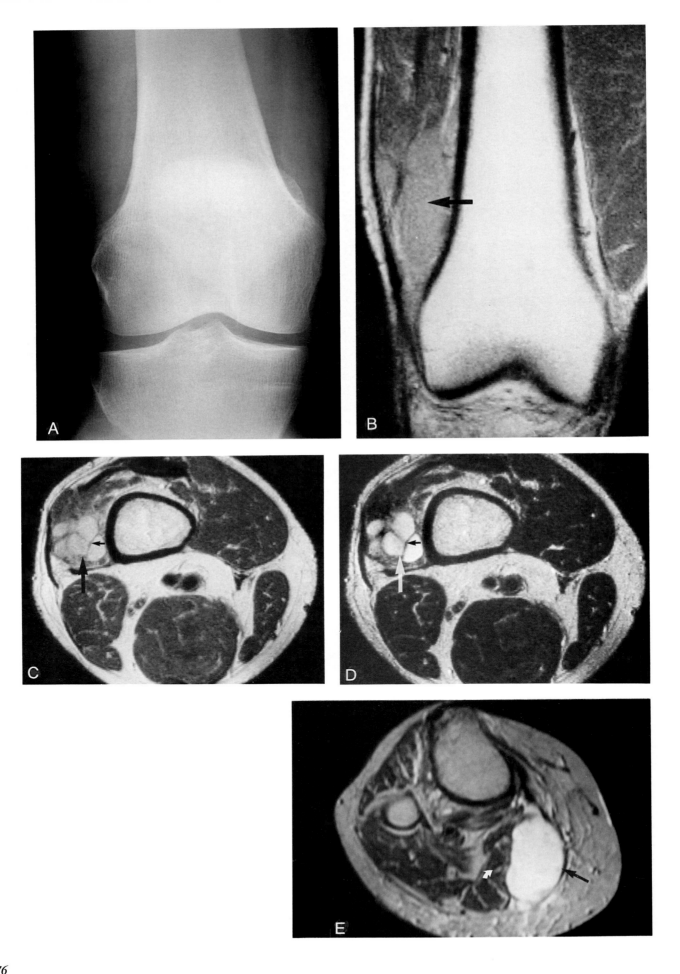

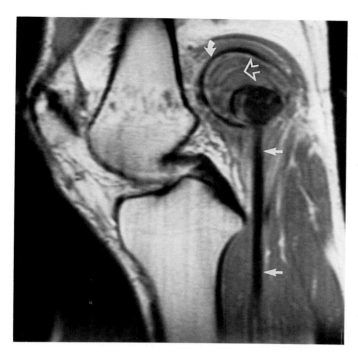

Figure 4-122

T1-weighted sagittal image demonstrating enlarged aneurysm of the popliteal artery. Native low signal intensity popliteal artery *(solid arrows)*, intermediate signal intensity thrombus *(open arrow)*, and low signal intensity peripheral rim of calcification *(curved arrow)* are identified. TR = 800 msec, TE = 20 msec.

◄ **Figure 4-121**

Atypical synovial cyst. *(A)* Unremarkable AP radiograph. *(B)* Corresponding intermediate weighted coronal image demonstrating synovial cyst tracking along the distal lateral femur *(arrow)*. Septated *(small arrow)* atypical popliteal cyst *(large arrow)* imaging with intermediate signal intensity on balanced weighted axial image *(C)* and with high signal intensity on T2-weighted axial image *(D)*. TR = 2000 msec, TE = 40, 80 msec. *(E)* In comparison, a more typical location of a popliteal cyst *(straight arrow)* medial to the medial head of the gastrocnemius muscle *(curved arrow)*. T2-weighted axial image; TR = 2000 msec, TE = 60 msec.

Figure 4-123

Venous malformation. *(A)* Serpiginous tangle of vessels on venous angiogram *(arrow)*. T1-weighted *(B)* and T2-weighted *(C)* coronal images demonstrating inhomogeneity with generalized increased signal intensity on T2-weighted image *(C)*. Low-signal intensity foci represent vessels with faster flowing blood *(curved arrow)*.

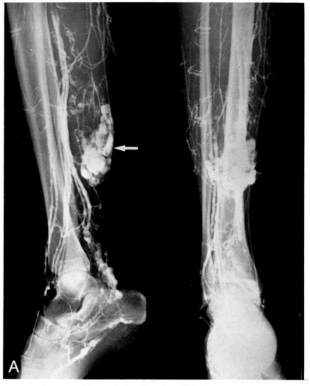

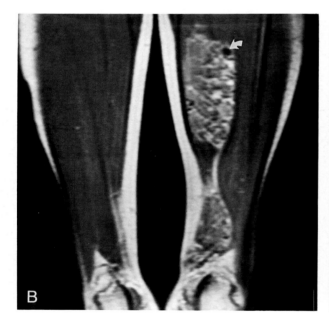

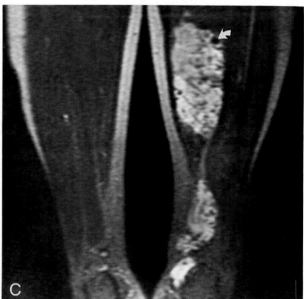

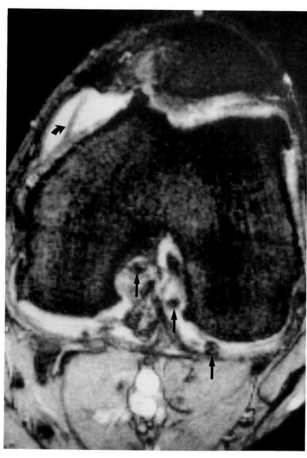

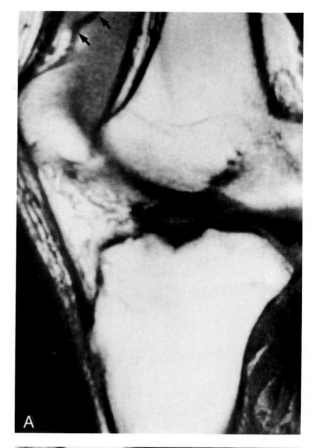

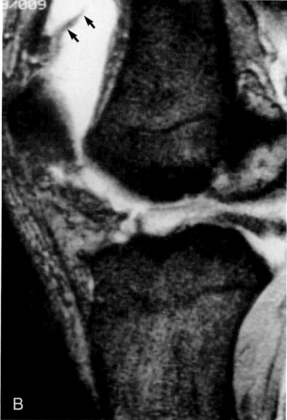

Figure 4-124

Low signal intensity incomplete medial patella plica is outlined by high signal intensity joint fluid on T2* axial image *(curved arrow)*. Loose osteochrondral fragments are identified posteriorly *(straight arrows)*. TR = 400 msec, TE = 30 msec; flip angle = 30°.

Figure 4-125

Low signal intensity suprapatellar plica *(arrows)* on T1-weighted *(A)* and T2* gradient echo *(B)* sagittal images. Effusion is shown as bright signal intensity on T2* weighted image. *(A)* TR = 600 msec, TE = 20 msec; *(B)* TR = 400 msec, TE = 30 msec; flip angle = 30°.

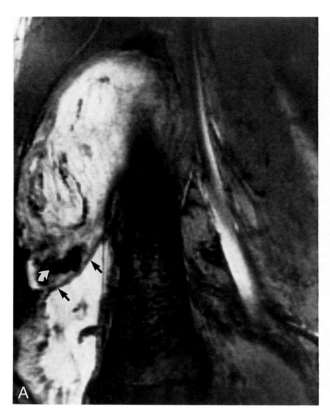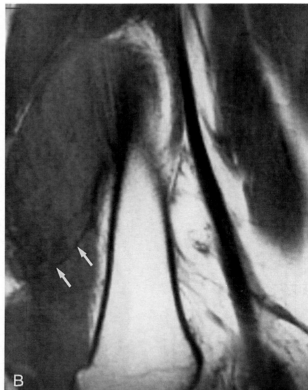

Figure 4-126

Complete suprapatellar plica. Division of the suprapatellar bursa into two compartments with an intact suprapatellar plica imaged as a low signal intensity band *(solid arrows)* on T2* gradient echo *(A)* and T1-weighted *(B)* sagittal images. Low signal intensity hemosiderin deposits *(curved arrow)* are contrasted with surrounding bright signal intensity hemorrhagic fluid *(A)*.

Figure 4-127

Surgically confirmed medial patella plica was responsible for localized fluid collection *(curved black arrow)* and medial facet cartilage erosions *(white arrows)*.

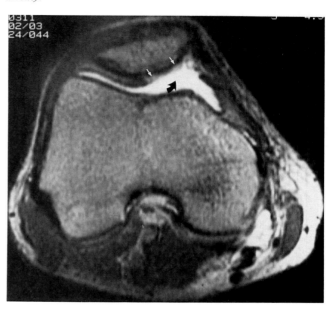

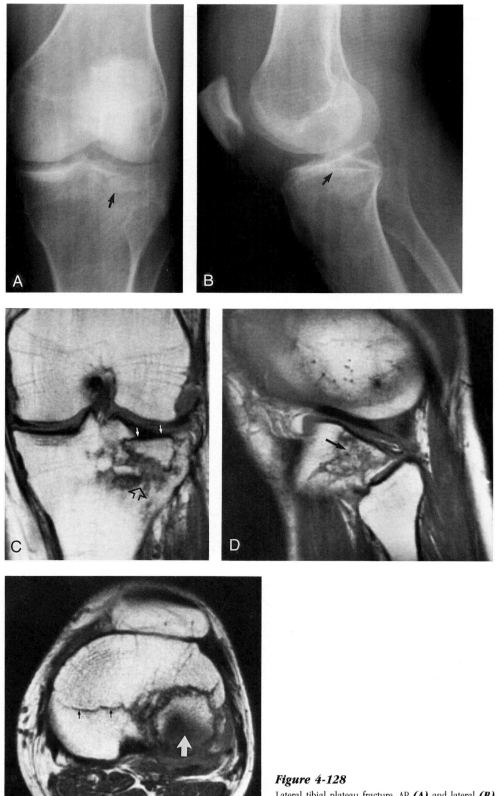

Figure 4-128

Lateral tibial plateau fracture. AP **(A)** and lateral **(B)** radiographs demonstrating disruption of lateral tibial plateau cortical surface *(arrow)*. **(C)** Coronal image identifying depressed plateau *(white arrows)* and associated edema *(open arrow)*. **(D)** Sagittal plane image displaying edematous fracture segment *(arrow)*. **(E)** Circular area of fracture impaction *(white arrow)* with radiating linear fracture extension *(black arrows)*.

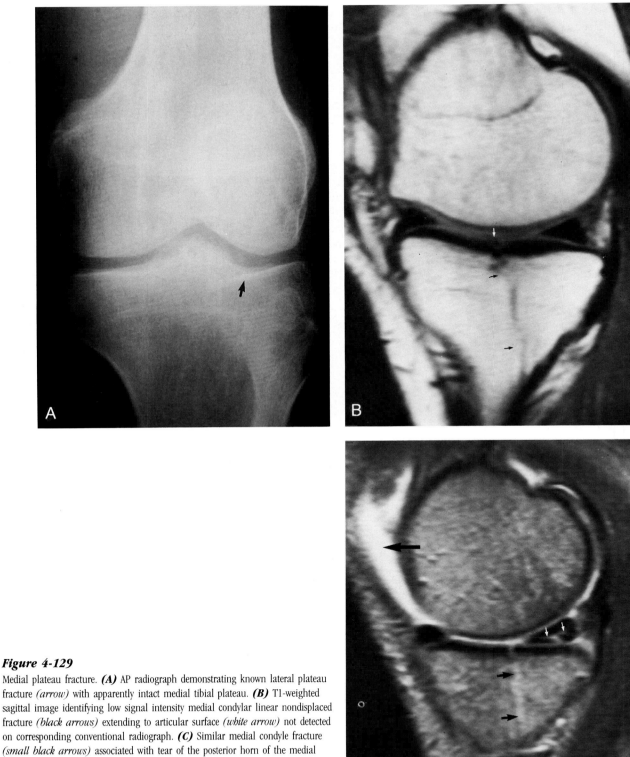

Figure 4-129

Medial plateau fracture. **(A)** AP radiograph demonstrating known lateral plateau fracture *(arrow)* with apparently intact medial tibial plateau. **(B)** T1-weighted sagittal image identifying low signal intensity medial condylar linear nondisplaced fracture *(black arrows)* extending to articular surface *(white arrow)* not detected on corresponding conventional radiograph. **(C)** Similar medial condyle fracture *(small black arrows)* associated with tear of the posterior horn of the medial meniscus *(white arrows)* in another patient. Fracture and effusion *(large black arrow)* image with bright signal intensity on T2-weighted sagittal image. TR = 2000 msec, TE = 60 msec.

Fractures about the knee can be identified on MR scans in patients with acute or chronic knee pain and negative conventional radiographs (Fig. 4-129). Subsequent radiography often shows areas of sclerosis or periosteal reaction at the fracture sites initially identified on MR. The most frequent MR pattern of fracture is sharp, well-defined linear segments of decreased signal intensity visualized in the distal femur or proximal tibia. In an acute fracture, associated fluid or hemorrhage images with increased signal intensity on T2-weighted images (Fig. 4-130). Fractures with diffuse areas of associated low signal intensity on T1-weighted images demonstrate increased signal intensity with long TR and TE settings, reflecting the prolonged T2 values in edematous marrow. Chronic fractures remain low in signal intensity with variable TR and TE parameters. The metaphyseal–epiphyseal junction of the physis should not be mistaken for a transverse linear fracture (Fig. 4-131). In the adult, the physeal line or scar does not demonstrate increased signal intensity on T2-weighted images. In a child, a chemical shift artifact may display bright signal intensity parallel to the physis.

MR imaging is also useful in the differentiation of stress fractures, common in the proximal tibia, from neoplastic processes (Fig. 4-132).[76] The linear segment of the stress fracture in the knee is usually accompanied by marrow edema. Lack of a soft tissue mass, cortical destruction, or characteristic marrow extension effectively excludes a tumor from the differential consideration. Rarely, a stress fracture is obscured on MR scans by reactive edema, and high resolution, thin section CT is required to define it.

A diffuse or localized pattern of low signal intensity on T1-weighted images without a defined fracture is seen with bone bruises or contusions at sites of impaction or repetitive trauma (Fig. 4-133). In an acute or subacute setting, increased signal intensity is visualized on T2-weighted images prior to the appearance of plain film sclerosis (Fig. 4-134). A pathologic fracture may be complicated by internal hemorrhage, obscuring the underlying lesion (Fig. 4-135). Compartment syndrome, a known complication of trauma including fracture, has been identified with edema limited to a specified muscle group (Fig. 4-136).[77] Sudeck's atrophy or reflex sympathetic dystrophy can occur as a complication of fracture. Diffuse juxtaarticular low signal intensity on

Figure 4-130

Fibular fracture. Nondisplaced fibular head fracture *(closed arrows)* with associated marrow edema *(open arrow)* images with low signal intensity on T1-weighted *(A)* and high signal intensity on T2-weighted *(B)* sagittal images. *(A)* TR = 600 msec, TE = 20 msec; *(B)* TR = 2000 msec, TE = 60 msec.

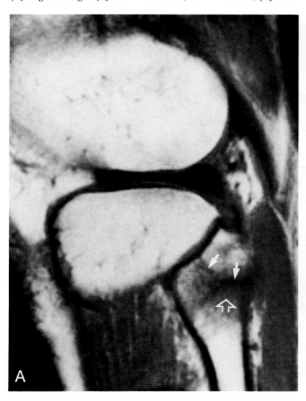
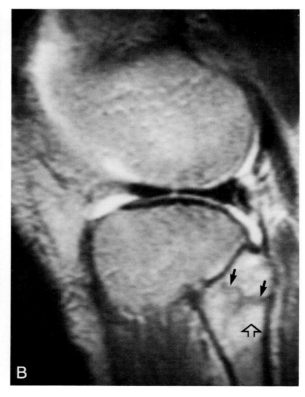

T1-weighted images was imaged in one patient who developed aggressive osteoporosis after sustaining a patellar fracture (Fig. 4-137).[78] Reflex sympathetic dystrophy has been shown to image with increased signal intensity on T2-weighted images secondary to hyperemic bone marrow edema.[79]

Infection

Capsular distension and joint effusion are identified on MR scans of joint infection, but are nonspecific.[80] A septic joint may be further characterized by intraarticular debris and synovitis from hematogenous seeding. In one child with staphylococcus *osteomyelitis,* a mottled pattern of the yellow marrow stores could be identified in the tibial epiphyseal center. This appearance should not be confused with the coarsened trabecular pattern

seen in Paget's disease. In a case of osteomyelitis involving the distal femur, collections of infected fluid confined by elevated periosteum were demonstrated on MR scans (Fig. 4-138). Plain film radiography and nuclear bone scans were negative in this case, which was surgically debrided on the basis of the MR findings.

An infectious tract with fluid may simulate a pathologic or stress fracture, and, when associated with extensive surrounding edema, can be confused with tumor (Fig. 4-139). In a patient with multifocal osteomyelitis, seeding of the distal femur and proximal humerus was identified on MR scans as a central nidus of high signal intensity marrow and calcified sequestra of low signal intensity (Fig. 4-140). Marrow infiltration and soft tissue extension of osteomyelitis have also been demonstrated using short TI inversion recovery (STIR) sequences (Fig. 4-141).

Text continues on p. 194

Figure 4-131

Normal low signal intensity physeal line imaged at the metaphyseal–epiphyseal junction *(arrows).*

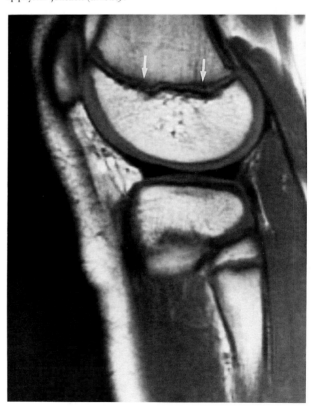

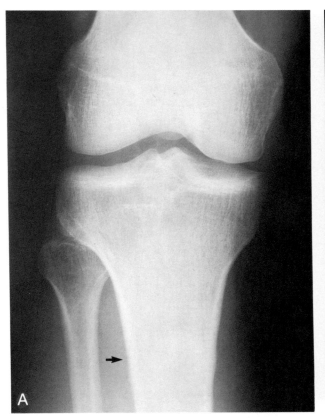

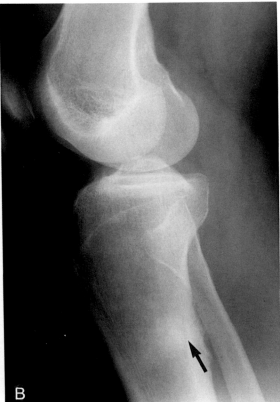

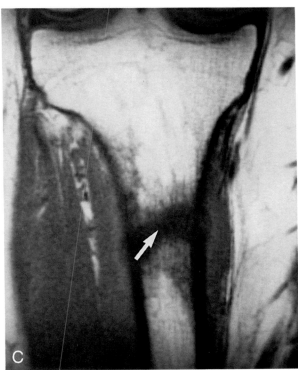

Figure 4-132

Stress fracture. Localized tibial sclerosis *(arrow)* shown on AP *(A)* and lateral *(B)* radiographs. *(C)* Low signal intensity transverse stress fracture *(arrow)* defined in proximal tibia on T1-weighted coronal image. TR = 600 msec, TE = 20 msec.

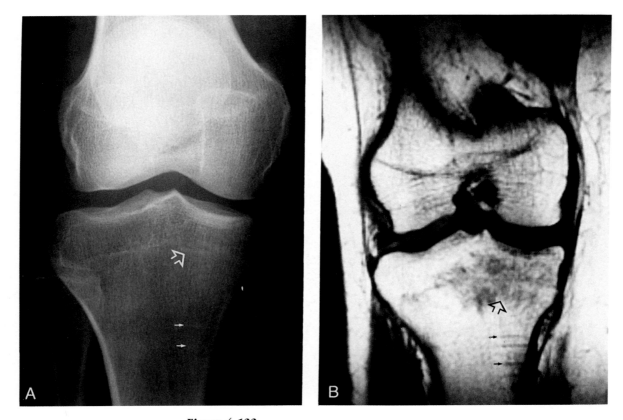

Figure 4-133

Bone contusion. **(A)** Minimal sclerosis in medial tibial condyle *(open arrow)*. Normal transverse growth lines of trabecular condensation are shown in the proximal tibia *(small solid arrows)*. **(B)** T1-weighted coronal image identifies diffuse region of low-signal intensity marrow edema in area of bone contusion without discrete fracture *(open arrow)*. Adjacent stress or growth lines are distinguished by their parallel arrangement and transverse orientation *(small solid arrows)*. TR = 600 msec, TE = 20 msec.

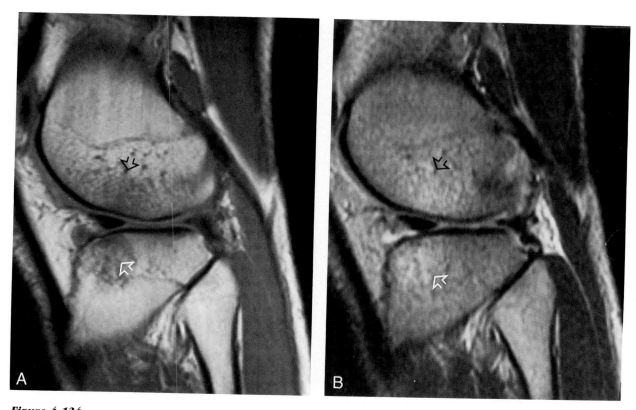

Figure 4-134

Bone contusion. T1-weighted **(A)** and T2-weighted **(B)** sagittal images demonstrating low and high signal intensity, respectively, in marrow edema-hemorrhage within the subchondral bone of the proximal tibia *(white arrow)* and distal femur *(black arrow)*. In the absence of any radiographic abnormality this appearance was consistent with the patient's history of trauma and corresponding pain and tenderness. **(A)** TR = 600 msec, TE = 20 msec; **(B)** TR = 2000 msec, TE = 80 msec.

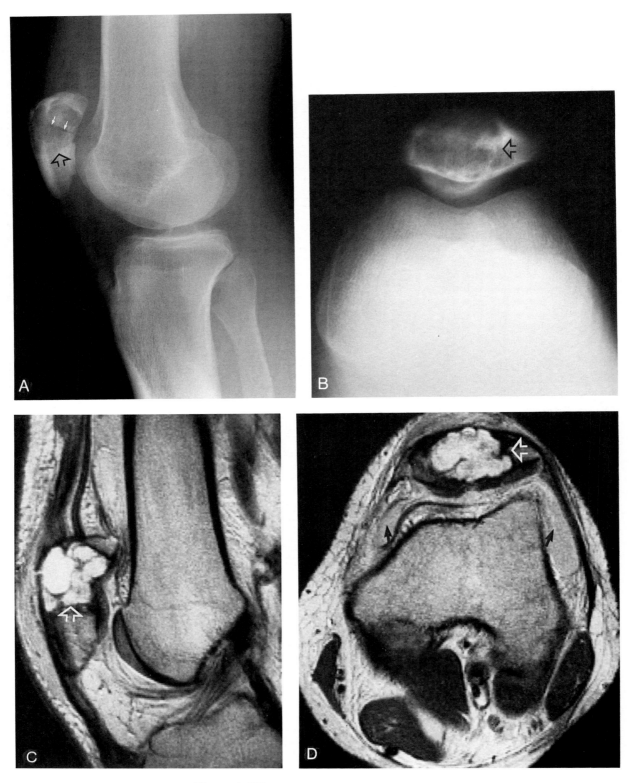

Figure 4-135

Pathologic fracture of the patella. Lateral *(A)* and patella view *(B)* radiographs showing lytic patellar lesion *(open arrow)* with pathologic fracture *(closed arrows)*. Intermediate-weighted sagittal *(C)* and axial *(D)* images demonstrating high signal intensity lesion *(open arrow)* with areas of internal septations. This was shown to represent organizing subacute hemorrhage and eosinophilic granuloma tissue after patellectomy. Associated joint effusion is indicated *(solid arrows)*. In the presence of extensive hemorrhage, MR failed to delineate the fracture segment.

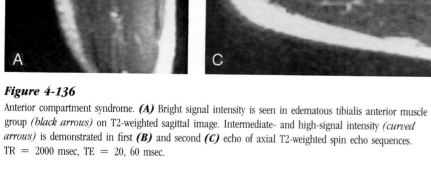

Figure 4-136

Anterior compartment syndrome. *(A)* Bright signal intensity is seen in edematous tibialis anterior muscle group *(black arrows)* on T2-weighted sagittal image. Intermediate- and high-signal intensity *(curved arrows)* is demonstrated in first *(B)* and second *(C)* echo of axial T2-weighted spin echo sequences. TR = 2000 msec, TE = 20, 60 msec.

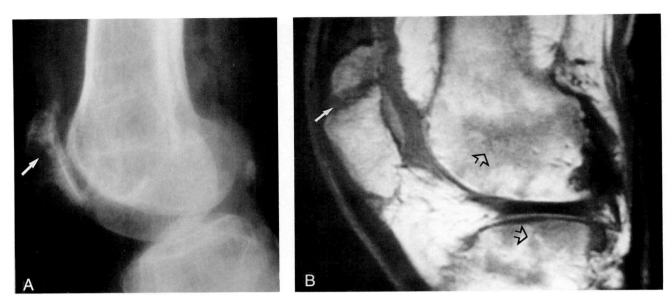

Figure 4-137
Reflex sympathetic dystrophy. **(A)** Patella fracture *(arrow)* and diffuse osteoporosis shown on lateral radiograph. **(B)** T1-weighted sagittal image identifying transverse patella fracture *(closed arrow)* and patchy juxtaarticular low signal intensity *(open arrows)* corresponding to aggressive osteoporosis in reflex sympathetic dystrophy.

Figure 4-138   ▶
Staphylococcal osteomyelitis with negative conventional radiographs **(A)** and bone scintigraphy **(B).** T2-weighted sagittal **(C)** and intermediate-weighted **(D)** and T2-weighted **(E)** axial images demonstrating purulent fluid *(white arrows)*, necrotic tissue *(small black arrows)*, and elevated low-signal intensity periosteum *(large black arrows)*. Purulent debris (fluid) images with increased signal intensity on T2-weighted images *(small white arrows)*.

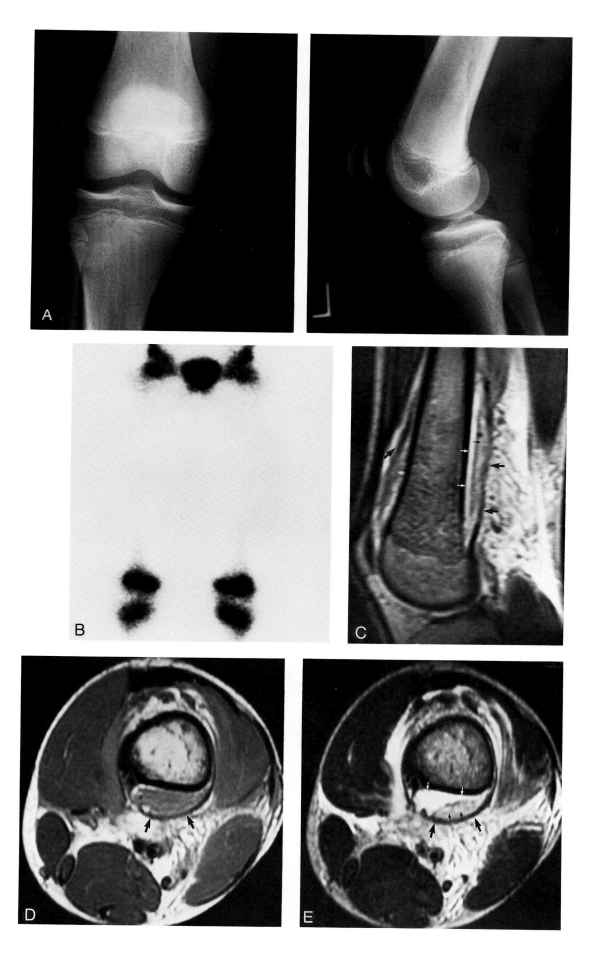

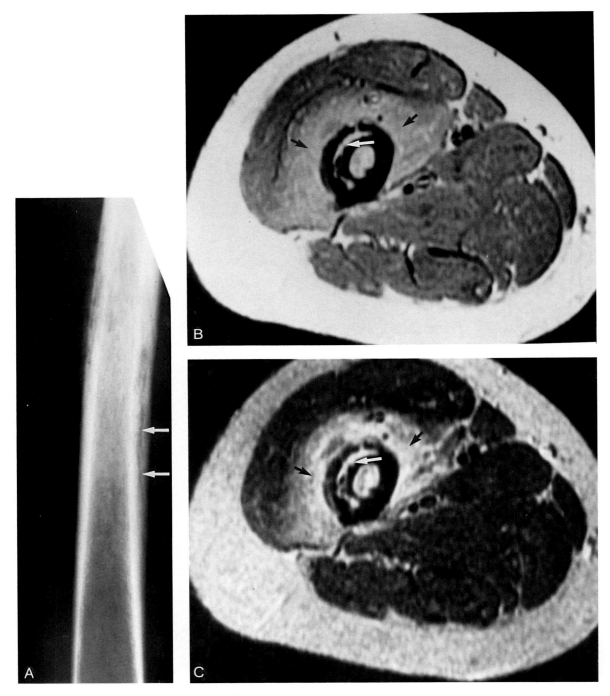

Figure 4-139

Osteomyelitis simulating Ewing sarcoma. *(A)* AP radiograph of the midfemur demonstrating periosteal reaction and longitudinal cortical lucency *(white arrows)*. Intermediate- *(B)* and T2-weighted *(C)* axial images identifying corresponding high-signal intensity infectious track *(white arrow)* with surrounding perilesional edema *(black arrows)*. Edema images with increased signal intensity on T2-weighted image. TR = 2000 msec, TE = 20, 60 msec.

Figure 4-140

Osteomyelitis with sequestration. **(A)** Axial CT of the femur identifies calcified sequestrum *(white open arrow)* with thickened periosteal and endosteal bone *(black arrows)*. Corresponding intermediate-weighted **(B)** and T2-weighted **(C)** axial images identifying infected fluid *(straight solid arrows)* and region of sequestrum *(curved arrow)* in staphylococcus osteomyelitis. Thickened periosteal bone is identified *(open arrow)*.

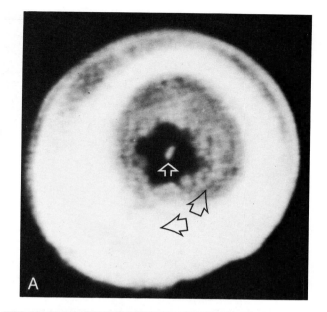

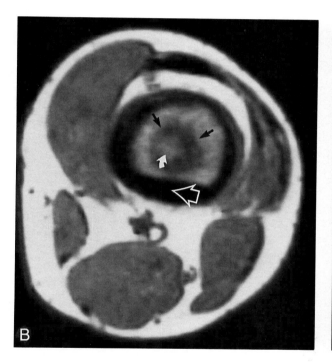

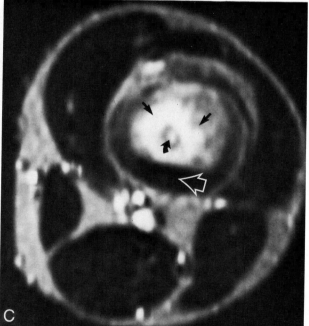

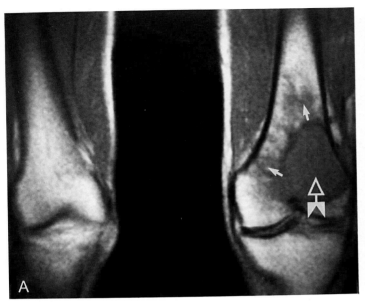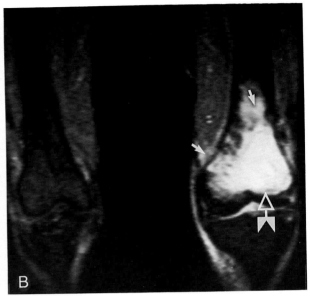

Figure 4-141

Osteomyelitis on (STIR) images. T1-weighted **(A)** and STIR **(B)** coronal images displaying focus of staphylococcal osteomyelitis in femoral metaphysis *(flagged arrow)*. Marrow infiltration and extension *(solid arrows)* are visualized as low signal intensity on T1-weighted image and as high signal intensity on STIR image.

Neoplastic Conditions

MR has been used to image benign and primary malignant tumors for staging, limb-salvage procedures, and to monitor chemotherapeutic response.[81–85] The longitudinal extent of marrow and cortical involvement is displayed on coronal or sagittal images, facilitating preoperative planning for allograft salvage techniques. T1- and T2-weighted axial images define intracompartmental extension and proximity to neurovascular structures. Interval response to preoperative chemotherapy can be assessed, and changes in tumor size; marrow infiltration; cortex, soft tissue, and muscle invasion; hemorrhage; calcification; and necrosis can be recorded. It is important to perform MR imaging studies prior to biopsy, in order to avoid postsurgical inflammation and edema that may prolong the T2 values of uninvolved tissues. Muscle edema is nonspecific, and has also been imaged with trauma, infection, and vascular insults. High signal intensity on T1-weighting in surrounding musculature can be seen in atrophy with fatty infiltration or neuromuscular disorders, and should not be mistaken for tumor (Figs. 4-142 and 4-143).

Venous varicosities may scallop subcutaneous tissue and image with low signal intensity on T1-weighted images. This appearance is characteristic and can be distinguished from neoplastic soft tissue extension or tumor vascularity (Fig. 4-144).

Red to yellow marrow conversion in middle-age female patients may be seen as low signal intensity in metaphyseal or diaphyseal locations without extension into the epiphysis (Fig. 4-145). These regions become isointense with the adjacent marrow on heavily T2-weighted images. Inhomogeneity of metaphyseal red and yellow marrow may also be observed in the immature skeleton (Fig. 4-146). Marrow infiltrative disorders such as leukemia, lymphoma, and Gaucher's disease, however, do extend into the epiphysis or subcondral bone (Figs. 4-147 to 4-149).[86,87] Leukemic infiltrates have been detected on MR examination of the knee, prior to clinical diagnosis and even before peripheral blood smears become abnormal. Coarsened nonuniformity of marrow signal intensity is characteristically imaged in Paget's disease (Fig. 4-150).

Many of the bone and soft tissue tumors that occur about the knee joint have already been addressed in Chapter 2. Several areas of emphasis, however, and certain additional tumors about the knee are discussed in this chapter.

Benign Lesions

In addition to their appearance in the calcaneus (see Chap. 3), *intraosseous lipomas* are known to affect the long tubular bones, including the fibula, tibia, and femur (Fig. 4-151).[88] Intraosseous lipomas image with the same signal intensity as that of fat—bright on T1-weighted images and intermediate on T2-weighted images.

Enchondromas may be difficult to evaluate for malignant change,[89–91] since benign lesions with chondroid matrix image with bright signal intensity on T2-weighted images (Fig. 4-152). The presence of a positive bone scan in the lack of pain cannot be used as a criterion for malignancy.

Fibrous cortical defects, histologically identical to the larger nonossifying fibroma, have been imaged with low to intermediate signal intensity on T1-weighted images and with increased signal intensity on T2- or T2*-weighted images (Fig. 4-153). The increased signal intensity observed on T2-weighted images may be secondary to tissue T2 prolongation in the varied cellular constituents including fibrous stroma, multinucleated giant cells, foam cells, cholesterol crystals, and stromal red blood cells in hemorrhage.[92]

The *desmoid tumor* of soft tissue may present in the popliteal fossa and infiltrate surrounding musculature (Fig. 4-154).[93,94] The desmoid tumor is characterized by low signal intensity fibrous bands traversing the tumor, which images with low to intermediate signal intensity on T1-weighted images and with high signal intensity on T2-weighted images. In contrast, the lesion of juvenile fibromatosis (discussed in Chap. 2) images with uniform low signal intensity on T1- and T2-weighted images.

Giant cell tumors commonly present about the knee (distal femur and proximal tibia) and abut the subchondral bone (Fig. 4-155).[95] Areas of necrosis (signal inhomogeneity), cortical erosion, and associated effusions may be characterized on MR imaging. Intratumoral hemorrhage may produce bright signal intensity on T1- and T2-weighted images, although the tumor generally images with low signal intensity on T1-weighted images and with increased signal intensity on T2-weighted sequences.

Text continues on p. 205

Figure 4-142

Diffuse fatty infiltration of leg musculature with high signal intensity bands of fat *(white arrows)* on T1-weighted image *(A)*, becoming less conspicuous on T2-weighted image *(B)*. Subcutaneous edema is visualized as low signal intensity on the T1-weighted image and as high signal intensity on T2-weighted image *(black arrow)*.

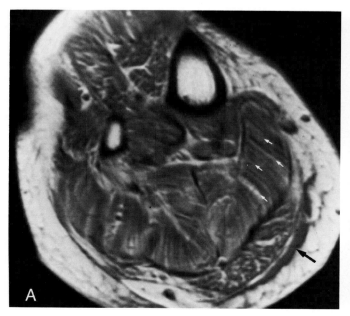
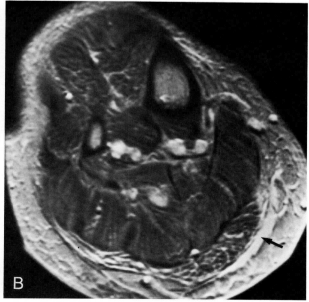

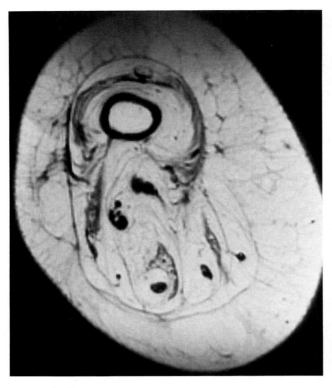

Figure 4-143

Diffuse muscle atrophy with high signal intensity fatty replacement on T1-weighted axial image in a patient with polio. TR = 600 msec, TE = 20 msec.

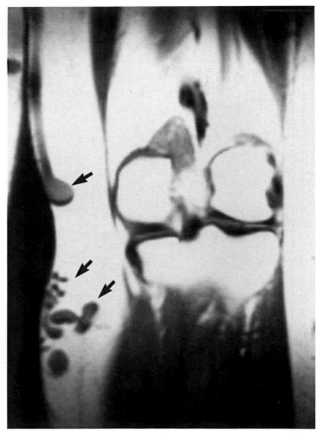

Figure 4-144

Low signal intensity venous varicosities *(arrows)* imaging with a lobulated, serpiginous contour scalloping the subcutaneous fat. TR = 800 msec, TE = 20 msec.

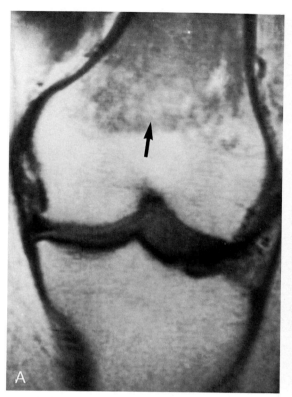

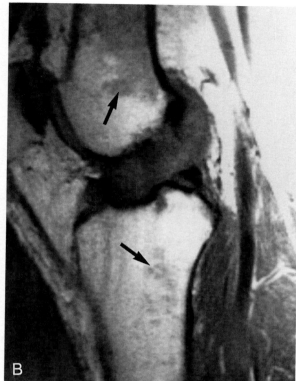

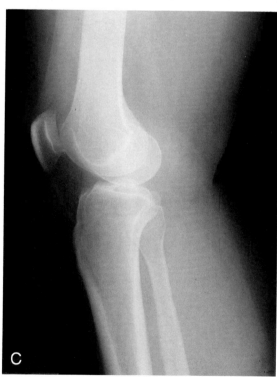

Figure 4-145

Red-yellow marrow. 50-year-old female with normal low signal intensity metadiaphyseal red marrow *(arrows)* seen in T1-weighted coronal *(A)* and sagittal *(B)* images. The epiphyseal regions image with uniform yellow marrow signal intensity. This finding of marrow inhomogeneity is considered a normal variant. *(C)* Negative conventional lateral radiograph shown for comparison.

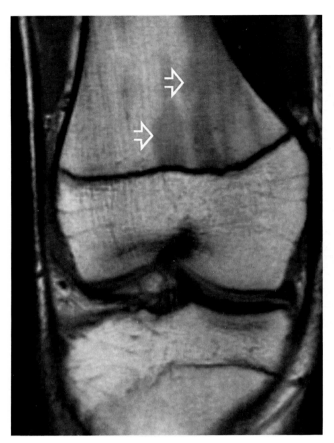

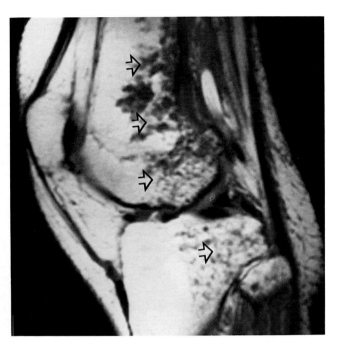

Figure 4-147

Low signal intensity leukemic infiltrates *(open arrows)*, extending into the epiphysis on T1-weighted sagittal image. TR = 600 msec, TE = 20 msec.

Figure 4-146

Residual metaphyseal red marrow in a child is visualized as patchy regions of low signal intensity *(open arrows)* on a T1-weighted coronal image. TR = 600 msec, TE = 20 msec.

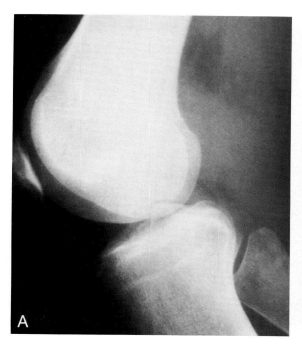
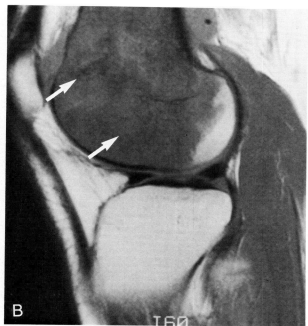

Figure 4-148

Lymphoma. **(A)** Negative lateral radiograph in a patient with osseous lymphoma. **(B)** Low signal intensity lymphomatous marrow replacement imaged crossing the physeal scar involving the subchondral bone *(arrows)*. T1-weighted sagittal image; TR = 800 msec, TE = 20 msec.

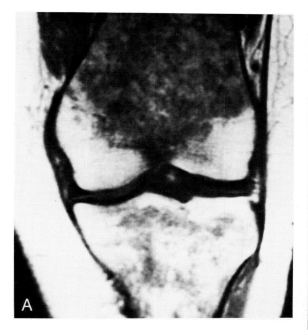
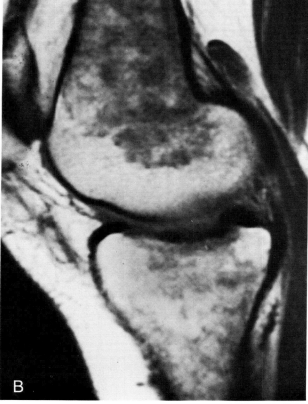
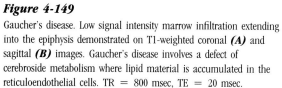

Figure 4-149

Gaucher's disease. Low signal intensity marrow infiltration extending into the epiphysis demonstrated on T1-weighted coronal **(A)** and sagittal **(B)** images. Gaucher's disease involves a defect of cerebroside metabolism where lipid material is accumulated in the reticuloendothelial cells. TR = 800 msec, TE = 20 msec.

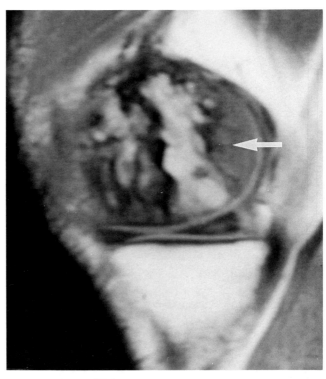

Figure 4-150

Coarse-fibered bone in Paget's disease is visualized as areas of low signal intensity intermixed with yellow marrow, creating an inhomogeneous appearance in the medial femoral condyle *(arrow)* on a T1-weighted sagittal image. TR = 800 msec, TE = 20 msec.

Figure 4-151

Intraosseous lipoma *(arrows)* of the distal femur is visualized as a lytic lesion with sclerotic borders on conventional radiograph *(A)* and high signal intensity focus on T1-weighted coronal image *(B)*.

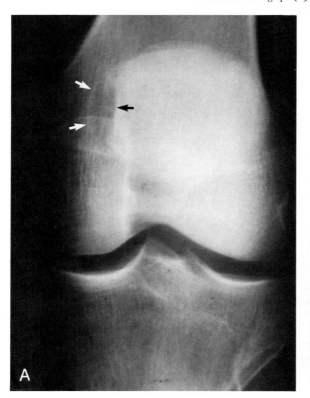

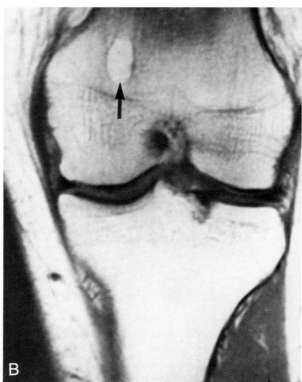

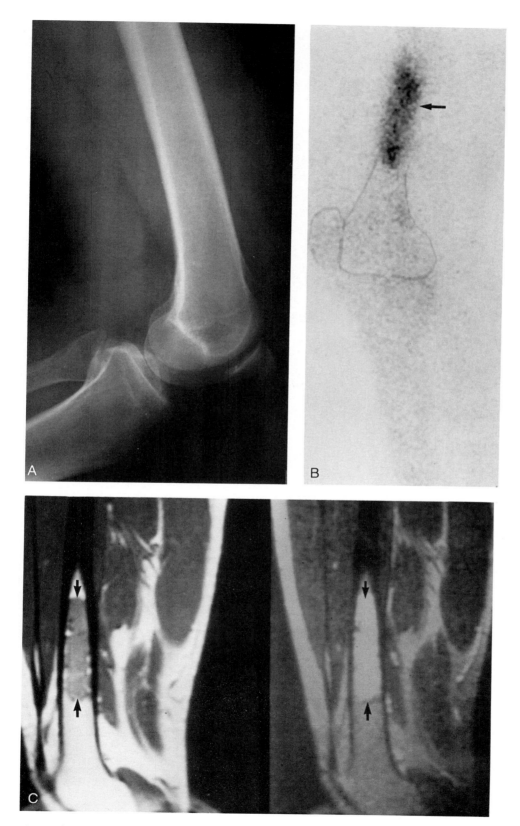

Figure 4-152

Enchondroma. **(A)** Unremarkable lateral radiograph. **(B)** Uptake of 99mTC-MDP bone tracer in distal femur *(arrow)*. **(C)** Benign enchondroma *(arrows)* imaging as low signal intensity on T1-weighted image *(left)* and as high signal intensity on T2-weighted image *(right)*. *Left*, TR = 1000 msec, TE = 20 msec; *right*, TR = 2000 msec, TE = 60 msec.

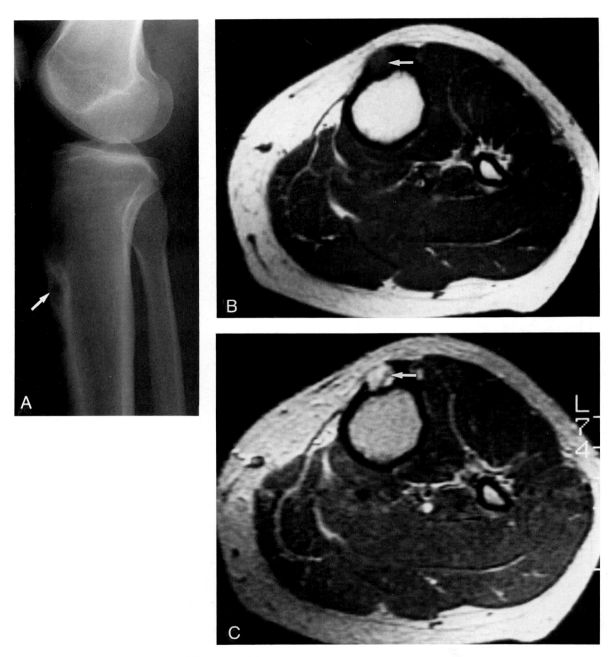

Figure 4-153

Fibrous cortical defect. *(A)* Sclerotic bordered fibrous cortical defect in anterior tibial cortex on lateral radiograph *(arrow)*. Fibrous cortical defect *(arrow)* images with low and high signal intensity on T1-weighted *(B)* and T2-weighted *(C)* axial images, respectively.

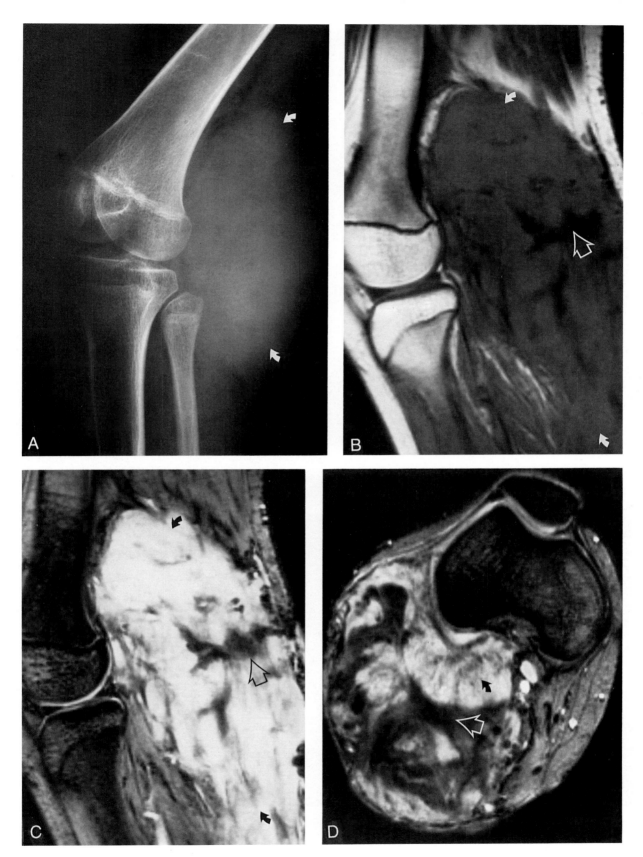

Figure 4-154

Desmoid tumor. **(A)** Popliteal soft tissue mass on lateral radiograph *(curved arrows)*. **(B)** Intermediate
signal intensity desmoid *(curved arrows)* with dark signal intensity fibrous bands *(open arrow)* on T1-
weighted sagittal image. TR = 600 msec, TE = 20 msec. T2* gradient echo image in the sagittal **(C)**
and axial **(D)** planes demonstrating high signal intensity tumor *(curved arrows)* with low signal
intensity fibrous stroma *(open arrow)*. TR = 400 msec, TE = 30 msec; flip angle = 30°.

Figure 4-155

Eccentric giant cell tumor *(arrow)* imaging with low signal intensity on T1-weighted coronal *(A)* and axial *(B)* images and with increased signal intensity on T2-weighted axial images *(C).* Necrotic areas of the tumor demonstrate signal inhomogeneity on the T2-weighted image. Joint effusion *(open arrows)* is identified as low and high signal intensity on T1- and T2-weighted images, respectively.

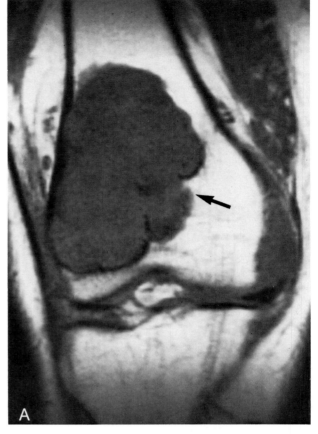

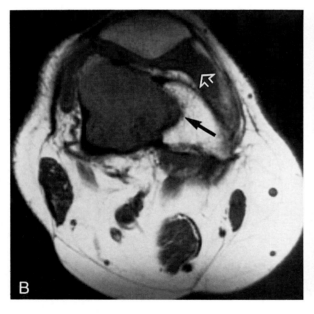

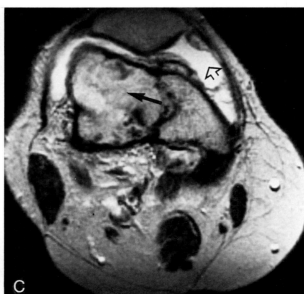

Malignant Lesions

Osteosarcoma in addition to occurring as a primary extremity neoplasm is a known complication of *osteogenesis imperfecta*. Tumoral callus may mimic the appearance of osteosarcoma (Fig. 4-156).[96] MR imaging can be used to differentiate exuberant bone, which is isointense with yellow marrow, from osteosarcoma, which causes both T1 and T2 prolongation.[97] As discussed in Chapter 2, MR offers superior soft tissue discrimination in the evaluation of osteosarcoma. Marrow, cortical, soft tissue, and muscle extension or invasion identified on MR imaging has correlated with surgical and gross specimens (Figs. 4-157 and 4-158).

Liposarcomas are frequently found in the extremities. The myxoid liposarcoma commonly involves the thigh and popliteal region (Fig. 4-159).[98] Whereas lipomas image with high signal intensity on T1-weighted images and with intermediate signal intensity on T2-weighted images, liposarcomas tend to demonstrate a greater degree of signal inhomogeneity.[99] Lipomas with focal areas of sarcomatous development have been visualized with lower signal intensity on T1-weighted images and inhomogeneous areas of high signal intensity on T2-weighted images.

Lymphoma of bone is also discussed in Chapters 2 and 5. In the knee, a soft tissue non-Hodgkin's histiocytic lymphoma was imaged with large lobulated soft tissue masses, demonstrating intermediate signal intensity on T1-weighted images and high signal intensity on T2-weighted images (Fig. 4-160). Marrow of adjacent tibia and fibula was unaffected.

Synovial sarcoma commonly involves the lower extremities in an extraarticular location.[100] Less than 10% of these tumors arise within the joint cavity. In one patient with recurrent intraarticular synovial sarcoma, a nodule of malignant tissue was imaged adjacent to the anterior horn of the lateral meniscus (Fig. 4-161). Infrapatellar fat edema as well as recurrent tumor imaged with increased signal intensity on T2-weighted images.

Figure 4-156

Osteogenesis imperfecta of the femur. Tumoral callus *(arrows)* in osteogenesis imperfecta seen on AP radiograph *(A)* and T1-weighted coronal image *(B)*. Normal yellow marrow signal intensity is visualized with exuberant osteoid tissue *(B)*.

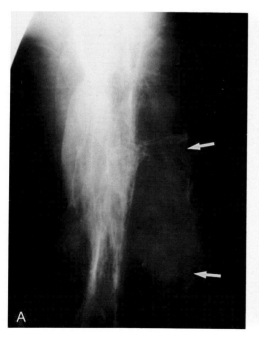
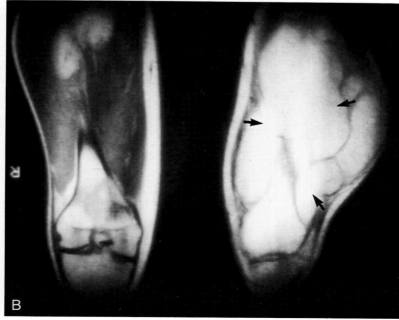

Artifacts

The presence of orthopedic hardware (including plates, screws, pins, and prostheses) is not a contraindication for MR imaging. Low signal intensity artifact is a function of the size, composition, orientation, and design of the device and of the number of devices present within the imaging field.[101–104] MR imaging has been successfully used to evaluate tumor recurrence in patients with limb salvage prostheses. A femoral rod or stem does not pre-clude evaluation of adjacent meniscal or ligamentous structures (Fig. 4-162).

MR is very sensitive to metallic foreign bodies. Even microscopic metallic shavings or residue from arthroscopy can be detected on MR as focal areas of low signal intensity with a high signal intensity peripheral or fringe border. In a patient with patellofemoral knee pain, MR scans revealed a large circular artifact, resulting from a needle lodged within the infrapatellar fat pad (Fig. 4-163).

Text continues on p. 212

Figure 4-157

Osteosarcoma. **(A)** T2-weighted sagittal image of osteosarcoma involving the femoral metaphysis *(small black arrows)*. Brighter contrast portions of the high signal intensity tumor represents necrosis with hemorrhage *(large arrow)*. TR = 2000 msec, TE = 60 msec. **(B)** Corresponding gross specimen identifying central tumor necrosis *(arrow)*.

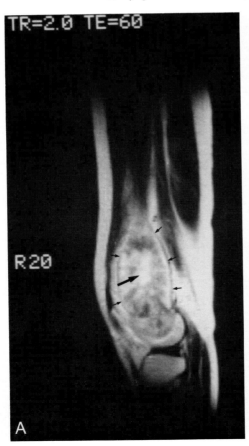
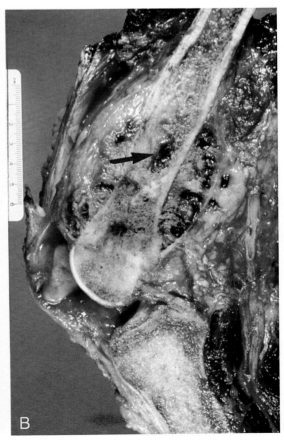

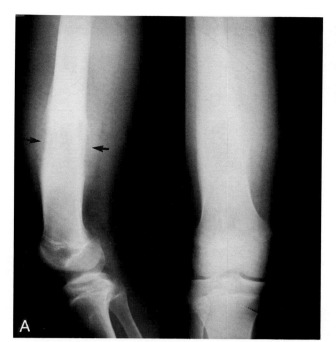

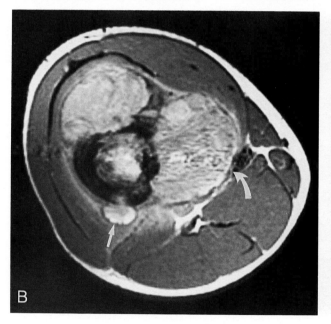

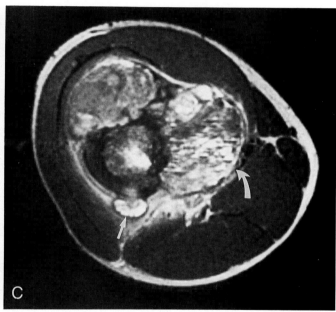

Figure 4-158

Osteosarcoma. **(A)** AP *(left)* and lateral *(right)* radiographs demonstrating aggressive cortical destruction with periosteal reaction *(arrow)*. Intermediate-weighted **(B)** and T2-weighted **(C)** axial images displaying high signal intensity tumor with cortical transgression *(curved arrow)* and soft tissue extension *(straight arrow)*.

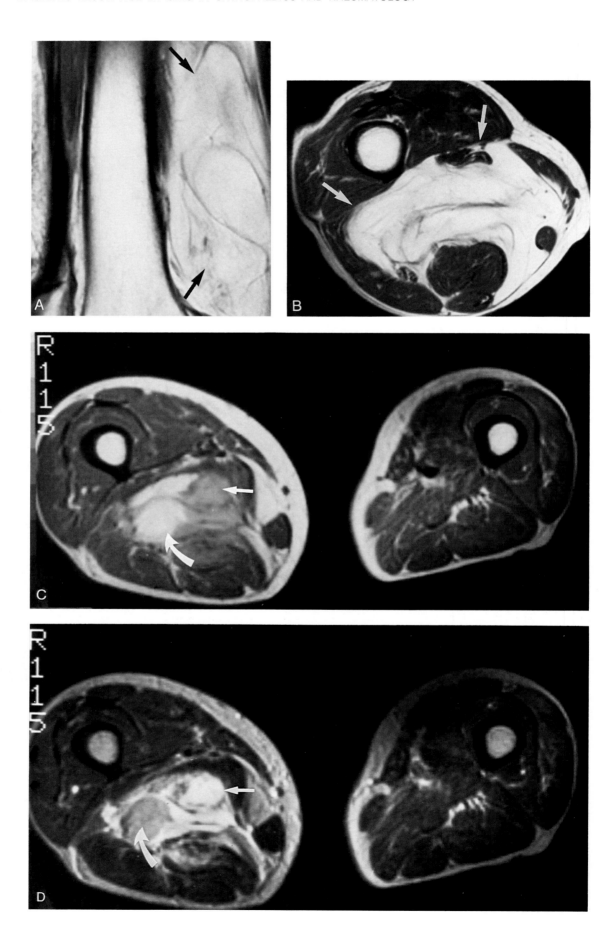

◄ *Figure 4-159*

Liposarcoma. T1-weighted sagittal *(A)* and axial *(B)* images through the distal femur display popliteal high signal intensity lipomatous tissue *(arrows)* in the popliteal fossa. *(C)* Intermediate-weighted axial image defines sarcomatous change as lower signal intensity *(straight arrow)* than adjacent lipomatous tissue *(curved arrow)*. TR = 2000 msec, TE = 20 msec. *(D)* Flip-flop of signal intensity on T2-weighted axial image. Liposarcoma demonstrates high signal intensity *(straight arrow)*, whereas adjacent lipoma is isointense with subcutaneous fat *(curved arrow)*. TR = 2000 msec, TE = 60 msec.

Figure 4-160

Histiocytic lymphoma. *(A)* Intermediate signal intensity soft tissue masses of lymphoma *(arrows)* are visualized on T1-weighted axial image. TR = 1000 msec, TE = 40 msec. *(B)* High signal intensity is demonstrated in histiocytic lymphoma *(arrows)* on T2-weighted sequence. TR = 2000 msec, TE = 80 msec.

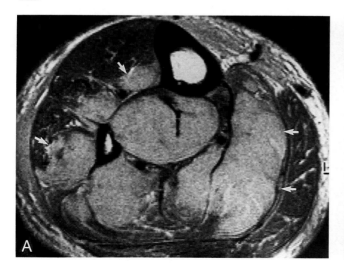
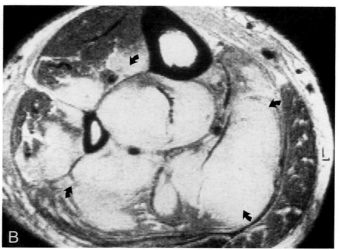

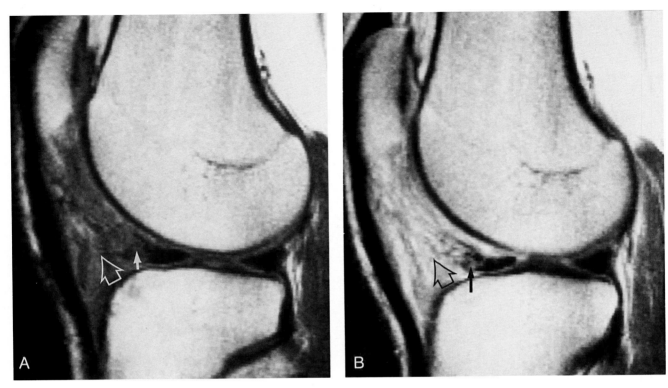

Figure 4-161

Intraarticular recurrent synovial sarcoma nodule adjacent to anterior horn of lateral meniscus on T1-weighed **(A)** and T2-weighted **(B)** sagittal images. Infrapatellar fat pad edema *(open arrow)* and sarcoma *(solid arrow)* image with low signal intensity on T1-weighted image and with high signal intensity on T2-weighted image.

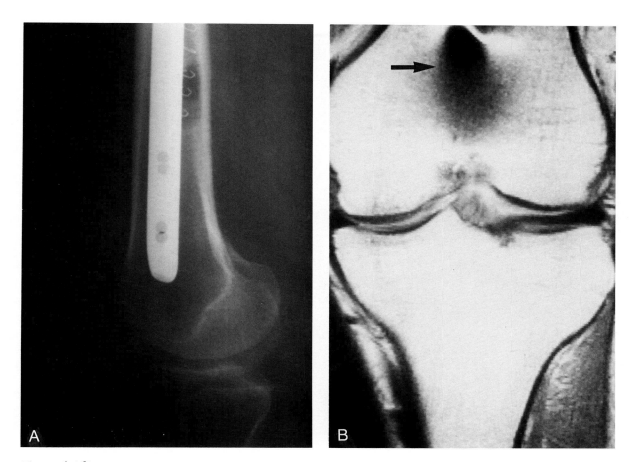

Figure 4-162
Metallic artifact. *(A)* Lateral radiograph showing the distal portion of a femoral prosthesis. *(B)* Local artifact created by metallic prosthesis *(arrow)* without interfering with joint visualization. T1-weighted coronal image; TR = 1000 msec, TE = 40 msec.

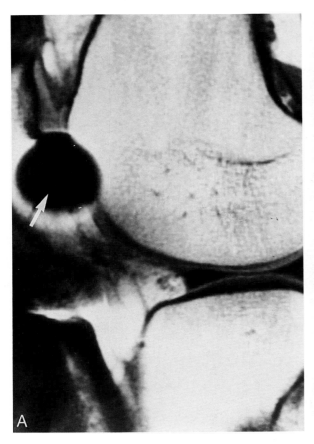 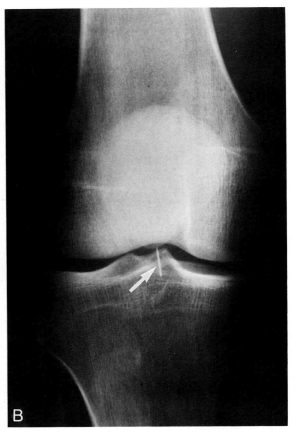

Figure 4-163

Foreign body artifact. **(A)** Circular area of signal void as seen on T1-weighted sagittal image *(arrow)*. TR = 600 msec, TE = 20 msec. **(B)** AP radiograph identifying small intraarticular needle *(arrow)*.

PERSPECTIVE ON MR IMAGING OF THE KNEE

For the diagnosis of meniscal and ligamentous injuries in internal knee derangements, imaging with MR has gained substantial acceptance by radiologists and orthopedists as a replacement for the more traditional techniques of arthrography and CT. Current recommendations for the use of MR in internal knee derangements include patients presenting with acute hemarthrosis and tibial collateral ligament injuries, both of which may have associated meniscal tears. Patients under 15 years of age and over 50 years of age are better evaluated with MR prior to arthroscopy. Negative arthroscopies should also be considered a basis for MR referral.

Noninvasive imaging with MR provides superior tissue characterization in evaluating arthritis, fractures, infection, and neoplasia, not possible with conventional radiographic techniques. Specificity in diagnostic interpretation of knee studies is also enhanced by direct multiplanar imaging, with T1, conventional T2, and T2* gradient echo contrast. With improved surface coils and

fast-scan techniques, routine knee examinations can be performed with 10 min of imaging time and have become more cost effective than arthrography.

REFERENCES

1. Reicher MA, et al: High resolution magnetic resonance imaging of the knee joint: Normal anatomy. AJR 145: 895, 1985

2. Reicher MA, et al: MR imaging of the knee, Part I: Traumatic disorders. Radiology 162:547, 1987

3. Hartzman MD, et al: MR imaging of the knee, Part II: Chronic disorders. Radiology 162:553, 1987

4. Mink JH, et al: Magnetic Resonance Imaging of the Knee. New York, Raven Press, 1987

5. Li DKB, et al: Magnetic resonance imaging of the ligaments and menisci of the knee. Radiol Clin North America 24:209, 1986

6. Stoller DW, et al: Meniscal tears: Pathologic correlation with MR imaging. Radiology 163:452, 1987

7. Stoller DW, et al: Gradient echo MR imaging of the knee. Radiology 165(P), 1987

8. Arnoczky SP, Warren, RF: Microvasculature of the human meniscus. Am J Sports Med 10:90, 1982

9. Turek SL: Orthopedics: Principles and Their Applications, 4th ed, pp 1269–1406. Philadelphia, JB Lippincott, 1984

10. Crues JV III, et al: Meniscal tears of the knee: Accuracy of MR imaging. Radiology 164:445, 1987

11. Mandelbaum BR, et al: Magnetic resonance imaging as a tool for evaluation of traumatic knee injuries: Anatomical and pathoanatomical correlations. Am J Sports Med 14:361, 1986

12. Mink JH, et al: MR imaging of the knee: Technical factors, diagnostic accuracy, and further pitfalls. Radiology 165(P):175, 1987

13. Tyrrell R, et al: Fast three-dimensional MR imaging of the knee: A comparison with arthroscopy. Radiology 165P, 1987

14. Beltran J, et al: Meniscal tears: MR demonstration of experimentally produced injuries. Radiology 158:691, 1986

15. Koenig SH, Brown RD: The importance of the motion of water for magnetic resonance imaging. Invest Radiology 20:297, 1985

16. Tobler TH: Makroskopische und histologische Befund am kniegelenk Meniscus in verschiedenen Lebensaitern. Schweiz Med Wschr 56:1359, 1926

17. Roca FO, Vilalta A: Lesions of the meniscus, I: Macroscopic and histologic findings. Clin Orthop 146:289, 1980

18. Roca FO, Vilalta A: Lesions of the meniscus, II: Horizontal cleavages and lateral cysts. Clin Orthop 146:301, 1980

19. Smillie LS: Diseases of the Knee Joint, 2nd ed, pp 340–347. London, Livingston, 1980

20. Ricklin P, et al: Meniscus Lesions: Diagnosis, Differential Diagnosis, and Therapy, 2nd ed. New York, Stratton, 1983

21. Levinsohn ME, Baker BE: Prearthrotomy diagnostic evaluation of the knee: Review of 100 cases diagnosed by arthrography and arthroscopy. AJR 134:107, 1980

22. Watts I, Tasker T: Pitfalls in double contrast knee arthrography. Br J Radiol 53:754, 1980

23. Mink JR, et al: MR imaging of the knee: Pitfalls in interpretation. Radiology 165(P):239, 1987

24. Burk DL, et al: 1.5T surface-coil MRI of the knee. AJR 147:293, 1986

25. Kaplan EB: Discoid lateral meniscus of the knee joint. J Bone Joint Surg 39:77, 1957

26. Dickason JM, et al: A series of ten discoid medial menisci. Clin Orthop 168:75, 1982

27. Weiner B, Rosenberg N: Discoid medial meniscus: Associations with bone changes in the tibia. J Bone Joint Surg 56:171, 1974

28. Gallimore GW, Harms SE: Knee injuries: High-resolution MR imaging. Radiology 160:457, 1986

29. Burk DL, et al: Meniscal and ganglion cysts of the knee: MR evaluation. AJR 150:331, 1988

30. Kennedy JC, et al: The anatomy and function of the anterior cruciate ligament. J Bone Joint Surg 56:223, 1974

31. Feagin JA, Curl WW: Isolated tear of the anterior cruciate ligament: 5-year follow-up study. Am J Sports Med 4:95, 1976

32. Indelicato PA, Bittar, ES: A perspective of lesions associated with ACL insufficiency of the knee: A review of 100 cases. Clin Orthop 198:77, 1985

33. Turner, et al: Acute injury of the ligaments of the knee: Magnetic resonance evaluation. Radiology 154:717, 1985

34. Stoller DW, Genant HK: MR Imaging of knee arthritides. Radiology 165(P):233, 1987

35. Arnoczky SP, Warren RF, Ashlock MA: Replacement of the anterior cruciate ligament using a patellar tendon allograft. J Bone Joint Surg 68:376, 1986

36. Fox JM, et al: Techniques and preliminary results in arthroscopic anterior cruciate prosthesis. Presented at the 53rd annual meeting of the American Academy of Orthopaedic Surgeons, New Orleans, February 20–25, 1986

37. Zarins B, Rowe CR: Combined anterior cruciate ligament reconstruction using semitendinosus tendon and iliotibial tract. J Bone Joint Surg 68:160, 1968

38. Hughston JC, et al: Classification of knee ligament instabilities, Part I: The medial compartment and cruciate ligaments. J Bone Joint Surg 58:159, 1976

39. Kennedy JC: The posterior cruciate ligament. J Trauma 7:367, 1967

40. Turner DA, et al: Acute injury of the ligaments of the knee: Magnetic resonance evaluation. Radiology 154:717, 1985

41. Anderson JE: Grant's Atlas of Anatomy. Baltimore, Williams & Wilkins, 1983

42. Stoller DW, Mink J: MRI detection of knee fractures. American Roentgen Ray Society (abstr.) Miami, Florida, April 15–May 1, 1987

43. Seebacher JR, et al: The structures of the postero-lateral aspect of the knee. J Bone Joint Surg 64:536, 1982

44. Arndt RE, et al: Clinical Arthrography, 2nd ed. Baltimore, Williams & Wilkins, 1985

45. Bentley, G.: Articular cartilage changes in chondromalacia patellae. J Bone Joint Surg 67:769, 1985

46. Dowd GS, Bentley G: Radiographic assessment in patellar instability and chondromalacia patellae. J Bone Joint Surg 68:297, 1986

47. Resnick D, Niwayama G: Diagnosis of Bone and Joint Disorders, 2nd ed, vol 3, pp 1455–1458. Philadelphia, WB Saunders, 1988

48. Stoller DW: MRI of the patella and patellofemoral joint. Presented to the American Roentgen Ray Society, San Francisco, California, May 8–13, 1988

49. Yulish BS, et al: Chondromalacia patellae: Assessment with MR imaging. Radiology 164:763, 1987

50. Resnick D, Niwayama G: Diagnosis of Bone and Joint Disorders, 2nd ed, vol 5, pp 2896–2897. Philadelphia, WB Saunders, 1988

51. Resnick D, Niwayama G: Diagnosis of Bone and Joint Disorders, 2nd ed, vol 2, pp 722–723. Philadelphia, WB Saunders, 1988

52. Rockwood CA, Green CP: Fractures. Philadelphia, JB Lippincott, 1975

53. Weissman BNW, Sledge CB: Orthopedic Radiology, pp 497–587. Philadelphia, WB Saunders, 1986

54. Stoller, DW: MRI in juvenile rheumatoid (chronic) arthritis. Presented to the Association of University Radiologists, Charleston, South Carolina, March 22–27, 1987

55. Stoller DW, Genant, HK: MRI of pigmented villonodular synovitis. American Roentgen Ray Society (abstr.) San Francisco, California, May 8–13, 1988

56. Kottal RA, et al: Pigmented villonodular synovitis: Report of MR imaging in two cases. Radiology 163:551, 1987

57. Kulkarni MV, et al: MR imaging of hemophiliac arthropathy. JCAT 10:445, 1986

58. Yulish BS, et al: Hemophilic arthropathy: Assessment with MR imaging. Radiology 164:759, 1987

59. Johnston YE, et al: Lyme arthritis: Spirochetes found in synovial microangiopathic lesions. Am J Pathol 118:26, 1985

60. Beltran J, et al: The knee: Surface-coil MR imaging at 1.5T. Radiology 159:747, 1986

61. Ahlback S, et al: Spontaneous osteonecrosis of the knee. Arthritis Rheum 11:705, 1968

62. Williams JL, et al: Spontaneous osteonecrosis of the knee. Radiology 107:15, 1973

63. Lotke PA, Ecker ML: Osteonecrosis-like syndrome of the medial tibial plateau. Clin Orthop Rel Res 176:148, 1983

64. Linden B: The incidence of osteochondritis dissecans in the condyles of the femur. Acta Orthop Scand 47:664, 1976

65. Mesgarzadeh M, et al: MR imaging of osteochondritis dissecans. Radiology 161(P):24.

66. Mesgarzadeh M, et al: Osteochondritis dissecans: Analysis of mechanical stability with radiography, scintigraphy, and MR imaging. Radiology 165:775, 1987

67. Resnick D, Niwayama G: Diagnosis of Bone and Joint Disorders, 2nd ed, vol 5, pp 3313–3316. Philadelphia, WB Saunders, 1988

68. Ehman RL, et al: MR imaging of the musculoskeletal system: A 5-year appraisal. Radiology 166:313, 1988

69. Beltran J, et al: Joint effusions: MR imaging. Radiology 158:133, 1986

70. Guerra J, et al: Gastrocnemio-semimembranosus bursal region of the knee. AJR 136:593, 1981

71. Lindgreen PG, Willen R: Gastrocnemius-semimembranosus bursa and its relation to the knee joint: Anatomy and histology. Acta Radiol (Diagn) 18:497, 1977

72. Edmonson AS, Crenshaw AH: Campbell's Operative Orthopedics, vol 2, pp 1408–1410. St. Louis, CV Mosby, 1980

73. Apple JS, et al: Synovial plicae of the knee. Skeletal Radiol 7:251, 1982

74. Passariello R, et al: CT and MR imaging of the knee joint in the "plica syndrome." Radiology 161(P):240, 1986

75. Berquist TH: Imaging of Orthopedic Trauma and Surgery, pp 293–392. Philadelphia, WB Saunders, 1986

76. Stafford SA, et al: MRI in stress fracture. AJR 147:553, 1986

77. Berquist TH, et al: Magnetic Resonance of the Musculoskeletal System, pp 127–164. New York, Raven Press, 1987

78. Kressel HY (ed): Magnetic Resonance Annual, pp1–36. New York, Raven Press, 1986

79. Resnick D, Niwayama G: Diagnosis of Bone and Joint Disorders, 2nd ed, vol 1, pp 228–229. Philadelphia, WB Saunders, 1988

80. Resnick D, Niwayama G: Diagnosis of Bone and Joint Disorders, 2nd ed, vol 1, chap 18. Philadelphia, WB Saunders, 1988

81. Stoller DW, et al: Comparison of Tl-201, GA-67, Tc-99m MDP, and MR imaging of musculoskeletal sarcoma. Radiology 165(P):223, 1987

82. Bloem JL, et al: Magnetic resonance imaging of primary malignant bone tumors. RadioGraphics 7:425, 1987

83. Wetzel LH, et al: A comparison of MR imaging and CT in the evaluation of musculoskeletal masses. RadioGraphics 7:851, 1987

84. Petasnick JP, et al: Soft-tissue masses of the locomotor system: Comparison of MR imaging with CT. Radiology 160:125, 1986

85. Totty WG, Murphy WA, Lee JKT: Soft-tissue tumors: MR imaging. Radiology 160:135, 1986

86. Lanir A, et al: Gaucher disease: Assessment with MR imaging. Radiology 161:239, 1986

87. Olson DO, et al: Magnetic resonance imaging of the bone marrow in patients with leukemia, aplastic anemia, and lymphoma. Invest Radiology 21:540, 1986

88. Ramos A, et al: Osseous lipoma: CT appearance. Radiology 157:615, 1985

89. Liu J, et al: Bone sarcoma associated with Ollier's disease. Radiology 165:589, 1987

90. Schwartz HS, et al: Malignant potential of enchondromatosis. Radiology 164:590, 1987

91. Cannon SR, Sweetnam DR: Multiple chondrosarcomas in dyschondroplasia (Ollier's disease). Radiology 156:565, 1985

92. Resnick D, Niwayama G: Diagnosis of Bone and Joint Disorders, 2nd ed, pp 3739–3746. Philadelphia, WB Saunders, 1988

93. Stoller DW, et al: MRI of popliteal masses of the knee. American Roentgen Ray Society (abstr.) San Francisco, California, May 8–13, 1988

94. Hamlin DJ, et al: Magnetic resonance characteristics of an abdominal desmoid tumor. Comput Radiol 10:11, 1986

95. Brady TJ, et al: NMR imaging of forearms in healthy volunteers and patients with giant-cell tumors of bone. Radiology 144:549, 1982

96. Resnick D, Niwayama G: Diagnosis of Bone and Joint Disorders, 2nd ed, vol 5, pp 3389–3400. Philadelphia, WB Saunders, 1988

97. Boyko OB, et al: MR imaging of osteogenic and Ewing's sarcoma. AJR, 148:317, 1987

98. Resnick D, Niwayama G: Diagnosis of Bone and Joint Disorders, 2nd ed, vol 6, pp 3916–3920. Philadelphia, WB Saunders, 1988

99. Dooms GC, et al: Lipomatous tumors and tumors with fatty component: MR imaging potential and comparison of MR and CT results. Radiology 157:479, 1985

100. Sundaram M, et al: Magnetic resonance imaging of lesions of synovial origin. Skeletal Radiol 15:10, 1986

101. Porter BA, et al: Classification and investigation of artifacts in magnetic resonance imaging. RadioGraphics 7:271, 1987

102. Pusey E, et al: Magnetic resonance imaging artifacts: Mechanism and clinical significance. RadioGraphics 6:891, 1986

103. Augustiny N, et al: MR imaging of large nonferromagnetic metallic implants at 1.5T. JACT 11:678, 1987

104. James R, et al: Unusual MR metallic artifact due to steel threads. JCAT 11:722, 1987

David W. Stoller
Harry K. Genant

Chapter 5 THE HIP

OUTLINE

The hip (including the acetabulum, femoral articulation, and supporting soft tissue, muscle, and cartilage structures) is a functionally and structurally complex joint. Disease processes involving the hip joint include trauma, osteonecrosis, arthritis, infection, and neoplasia—which are frequently not detected by conventional radiographic techniques until in an advanced clinical stage. Plain film radiography is of limited usefulness for assessment of soft tissue and articular surfaces. Contrast arthrography is useful in evaluation of the joint space and sampling of synovial fluid in cases of suspected infection. Computer tomography (CT), by the generation of axial scans with sufficient bone detail to perform sag-

ittal and coronal reconstructions, has played an important role in developing a multiplanar three dimensional perspective on hip disease.[1]

Magnetic resonance (MR) imaging has been successfully used to evaluate several pathologic processes in the hip. The excellent spatial and contrast resolution facilitates early detection and evaluation of femoral head osteonecrosis, definition of hyaline articular cartilage in arthritis, identification of joint effusions, and characterization of osseous and soft tissue tumors about the hip. Direct, noninvasive imaging of bone marrow with MR has allowed identification of fractures and infiltrative diseases, including leukemias, prior to radiographic detection. In addition, the cartilaginous epiphysis in an infant or a child, not yet visible on routine radiographs, can be demonstrated on MR images (see also Chap. 2).

IMAGING PROTOCOLS FOR THE HIP

The body coil is used in most MR examinations of the hip, allowing comparison of both hips when large (32 to 40 cm) fields of view (FOVs) are used (Fig. 5-1). T1-weighted images can be acquired in the axial, sagittal, or coronal plane with a recovery time (TR) of 600 msec and an echo time (TE) of 20 msec, in a 256 × 256 acquisition matrix, from two signal averages or excitations (NEX). Thin (5 mm) sections are obtained either contiguously or with a minimal interslice gap. Three-millimeter sections are preferred in pediatric patients, or when precise assessments are required to image thin articular cartilage surfaces and labrum. T2-weighted images are acquired with a TR of 1500 to 2000 msec and a TE of 20 and 60 to 80 msec. T2-weighted images are particularly useful when evaluating arthritis, infection, and neoplasia. T2* gradient echo and short TI inversion recovery (STIR) sequences can be used to supplement conventional spin echo images in the evaluation of neoplastic and marrow disorders.[2-4] Smaller (24 cm) FOVs should be used to obtain high spatial resolution when imaging a single hip in the sagittal plane.

Figure 5-1

Body coil for MR imaging of the hip.

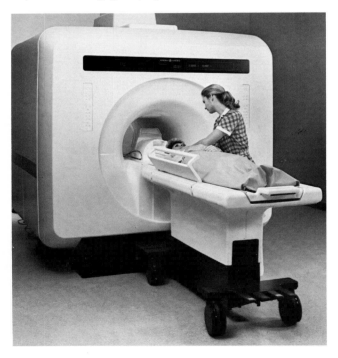

NORMAL MR ANATOMY OF THE HIP

Axial Images

At the level of the acetabular roof, there may be partial voluming with the femoral head. Signal intensity in the acetabulum and femoral head is bright because of yellow and red marrow fat (Fig. 5-2). The muscles of the hip joint image with intermediate signal intensity. The gluteal muscles—the gluteus medius (laterally), the gluteus minimus (deep), and the gluteus maximus (posteriorly)—can be differentiated from one another by high signal intensity fat along fascial divisions. The tensor fasciae latae muscle is seen anterior to the gluteus medius, and is bordered anteriorly by subcutaneous fat that images with high signal intensity. The iliopsoas muscle group is directly anterior to the femoral head in a 12 o'clock position. The sartorius muscle is the most anterior, whereas the rectus femoris is positioned between the more lateral tensor fasciae latae and the medial iliopsoas. The obturator internus muscle is visualized medial to the anterior and posterior acetabular columns. The sciatic nerve images with intermediate signal intensity and is located directly posterior to the posterior column of the acetabulum. The external iliac vessels, which are of low signal intensity, are medial to the iliopsoas muscle and anterior to the anterior acetabular column.

At the level of the femoral head, the more distal femoral artery and vein are visualized. Femoral head articular cartilage images with intermediate signal intensity.

At the level of the greater trochanter and femoral-neck, the obturator internus is identified and extends between the pubis and ischium. The iliofemoral ligament images with low signal intensity and blends with the dark (low spin density) cortex of the anterior femoral neck. At this level the sciatic nerve courses posterior to the ischium. The iliotibial tract can be seen peripherally, identified as a thin low signal intensity band surrounded by high signal intensity fat on its medial and lateral surfaces. The obturator vessels also image with low signal intensity, encased in high signal intensity fat, and can be identified posterolaterally to the pubic bone, between the pectineus and obturator internus muscles. The adductor muscles (anteromedially), the obturator externus and quadratus femoris (medially), the ischial tuberosity attachment of the long head of the biceps femoris, and the semitendinosus tendon can be visualized posteriorly at the level of the proximal femur.

Sagittal Images

On lateral sagittal images the femoral head, greater trochanter, and proximal femur can be seen on the same section (Fig. 5-3). The femoral physeal scar is identified as a horizontal band of low signal intensity, directed in an anterior to posterior orientation (Fig. 5-4). In the sag-

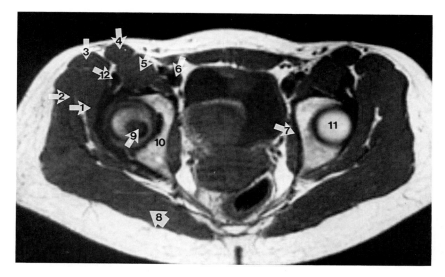

Figure 5-2

Axial image through the femoral heads: gluteus minimus muscle *(1)*, gluteus medius muscle *(2)*, tensor fasciae latae muscle *(3)*, sartorius muscle *(4)*, iliopsoas muscle *(5)*, femoral vessels *(6)*, obturator internus muscle *(7)*, gluteus maximus muscle *(8)*, femoral head cyst *(9)*, acetabulum *(10)*, femoral head *(11)*, rectus femoris tendon *(12)*. T1-weighted image; TR = 600 msec, TE = 20 msec.

Figure 5-3

Sagittal image through the femoral head: acetabular labrum *(1)*, iliacus muscle *(2)*, gluteus minimus muscle *(3)*, gluteus medius muscle *(4)*, gluteus maximus muscle *(5)*, obturator externus muscle *(6)*, guadratus femoris muscle *(7)*, adductor muscle *(8)*, femoral head *(9)*, acetabulum *(10)*. T1-weighted image; TR = 600 msec, TE = 20 msec.

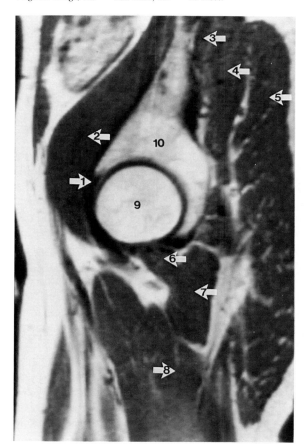

ittal plane the intermediate signal hyaline articular cartilage of the femoral head and acetabulum can be separately defined, and the posterior gluteal and anterior rectus femoris muscles are displayed in long axis (Fig. 5-5). Distally, the vastus musculature is imaged anteriorly to the proximal femoral diaphysis and the biceps

Figure 5-4

Sagittal image at the level of the femoral head in a young adult identifying the physeal scar *(open arrow)* separating epiphyseal yellow marrow and metaphyseal red marrow. Intermediate signal intensity articular cartilage of the acetabulum *(long solid arrow)* and femoral head *(small arrows)* is defined. T1-weighted image; TR = 600 msec, TE = 20 msec.

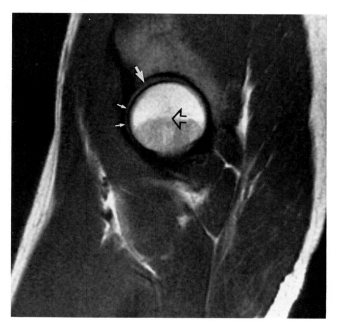

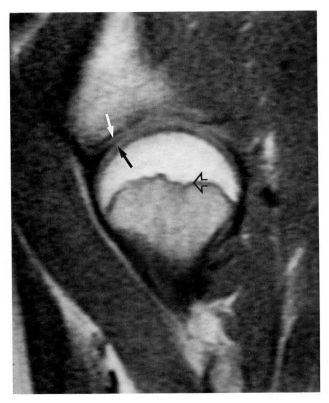

Figure 5-5
Sagittal image of the femoral head in a 12-year-old child showing separation of hyaline articular cartilage in the acetabulum *(white arrow)* and femoral head *(black arrow)*. Open physis (low signal intensity) is transversely oriented *(open arrow)*. T1-weighted image; TR = 600 msec, TE = 20 msec.

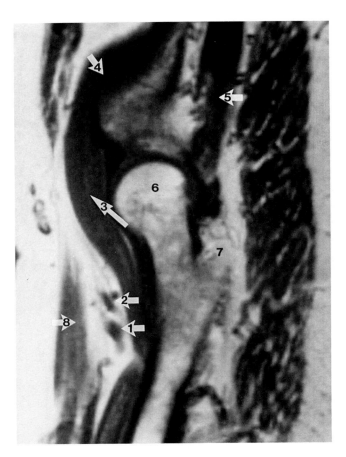

Figure 5-6
Sagittal image of the lateral hip: femoral vein *(1)*, femoral artery *(2)*, iliopsoas muscle *(3)*, iliacus muscle *(4)*, gluteus medius muscle *(5)*, femoral head *(6)*, greater trochanter *(7)*, sartorius muscle *(8)*. T1-weighted image; TR = 600 msec, TE = 20 msec.

femoris is viewed posteriorly. The sciatic nerve can be followed longitudinally between the anterior quadratus femoris and the posterior gluteus maximus. The low signal intensity attachment of the sartorius to the anterosuperior iliac spine is shown anteriorly on sagittal images. The low signal intensity iliopsoas tendon spans the hip joint anteriorly, crossing to its insertion on the lesser trochanter. The adductor muscle group is imaged inferior and medial to the iliopsoas tendon and pectineus muscle.

On medial sagittal images the acetabulum encompasses 75% of the femoral head, and the low signal intensity transverse acetabular ligament bridges the uncovered anterior–inferior gap (Fig. 5-6).

Coronal Images

It may be more difficult to differentiate acetabular and femoral head articular cartilage on coronal planar images than on sagittal planar images. The fibrocartilaginous limbus, or acetabular labrum, is visualized as a low signal intensity triangle interposed between the supero-lateral aspect of the femoral head and the inferolateral aspect of the acetabulum. The joint capsule is visualized as a low signal intensity structure circumscribing the femoral neck. In the presence of fluid, the capsule distends and the lateral and medial margins become convex.

Anterior coronal images show the iliac crest in continuity with the acetabulum (Figs. 5-7 and 5-8). A defect in the articular cartilage of the femoral head can be seen medially at the ligamentum teres insertion site. The low signal intensity iliofemoral ligament is present on the lateral aspect of the femoral neck near the greater trochanter. The orbicular zone may be identified as a small outpouching on the medial aspect of the junction of the femoral head and neck. The intraarticular femoral fat pad is located between the medial femoral head and the acetabulum and generates increased signal intensity on T1-weighted images. The obturator externus muscle crosses the femoral neck on posterior coronal images.

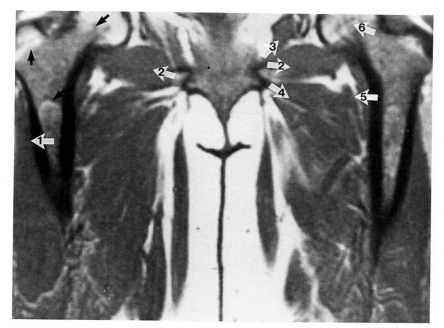

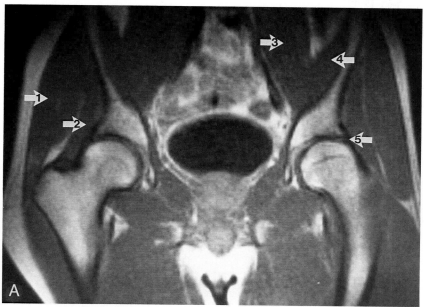

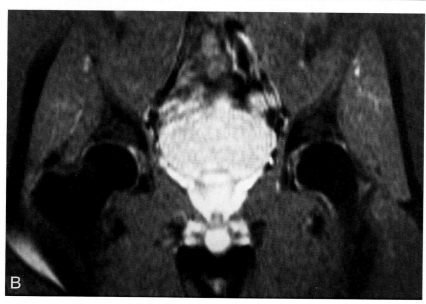

Figure 5-7

Coronal image through the hips: vastus lateralis muscle *(1)*, obturator externus muscle *(2)*, obturator internus muscle *(3)*, adductor magnus muscle *(4)*, iliopsoas muscle *(5)*, femoral head *(6)*. Normal red marrow (low signal intensity) and yellow marrow (bright signal intensity) inhomogeneity is indicated *(black arrows)*. T1-weighted image; TR = 600 msec, TE = 20 msec.

Figure 5-8

Coronal image through the midhips. *(A)* Gluteus medius muscle *(1)*, gluteus minimus muscle *(2)*, psoas muscle *(3)*, iliacus *(4)*, labrum *(5)*. T1-weighted image; TR = 600 msec, TE = 20 msec. *(B)* Corresponding STIR image demonstrating dark signal from areas of nulled fat signal intensity. TR = 1400 msec, TI = 125 msec, TE = 40 msec.

Inhomogeneity of acetabular marrow signal intensity can be a normal finding on T1-weighted images.

PATHOLOGY OF THE HIP

Osteonecrosis and Avascular Necrosis

Osteonecrosis of the femoral head is associated with a variety of causes including fractures (usually of the subcapital femoral neck), dislocations, sickle cell disease, steroid treatment, Cushing's disease, alcoholism, Gaucher's disease, irradiation, gout, and dysbaric disorders.[5] Although the terms osteonecrosis and *avascular necrosis* (AVN) are often used interchangeably, the latter term is more accurately reserved for osteonecrosis associated with an interruption of major nutrient arteries leading to ischemia. Osteonecrosis occurs most frequently in 30 to 50-year-old individuals, and is bilateral in 30% to 80% of cases. Resultant fragmentation and superimposed degenerative arthritis can lead to early pain and disability.

Assessment of AVN

A system of staging for osteonecrosis, using conventional *plain film radiographs*, classifies osteonecrotic changes into five stages.[6] These changes, however, occur late in the disease process and reflect alterations in bone density (mineral content), collapse, sequestra formation, and degenerative arthritis. In stage 1, radiographs are normal, but bone scans are positive. Stage 2 is characterized by visible sclerosis or cystic changes. Subchondral lucency and fracture, with loss of the normal femoral contour (structural integrity), occur in stage 3. In stage 4, abnormalities are detected in both femoral and acetabular structure with subchondral collapse. Narrowing of the hip joint occurs in stage 5 disease.

The specificity of radiographic staging of osteonecrosis is upgraded by the use of CT that has also been used to define the associated sclerotic arc, to detect acetabular dome and femoral head contour changes, to assess the joint space, and to evaluate the extent or volume of femoral head involvement.[1] These changes, however, do not reflect the early vascular and marrow histologic processes in osteonecrosis.

Nuclear scintigraphy with technetium-labeled phosphate analogues such as methylene diphosphonate (99mTC-MDP) has been used for the early detection of osteonecrosis.[7] During the acute phase of the disease, decreased uptake of bone tracer is associated with vascular compromise. Increased radiopharmaceutical accumulation occurs with chronic vascular stasis, in repair and in revascularization. Blood flow (dynamic) scanning has been used to assess regional blood flow. The specificity of marrow scanning with technetium sulfur colloid (99mTC-sulfur colloid) is variable, depending on underlying disease states and the normal pattern of marrow distribution.

The sensitivity of *MR imaging* for detection of AVN of the hip has been reported to exceed corresponding CT and radionuclide bone scintigraphy.[8,9] MR images are also effective in assessing joint effusions, marrow conversion, edema, and articular cartilage congruity, not possible with bone scintigraphy, plain film, or CT.

Treatment of AVN

Present treatment includes core decompression, bone grafting, and rotational osteotomies (Sugioka procedure).[10] In the advanced stages of osteonecrosis, with significant segmental collapse and pain, total hip arthroplasty is often required. Selection of the correct treatment option is influenced by the extent of necrosis and reactive repair. Core decompressions are recommended in the early stages of osteonecrosis (radiographic stages 1 and 2). Rotational osteotomies may be used in stage 2 disease, whereas advanced (stages 4 or 5) disease is best treated by total hip replacement.

MR Imaging Techniques for AVN

Evaluation of patients with osteonecrosis can be accomplished with a T1-weighted axial localizer and either a

Figure 5-9
Femoral head osteonecrosis images with low signal intensity on T1-weighted sagittal image *(arrow)*. The sagittal imaging plane displays anterior to posterior relationships in determining the extent of femoral head involvement. TR = 600 msec, TE = 20 msec.

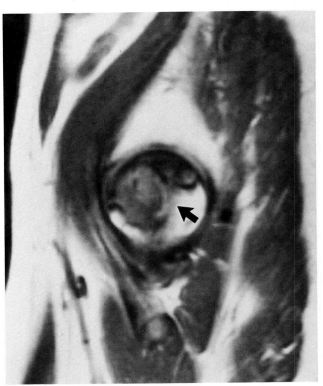

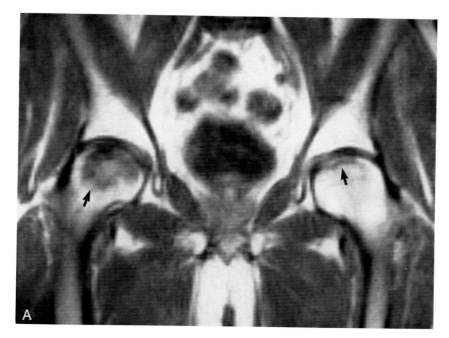

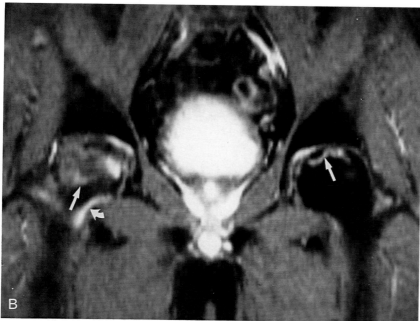

Figure 5-10

Avascular necrosis (AVN). *(A)* Bilateral osteonecrosis of the hips images with low signal intensity *(arrows)* on T1-weighted image. TR = 600 msec, TE = 20 msec. *(B)* On STIR images, AVN *(straight arrows)* and associated joint effusion *(curved arrow)* are visualized with bright signal intensity. TR = 1400 msec, TI = 125 msec, TE = 40 msec.

T1- or T2-weighted spin echo coronal sequence. Imaging in the sagittal plane is optional (Fig. 5-9). STIR pulse sequences, which negate yellow marrow fat signal, provide excellent contrast for the detection of marrow replacement, fluid, and necrotic tissue (Fig. 5-10).[11] Premature fatty marrow conversion associated with osteonecrosis can be detected using chemical shift imaging techniques.[12] On fat-selective and water-selective images, fatty and hematopoietic marrow and distribution of water within the ischemic focus can be differentiated.

MR Staging of AVN

Mitchell et al have described an MR classification system for AVN based on alterations in the central region of MR signal intensity in the osteonecrotic focus.[7,13] In MR class A, the osteonecrotic lesion demonstrates signal characteristics analogous to fat—a central region of high signal intensity on short TR/TE settings (T1-weighted) and intermediate signal intensity on long TR/TE settings (T2-weighted; Fig. 5-11). Class B hips image with the signal

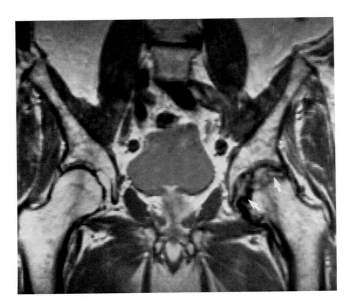

Figure 5-11

Osteonecrosis of the left femoral head is visualized with a central focus of high signal intensity on a T1-weighted coronal image *(arrows)*. TR = 600 msec, TE = 20 msec.

characteristics of blood or hemorrhage—high signal intensity on both short and long TR/TE images (Fig. 5-12). Hips identified as class C demonstrate fluid signal properties—low signal intensity on short TR/TE images and high signal intensity on long TR/TE images (Fig. 5-13). Class D hips image with the signal characteristics of fibrous tissue—low signal intensity on short and long TR/TE sequences (Fig. 5-14). A peripheral band of low signal intensity demarcates the central focus of avascular necrosis in class A through class D hips. This border is most visible on T1-weighted images of class A and B hips, where the central focus is on high signal intensity and on T2-weighted images of class C hips. Manipulation of TR/TE pulse parameters does not affect the low signal intensity border.

A characteristic *double line sign* can be observed in up to 80% of lesions and is not attributed to a chemical shift artifact or misrepresentation. On T2-weighted images it is visualized as an inner border of high signal intensity, paralleling the low signal intensity periphery (Fig. 5-15).

Clinical and Pathologic Correlation with MR Findings

Patient symptoms correlate with MR classification and are least severe in class A hips and most severe in class D hips. MR signal intensity, therefore, can be seen to follow a chronologic progression from acute (class A) to chronic (class D) osteonecrosis.

When compared with conventional radiographic findings, 50% of radiographic stage 1 and 83% of stage 2 lesions imaged with fatlike central signal intensity and were classified as MR class A. Class A lesions were infrequent in more advanced radiographic stages (3–4).

MR findings can also be correlated with histologic changes (Fig. 5-16). The central region of high signal intensity corresponds to necrosis of bone and marrow, prior to development of capillary and mesenchymal ingrowth.[14] The low signal intensity peripheral band corresponds to a sclerotic margin of reactive tissue at the interface between necrotic and viable bone. Low signal intensity on T1-weighted images and intermediate to high signal intensity on T2-weighted images can be attributed to the high water content of mesenchymal tissue and thickened trabecular bone. The double line sign is thought to represent a hyperemic or inflammatory response causing granulation tissue inside the reactive bone interface.[7] A second pattern of MR signal intensity, diffuse low signal intensity on T1-weighted images with isointense or increased signal intensity on T2-weighted images, is associated with marrow edema in the femoral head and neck (Fig. 5-17).

Decreased signal intensity on T2-weighted images, in areas of proposed vascular engorgement and inflammation, has been associated with successful core decompression treatments (Fig. 5-18).[7] In one case of osteonecrosis in Legg–Calvè–Perthe's disease, return of yellow marrow signal intensity was recorded 8 months following a varus osteotomy.[15] Joint effusions of low signal intensity on T1-weighted images and of high signal intensity on T2-weighted images were commonly associated with more advanced stages of avascular necrosis (Fig. 5-19).[16] It is not known whether the presence or absence of a joint effusion is of prognostic significance for the course and treatment of the disease.

The most important contribution of MR imaging to the early detection of avascular necrosis is identification of the osteonecrotic lesion in patients with normal bone scintigraphy and conventional radiographs. Chronological staging and accurate assessment of involvement of the marrow of the femoral head offer additional information and facilitate the proper choice of therapeutic modality, prior to reactive bone changes such as subchondral fracture, collapse, and fragmentation.

Trauma

Fractures

Fractures about the hip and pelvis may be associated with significant morbidity, especially when diagnosis and treatment are delayed.[17–19] Femoral fractures are classified as either intra- or extracapsular. Intracapsular femoral neck fractures are subcapital, transcervical, or basicervical in location (Fig. 5-20).[6,10] The incidence of posttraumatic osteonecrosis increases as the fracture site nears the femoral head, culminating in a 30% incidence

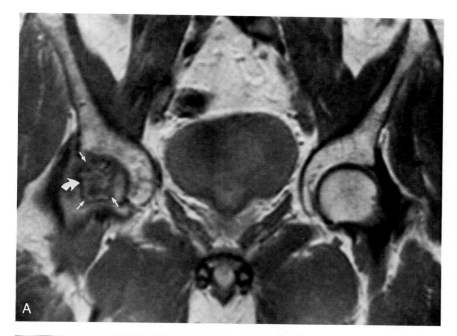

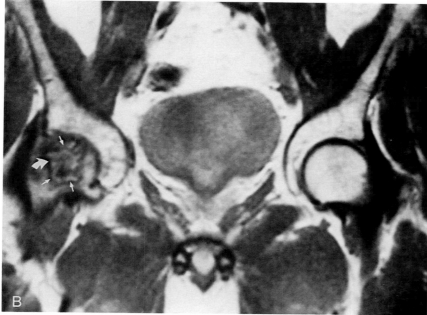

Figure 5-12

Right femoral head osteonecrosis *(straight arrows)* is visualized with intermediate to high signal intensity on T1-weighted *(A)* and T2 intermediate-weighted *(B)* images. The lesion is demarcated by a peripheral rim of low signal intensity *(curved arrow)*.

for fractures in closest proximity to the femoral head (Fig. 5-21).

Radiographic signs of cortical disruption may be subtle in femoral neck fractures, especially if there is either an incomplete or complete fracture without displacement of the medial trabeculae (Fig. 5-22). MR imaging has been particularly useful in identifying *nondisplaced femoral neck fractures* that require surgical treatment but which are not detected on routine radiography (Fig. 5-23). Bone scintigraphy is sensitive to fracture, but not specific, yet with MR it is possible to demonstrate the morphology of the fracture segment, not

seen on bone scans. In *displaced fractures*, complicating osteonecrosis can be excluded on an MR image and viability of the femoral head can be assessed.

The differential diagnosis of fatigue and insufficiency *stress fractures* may be difficult, and both infection and neoplasia need to be ruled out.[20] Stress fractures about the acetabulum, ilium, and femur may be associated with extensive edema, which images with low signal intensity on T1-weighted images and with high signal intensity on T2-weighted images, when there is no identifiable fracture segments. Thin section, high resolution CT may be necessary to achieve the precise cor-

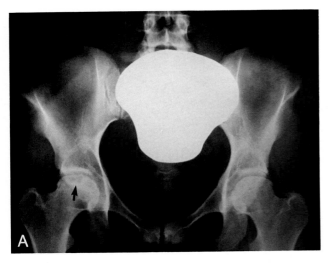

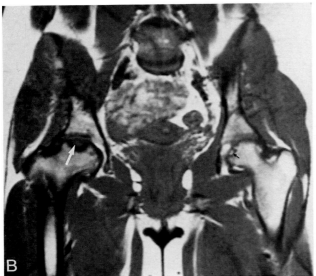

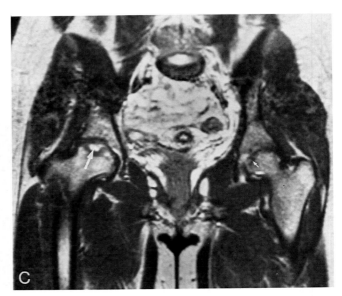

Figure 5-13

Bilateral AVN (class C). ***(A)*** A focus of osteonecrosis with a sclerotic border *(arrow)* is seen in the right femoral head on an AP radiograph. The left femoral head is without visible defect. Focus of osteonecrosis *(large arrow)* images with low to intermediate signal intensity on corresponding intermediate-weighted image ***(B)*** and with high signal intensity on T2-weighted image ***(C),*** characteristic of class C AVN. Associated focus of AVN is seen in contralateral hip *(small arrow).*

tical detail needed to display subtle cortical discontinuities (Figs. 5-24 and 5-25).

Dislocations

Posterior hip dislocations are more common than anterior dislocations, and fractures of the femoral head and acetabulum may be associated with either.[6,20] In one case of posterior fracture dislocation of the hip, MR imaging revealed an impacted femoral head fracture (of low signal intensity on T1-weighted images), an acetabular rim fracture (high signal intensity hemorrhage), and multiple intraarticular fragments that were subsequently removed through an arthroscope (Fig. 5-26).

Followup imaging with MR revealed the development of osteonecrosis at the site of fracture.

Congenital dislocation of the hip (CDH) is discussed in Chapter 2.

Labral Tears

It is now possible to resolve anatomic detail in the acetabular labrum with high spatial resolution MR capability. The normal labrum, triangular on cross section, is visualized on coronal planar images as a low signal intensity triangle, located between the lateral acetabulum and femoral head. Labral tears present with symptoms of pain, decreased range of motion, and clicking. Conventional radiographs and even arthrography are not satisfactory for accurate identification of labral defects. Our experience with MR evaluation of labral tears is limited, but in one patient having persistent pain and clicking with hip flexion and rotation, increased signal intensity within the labrum could be identified on T2-weighted MR images. An abnormal labrum with tear was surgically confirmed by subsequent arthroscopy.

Muscle Trauma

Muscle tears and avulsions image with high signal intensity on T2-weighted images in areas of edema or hemorrhage (Fig. 5-27).[21-23] MR axial imaging is useful for the demonstration of associated muscle retraction and

atrophy (high signal intensity on T1-weighted images; Fig. 5-28). Coronal or sagittal images provide a longitudinal display of the entire muscle on a single image.

Although conventional radiography should remain the initial diagnostic examination in excluding *posttraumatic myositis ossificans*, MR scans have imaged small areas of calcification or ossification as signal void or low signal intensity on T1- and T2-weighted images (Fig. 5-29).

Intramuscular hemorrhage may occur spontaneously or with minimal trauma in patients on anticoagulants (Fig. 5-30). On MR examination of a diabetic patient, intramuscular hemosiderin deposition in sites of insulin injections could be identified (Fig. 5-31).

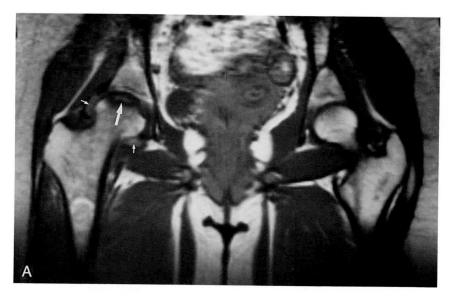

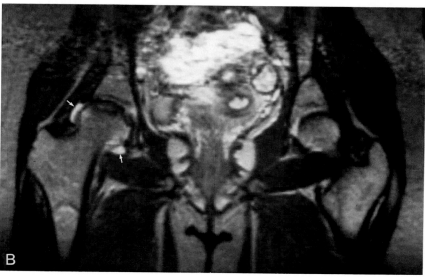

Figure 5-14

Osteonecrosis (class D). Right femoral head osteonecrosis with low signal intensity focus *(large arrow)* on T1-weighted *(A)* and on T2-weighted *(B)* image. Associated capsular effusion demonstrates increased signal intensity on T1-weighted image *(small arrows)*. *(A)* TR = 800 msec, TE = 20 msec; *(B)* TR = 2000 msec, TE = 60 msec.

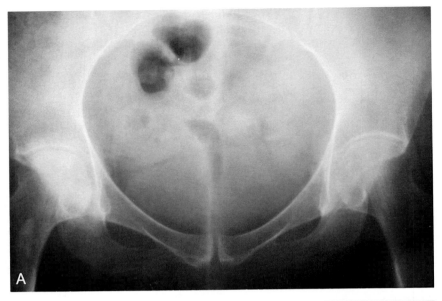

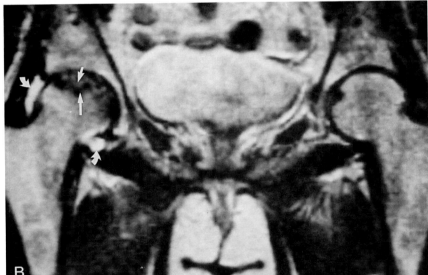

Figure 5-15

Double line sign. *(A)* Unremarkable AP radiograph in a patient with right hip pain. *(B)* Right femoral head osteonecrosis with characteristic double line sign on T2-weighted coronal image. Low signal intensity periphery *(large straight arrow)* and high signal intensity inner border *(short straight arrow)* are differentiated. Hip effusion is shown as bright signal intensity *(curved arrows)*. TR = 2000 msec, TE = 60 msec.

Arthritis

Joint Effusions

The volume of joint fluid in the normal hip is small, and it does not generate sufficient signal for detection. Small effusions, however, demonstrate low signal intensity on T1-weighted images and increased signal intensity on T2-weighted images.[16] On coronal images, joint fluid first accumulates in the recess bordered superiorly by the labrum of the acetabulum and inferomedially by the transverse ligament. With larger effusions the medial and lateral joint capsule is distended and images with convex margins (see Figs. 5-26A and 5-26B). Joint effu-

sions are also easily identified on axial and sagittal images.

Osteoarthritis

T1-weighted images of the hip are used to detect the early changes of osteoarthritis (Fig. 5-32). Articular cartilage attenuation is best demonstrated on either sagittal or coronal images, but separation of acetabular and femoral head articular cartilage is better displayed in the sagittal plane. Trabeculae thickened by stress can be seen with low signal intensity on T1- and T2-weighted images before there is evidence of subchondral sclerosis on conventional radiographs. Small subchondral

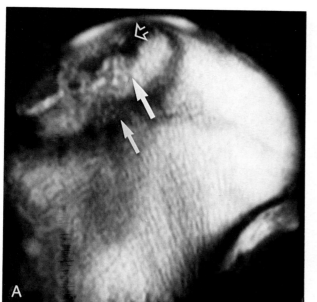

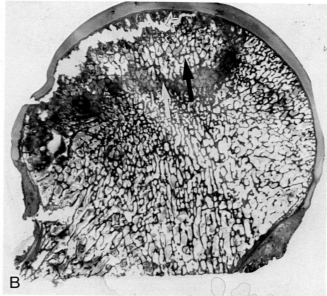

Figure 5-16

Osteonecrosis. *(A)* T1-weighted coronal image demonstrating high signal intensity cortical necrosis *(large arrow),* low signal intensity sclerotic peripheral interface between necrosis and viable marrow *(small arrow),* and low signal intensity subchondral fracture *(open arrow).* TR = 600 msec, TE = 20 msec. *(B)* Macroslide of gross specimen identifying corresponding subchondral collapse *(open arrow),* reactive periphery *(white arrow),* and cortical necrosis *(black arrow).*

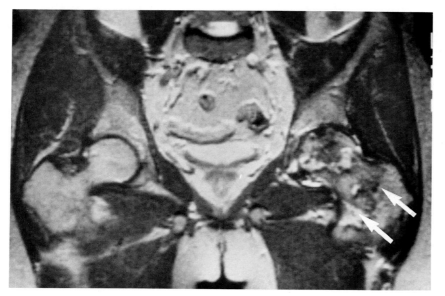

Figure 5-17

Diffuse pattern of osteonecrosis in the femoral head and neck *(arrows)* with high signal intensity area of marrow edema. T2-weighted coronal image; TR = 2000 msec, TE = 60 msec.

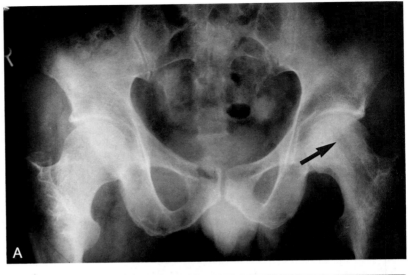

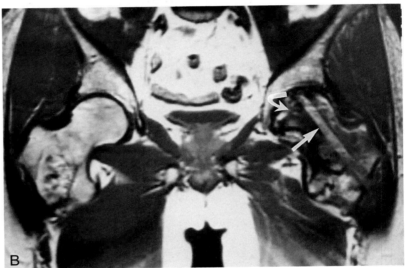

Figure 5-18

Core decompression. **(A)** AP radiograph identifying core decompression tract for osteonecrosis *(arrow)*. Unsuccessful core decompression for left femoral head osteonecrosis *(straight arrow)* with diffuse vascular edema visualized with low signal intensity on T1-weighted image **(B)** and high signal intensity on T2-weighted image **(C)**. Core tract *(straight arrow)* displays increased signal intensity from fluid contents on T2-weighted image. **(B)** TR = 600 msec, TE = 20 msec; **(C)** TR = 2000 msec, TE = 60 msec.

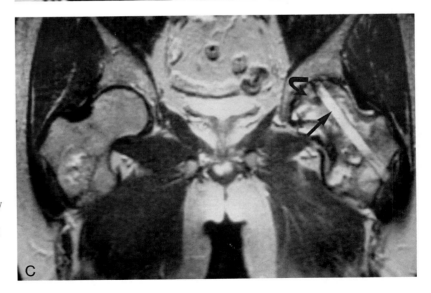

cystic lesions can be identified on MR scans before there is superior joint space narrowing, lateral acetabular and femoral head osteophytes, and medial femoral buttressing. Synovium-filled degenerative cysts about the hip image with low signal intensity on T1-weighted images and with uniform high signal intensity on T2-weighted images (Fig. 5-33). Osteoarthritis may also be associated with or superimposed on osteonecrosis of the femoral head (Fig. 5-34).

Synovial Chondromatosis and Loose Bodies

The hip is commonly involved in synovial (osteo-) chondromatosis, a monoarticular synovium-based cartilage metaplasia.[24] The development of intraarticular loose bodies may result in destruction of hyaline articular cartilage and progress to osteoarthritis. On T2-weighted MR imaging, the multiple, ossified loose bodies in synovial chondromatosis are visualized as foci of intermediate signal intensity, bathed in the surrounding joint effusion,

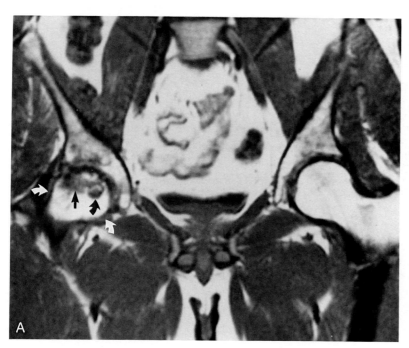

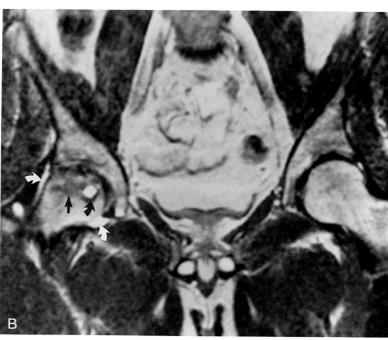

Figure 5-19

Advanced osteonecrosis with low signal intensity central cortical focus *(straight arrow)* on T1-weighted *(A)* and T2-weighted *(B)* images. Associated joint space narrowing, degenerative cyst *(curved black arrow)*, and effusion *(curved white arrow)*, are indicated. Cyst and hip effusion image with low signal intensity on T1-weighted sequences and with bright signal intensity on T2-weighted sequences. *(A)* TR = 800 msec, TE = 20 msec; *(B)* TR = 1500 msec, TE = 80 msec.

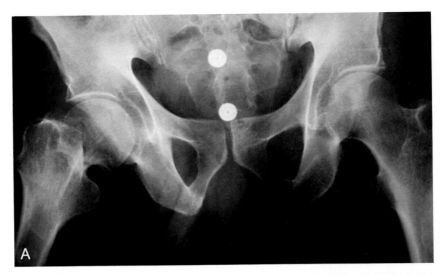

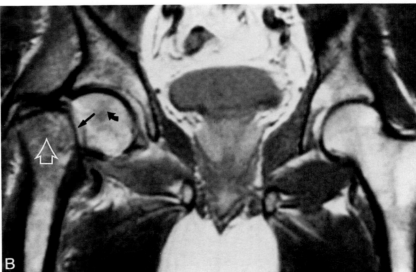

Figure 5-20

Femoral neck fracture. **(A)** AP radiograph demonstrating right femoral neck fracture in varus deformation. **(B)** T1-weighted coronal image identifies linear cervical neck fracture and low signal intensity proximal femoral marrow edema *(open arrow)*. Mild asymmetry in femoral head marrow signal intensity is observed at this stage *(curved arrow)*. TR = 600 msec, TE = 20 msec.

which images with bright signal intensity. These nodules may demonstrate the high signal intensity characteristics of fatty marrow on T1- and T2-weighted images (Fig. 5-35).

Rheumatoid Disease

MR examination of the hip joint in patients with juvenile rheumatoid (chronic) arthritis (see also Chap. 2) has revealed irregularities of the femoral capital epiphyses and growth plate, as well as osseous erosions that were underestimated on conventional radiographs.[25] Thinning of the hyaline articular cartilage can be identified on coronal and sagittal images, before there is radiographic evidence of joint space narrowing. Synovial hypertrophy, visualized as areas of low to intermediate signal intensity, has not been a frequent finding. With MR imaging, patients on corticosteroid therapy, who are at risk

for osteonecrosis, can be evaluated during acute episodes of pain.

Amyloid

Patients on long-term hemodialysis are at risk for an osteoarthropathy that has been reported to affect the hand, wrists, and less commonly, the spine.[26] Large cystic erosions have also been observed in the hip. These lesions are thought to represent a spectrum of amyloid (beta-microglobulin) deposition occurring in synovium, tendons, and cysts. In a chronic hemodialysis patient with amyloid of the hips, MR examination demonstrated intermediate signal intensity masses in the femoral head and neck on T1-weighted images (Fig. 5-36). Only minimal increase in signal intensity was observed on T2-weighted images. The lesions were imaged with an associated soft tissue component, not appreciated on plain film radiographs.

Joint Prostheses

Metallic total joint prostheses or arthroplasties generate sufficient low signal intensity artifact to prevent an accurate determination of component loosening or infection (Fig. 5-37).[27,28] Proximal and medial migration of the prosthesis into the pelvis, however, which complicates prosthetic revision and replacement, can be assessed by MR. In such instances, proximity to neurovascular structures can be assessed without invasive angiography.

Neoplastic and Marrow Disorders

Tumors about the hip are evaluated with T1-weighted coronal or sagittal images and with T2-weighted spin echo axial images. On STIR sequences, areas of marrow replacement and infiltration image as regions of increased signal intensity in contrast to dark (nulled) signal from fat.

Benign Lesions

The femur is the most common site of involvement for *osteoid osteomas*. On T1-weighted images the nidus of the lesion images with intermediate signal intensity, and thickened cortex or reactive bone maintains low signal intensity (Fig. 5-38). On T2-weighted images the central nidus demonstrates moderate to increased signal intensity.[29] Intraarticular osteoid osteomas of the hip usually cause a synovial inflammatory response, and are associated with joint effusions.

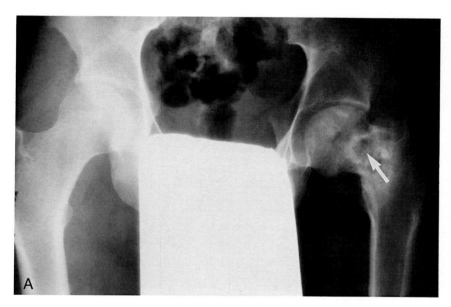

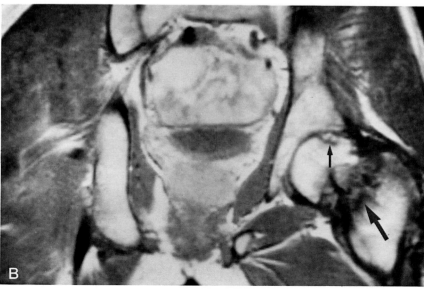

Figure 5-21

Femoral neck fracture. *(A)* AP radiograph of untreated left femoral neck fracture *(arrow)*. *(B)* Corresponding T1-weighted coronal image demonstrating low signal intensity sclerotic fracture site *(large arrow)* and associated focus of femoral head osteonecrosis *(small arrow)*. TR = 800 msec, TE = 20 msec.

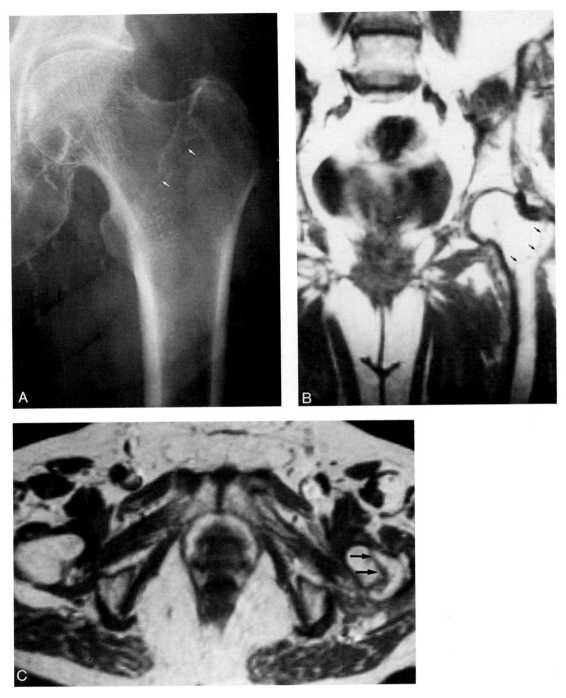

Figure 5-22

Femoral trochanteric fracture. *(A)* Nondisplaced intertrochanteric fracture missed on initial AP radiograph *(arrows)*. Corresponding T1-weighted coronal *(B)* and axial *(C)* images demonstrate low signal intensity fracture segment *(arrows)*. TR = 1000 msec, TE = 40 msec.

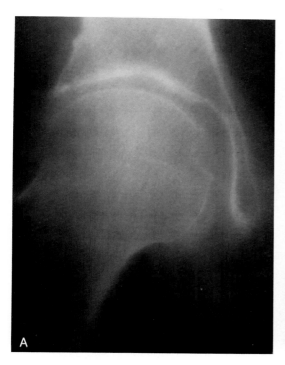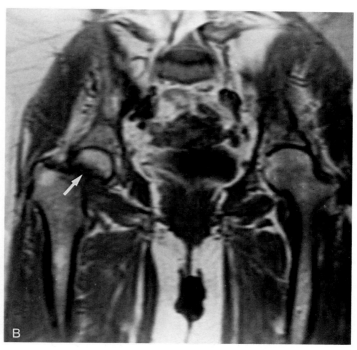

Figure 5-23

Nondisplaced femoral neck fracture missed on plain film tomography *(A)* and detected as low signal intensity segment *(arrow)* on T1-weighted coronal image *(B)*. Patient's fracture was subsequently pinned at surgery. TR = 800 msec, TE = 20 msec.

Aneurysmal bone cysts are reported to involve the femur in 13% of cases and the innominate bone in 9% of cases.[30] The aneurysmal bone cyst is an expansile, blood-filled lesion that is osteolytic on conventional radiographs. In the hip or pelvis, aggressive cortical expansion and soft tissue extension may simulate a malignant process. Inhomogeneity of signal intensity, with bright areas on T1- and T2-weighted images, with or without fluid levels is characteristic (Fig. 5-39).[31]

The femur is the site of involvement in 33% of cases of *chondroblastoma*.[30] It can arise in the epiphysis or trochanter apophysis. Primary or recurrent chondroblastoma images with low signal intensity on T1-weighted images and with nonuniform areas of increased signal intensity on T2-weighted images (Fig. 5-40).

Hemangiomas about the thigh are visualized with intermediate signal intensity on T1-weighted images and with high signal intensity on T2-weighted images.[32] Using STIR images, we have been able to map out feeding vessels in selected cases (Fig. 5-41).

Lipomas often present as a mass lesion in the thigh. They image with bright signal intensity on T1-weighted images without demonstrating an increase in signal intensity on T2-weighted sequences.[33] The fat signal can be nulled in these lesions when using STIR contrast (Fig. 5-42).

Enchondromas are visualized as well-defined lesions, with low signal intensity on T1-weighted images, and with nonuniform to homogeneous increased signal intensity on T2-weighted images (Fig. 5-43). On MR imaging, satellite cartilaginous foci are often seen in association with an enchondroma.

Hemangiopericytomas are hypervascular soft tissue tumors thought to originate from the capillary cell wall.[30] The hemangiopericytoma usually presents as a benign, deep, soft tissue mass of the thigh. The peripheral arterial branching seen on angiograms is visualized on MR images as an intricately packed network of vessels, imaging with signal void, whereas adjacent tumor is bright on T2-weighted images (Fig. 5-44).

The MR appearance of *giant cell tumor* of the long bones (described in detail in Chap. 2) is generally well defined and uniform.[34] In contrast, a more inhomogeneous and multilobular configuration was imaged in one case of giant cell tumor involving the flat pubic bone of the pelvis (Fig. 5-45). Low signal intensity on T1-weighted images and high signal intensity on T2-weighted images is demonstrated in both locations.

Malignant Lesions

Primary Malignancies. *Malignant fibrous histiocytoma* (MFH) of both bone and soft tissue has been char-

Text continues on p. 240

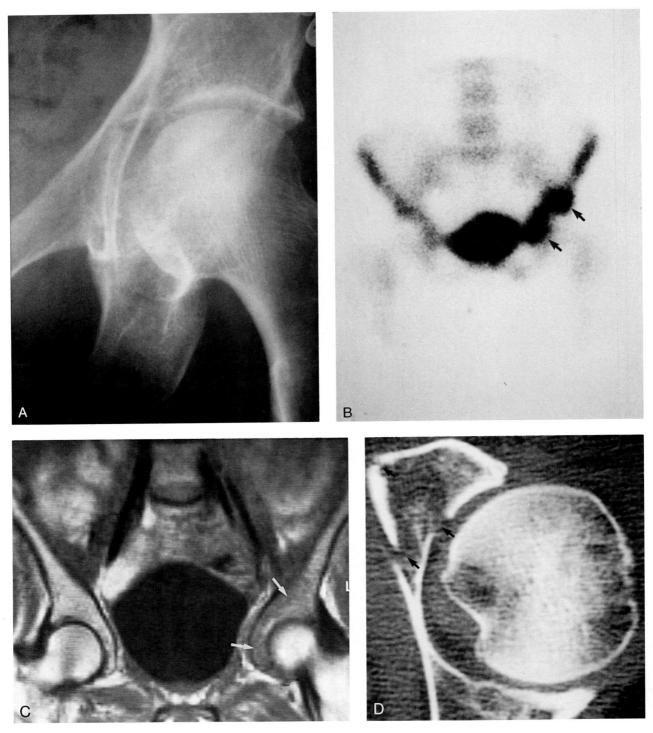

Figure 5-24

Acetabular stress fracture. **(A)** Negative AP radiograph in a patient with primary biliary cirrhosis and hip pain. **(B)** Positive 99mTC-MDP bone scan showing uptake in the left supraacetabular area *(arrows)*. **(C)** T1-weighted coronal image with diffuse low signal intensity marrow edema in left acetabular roof *(arrows)*. TR = 1000 msec, TE = 40 msec. **(D)** Multiple sites of cortical disruption in anterior column stress fracture *(arrows)* as displayed on thin section CT.

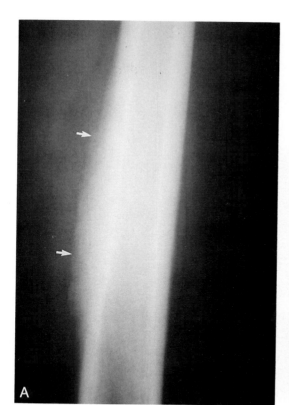

Figure 5-25

Femoral shaft stress fracture. *(A)* AP radiograph showing thickened periosteal reaction in the medial femoral shaft *(arrows)*. *(B)* Corresponding T1-weighted coronal MR image demonstrating thickened medial cortex *(black arrows)* and marrow edema *(white arrow)* as low signal intensity. TR = 1000 msec, TE = 20 msec. *(C)* Axial CT identifies stress fracture *(small arrows)* and adjacent periosteal reaction *(large arrows)*.

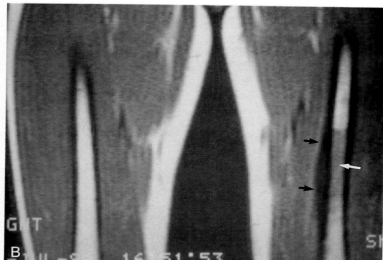

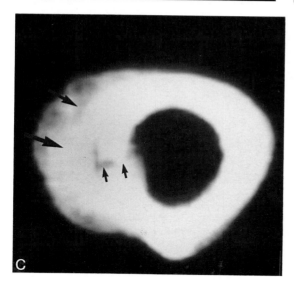

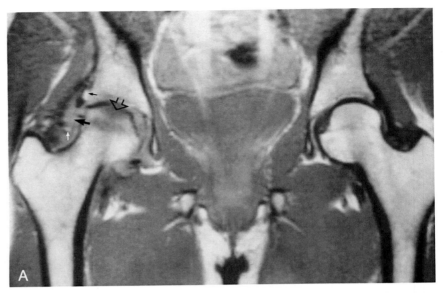

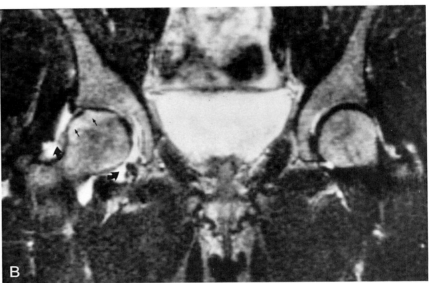

Figure 5-26

Posterior hip dislocation after reduction. **(A)** T1-weighted coronal image demonstrating femoral head compression fracture *(open arrow)*, acetabular rim fracture *(small black arrow)*, joint effusion *(large black arrow)*, and intraarticular loose bodies *(small white arrow)*. TR = 1000 msec, TE = 20 msec. **(B)** Corresponding T2-weighted coronal image displaying high signal intensity capsular effusion *(curved arrows)* and edema in area of compression fracture *(small straight arrows)*. TR = 2000 msec, TE = 60 msec. **(C)** Hip arthroscopy identifying acetabular fracture *(Ac)*, loose body *(LB)* and femoral head *(FH)*. A = anterior, P = posterior. **(D)** Follow-up radiograph at 6 months showing sclerotic focus within femoral head *(large arrow)*. Site of old acetabular rim fracture marked *(small arrow)*. Corresponding T1-weighted **(E)** and T2-weighted **(F)** coronal images demonstrate interval progression of osteonecrosis at 6 months *(arrow)*. **(E)** TR = 600 msec, TE = 20 msec; **(F)** TR = 2000 msec, TE = 60 msec.

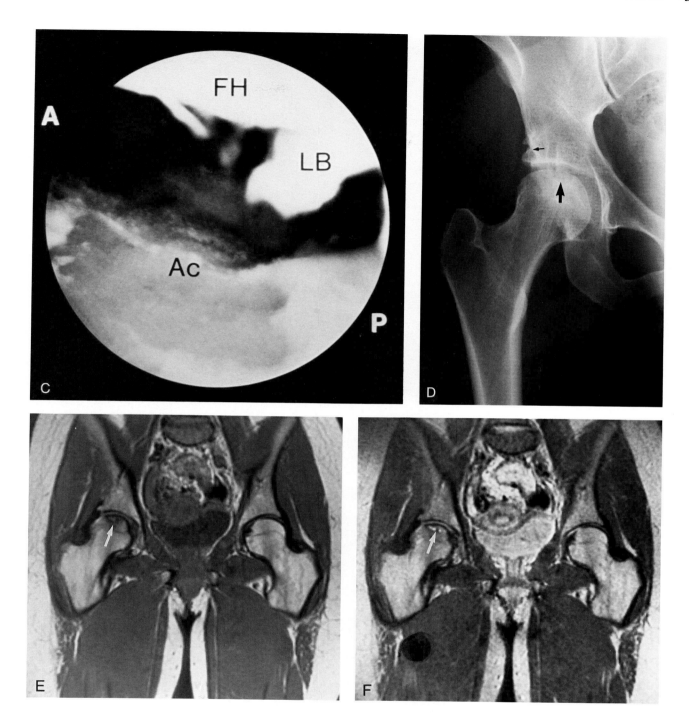

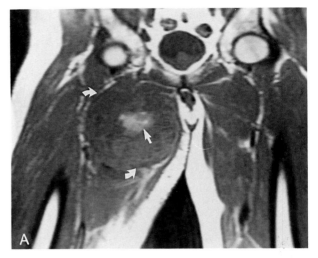

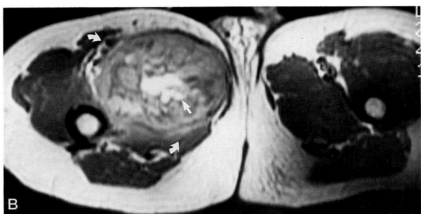

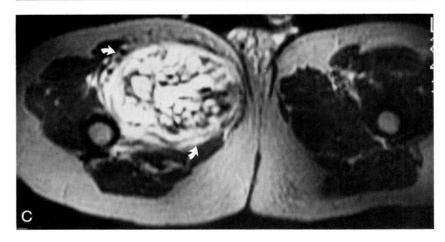

Figure 5-27

Adductor magnus rupture. *(A)* Complete rupture of the adductor magnus muscle *(curved arrow)* with central hemorrhagic component (subacute) visualized as bright signal intensity on T1-weighted image. TR = 600 msec, TE = 20 msec. Axial images demonstrate increasing signal intensity within edematous muscle fibers *(curved arrows)* on intermediate-weighted *(B)* and T2-weighted *(C)* images. Central hemorrhagic component *(straight arrow in B)* becomes isointense with surrounding edema on T2-weighted image *(C)*. TR = 2000 msec, TE = 20, 80 msec.

acterized on MR images (Fig. 5-46).[33] MFH is a soft tissue sarcoma occurring most frequently in the 50- to 70-year-old age group. Areas of hemorrhage and necrosis are common within this often large, multinodular, and hypervascular tumor. MR imaging characteristics, while not specific, have certain common features. Mixed inhomogeneity with low to intermediate signal intensity on T1-weighted images and with high signal intensity on T2-weighted images reflects the distribution of hemorrhage, necrosis, and calcification. Low signal intensity vessels correspond to hypervascular regions of the tumor.

Plasmacytoma is a solitary form of multiple myeloma that sometimes converts into multiple myeloma.[30] Solitary plasmacytomas affect a younger age group (50 years), and frequently target the spine and pelvis. A solitary lytic or expansile lesion is common, although an ivory vertebrae pattern has been reported in the spine. MR characteristics of plasmacytoma are nonspecific— low to intermediate signal intensity on T1-weighted images and high signal intensity on T2-weighted images (Fig. 5-47). Aggressive cortical disruption and infiltration into soft tissue and adjacent structures, with discontinuity of adjacent low signal intensity cortical bone, can be identified on MR examination.

Metastases. The MR appearance of metastatic lesions about the hip and pelvis is nonspecific for site of

Text continues on p. 245

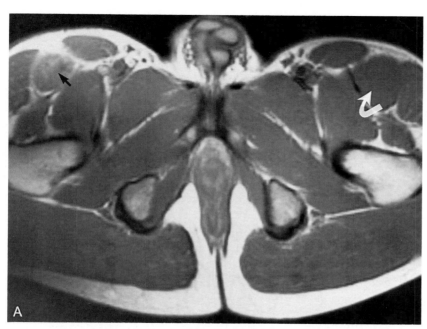

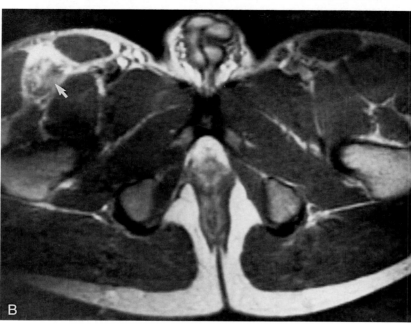

Figure 5-28

Torn right rectus femoris muscle with atrophy and edema *(arrow)* on intermediate-weighted *(A)* and T2-weighted *(B)* axial images. Edematous muscle fibers display increased signal intensity on T2-weighted image. Normal size left rectus femoris shown for comparison *(curved arrow)*. TR = 2000 msec, TE = 20, 80 msec.

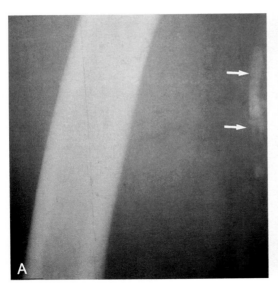
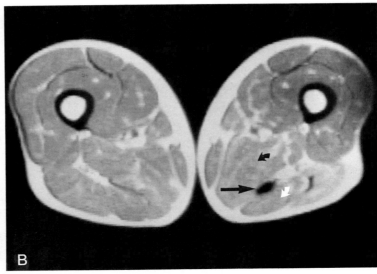

Figure 5-29

Myositis ossificans. **(A)** Myositis ossificans demonstrating linear calcification *(arrows)* on lateral radiograph of the thigh. **(B)** T1-weighted axial image identifying low signal intensity calcific deposits *(straight arrow)* in fascial plane between the semitendinosus *(curved white arrow)* and semimembranosus *(curved black arrow)* muscles. TR = 800 msec, TE = 20 msec.

Figure 5-30

Anterior thigh hemorrhage. **(A)** AP radiograph identifying focal soft tissue calcific deposits *(arrows)*. **(B)** T1-weighted coronal image delineates high signal intensity hemorrhage (subacute) in the region of the vastus lateralis muscle *(white arrows)*. Low signal intensity hemosiderin periphery *(small black arrows)* and internal septations *(curved arrow)* are shown. TR = 800 msec, TE = 20 msec.

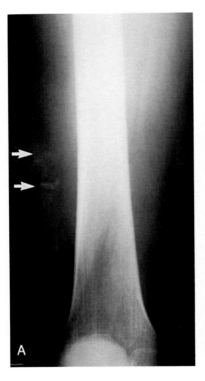
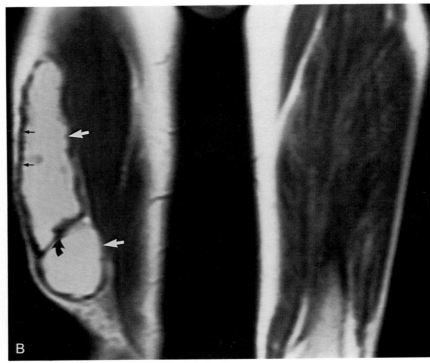

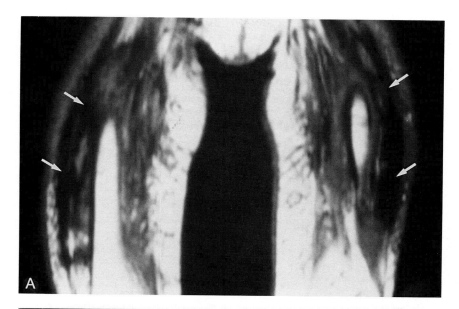

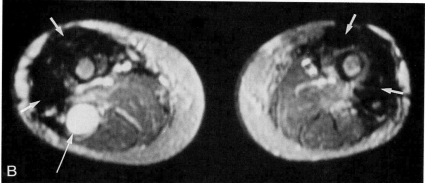

Figure 5-31

Chronic intramuscular hemorrhage from repeated injections of insulin in a diabetic patient. Low signal intensity paramagnetic hemosiderin deposition *(short arrows)* in vastus lateralis and intermedius muscles on T1-weighted coronal *(A)* and axial *(B)* images. High signal intensity focal hemorrhage (subacute) is visualized on axial image within the long head of the biceps femoris muscle *(long arrow)*. TR = 600 msec, TE = 20 msec.

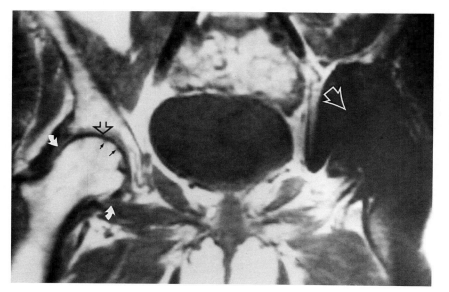

Figure 5-32

Degenerative osteoarthritis of the right hip with superior joint space narrowing, attenuated intermediate signal intensity articular cartilage *(open black arrow)*, and small low signal intensity subchondral cysts *(solid arrows)*. Signal void from total hip prosthesis is visualized *(open white arrow)*. Minimal joint effusion is imaged with intermediate signal intensity *(curved arrows)*. T1-weighted image; TR = 600 msec, TE = 20 msec.

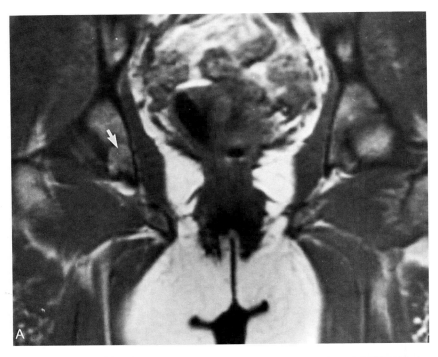

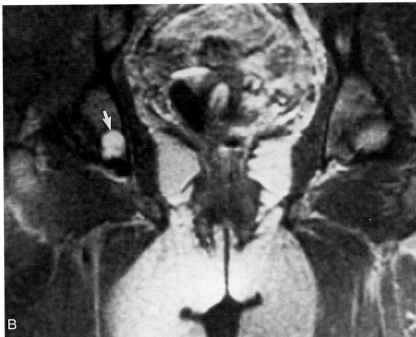

Figure 5-33

Degenerative cyst of the posterior acetabulum
(arrow) is isointense with marrow on T1-weighted
image ***(A)*** and is of uniform high signal intensity
on T2-weighted image ***(B)***. ***(A)*** TR = 600 msec,
TE = 20 msec; ***(B)*** TR = 2000 msec, TE = 60
msec.

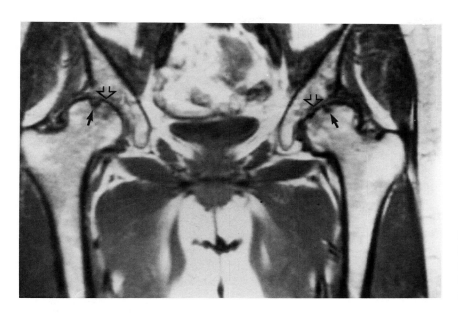

Figure 5-34
Secondary osteoarthritis of the hips with joint space narrowing, denuded cartilage *(open arrows),* irregular femoral heads, and bilateral AVN *(closed arrows).* TR = 600 msec, TE = 20 msec.

origin (Fig. 5-48).[3] Peritumoral soft tissue edema may be observed in the absence of a soft tissue mass (Fig. 5-49). Osteolytic metastatic lesions (commonly from carcinoma of the lung or breast) often image with a more uniform signal intensity on T1- and T2-weighted images than do mixed sclerotic or osteoblastic deposits (from carcinoma of the prostate or from medulloblastoma; Fig. 5-50).

Lymphoma. Lymphoreticular neoplasms of the reticuloendothelial system are classified as non-Hodgkin's or Hodgkin's lymphomas.[30] Conventional radiographic techniques underestimate the degree of bone involvement by lymphoma—for example, twice the incidence of bone involvement in patients with Hodgkin's disease is determined at autopsy (50%) than is detected by standard radiographic examinations (10% to 25%). Localization of potential biopsy sites is important in reaching proper histologic or cytologic diagnosis; and staging of the disease, evaluating extent and multiple sites of involvement, has a direct relationship on patient prognosis (Fig. 5-51).

Lymphoma has a propensity to develop into focal nodules of tumor (Fig. 5-52). This has been substantiated by marrow biopsy. MR has been used to detect focal marrow involvement, prior to the diffuse dissemination or infiltration of disease.[35] Of all the current imaging modalities, MR has the potential to be more sensitive than others, including bone scintigraphy (which is often negative in patients with affected marrow) and marrow biopsy (which may not accurately sample focal marrow deposits in early disease). MR is, however, limited in specificity of diagnosis. Infection, primary tumors, and metastasis can also image with low signal intensity on T1-weighted images and with high signal intensity on T2-weighted or STIR sequences, where T1 and T2 contrast is additive for processes that replace yellow or fatty bone marrow. Although focal areas of yellow to red marrow conversion may mimic lymphoma involvement on STIR images, red marrow does not generate increased signal intensity on conventional T2-weighted or T2* gradient echo images.

Leukemia. On T1-weighted images, chronic leukemias in adults tend to image with decreased marrow signal intensity in areas of previous red marrow distribution (Fig. 5-53).[35–37] This decreased signal intensity in leukemic infiltrates usually demonstrates a homogeneous, symmetric, and confluent distribution within the hips and pelvis. Most chronic leukemias tend to spare yellow marrow sites, such as those in the apophysis of the greater trochanter and femoral epiphysis. In patients in blast crisis (e.g., chronic myelogenous leukemia or CML) or in an acute phase of leukemia, replacement of both red and yellow marrow stores may be seen. The decreased signal intensity seen on T1-weighted images reflects the longer T1 value of leukemic infiltrates, which possess a higher water content than normal fatty or yellow marrow (short T1 and a relatively long T2). The STIR sequence is especially sensitive to this T1 prolongation, and leukemic marrow replacement images with bright signal intensity in contrast to normal dark (nulled) fatty marrow signal intensity. Hairy cell leukemia demonstrates a more patchy or less uniform pattern of involvement, similar to that described with lymphoma (Fig. 5-54).[37] Hairy cell leukemias have also been diagnosed on MR prior to the appearance of an abnormal peripheral blood smear.

Text continues on p. 264

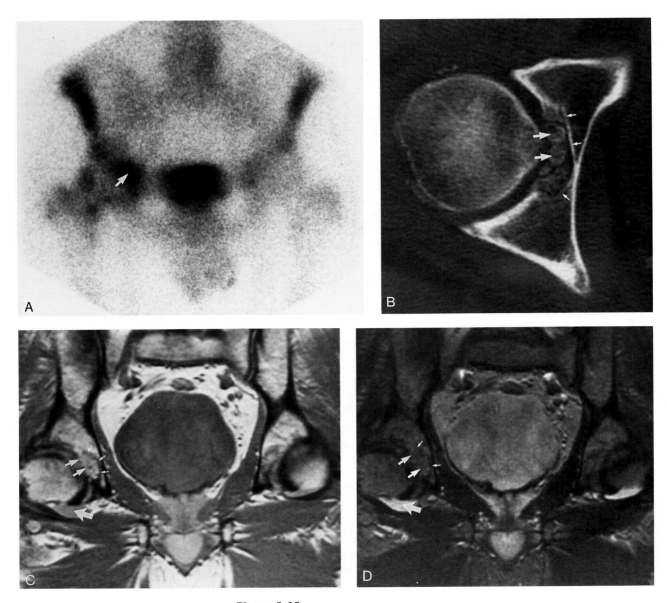

Figure 5-35

Synovial chondromatosis (osteochondromatosis). **(A)** Uptake of bone tracer in right hip *(arrow)* shown on 99mTC-MDP bone scan. **(B)** Axial CT scan identifying multiple intraarticular loose bodies *(large arrows)* contained within the acetabular convexity *(small arrows)*. Corresponding coronal images demonstrating marrow signal intensity in synovium-based free fragments *(medium arrows)* on T1-weighted **(C)** and T2-weighted **(D)** images. Inner wall of acetabulum is demarcated *(small arrows)*. Joint effusion *(large arrow)* generates increased signal intensity on T2-weighting.

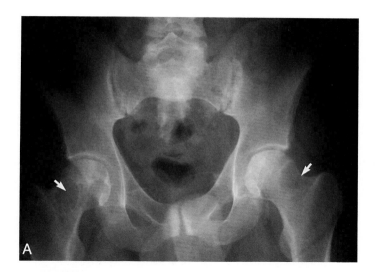

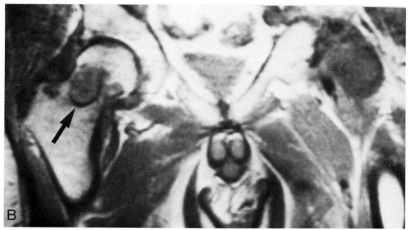

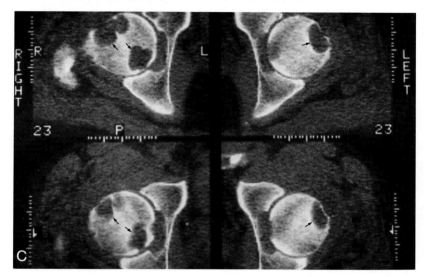

Figure 5-36

Amyloid hips. *(A)* Large cystic erosions of the femoral neck on AP radiograph in a patient on chronic renal dialysis *(arrows)*. *(B)* T1-weighted coronal image identifying intermediate signal intensity amyloid deposits in femoral head and neck *(arrow)*. TR = 600 msec, TE = 20 msec. *(C)* Axial CT displaying multiple cystic erosions of the femoral head *(arrows)*.

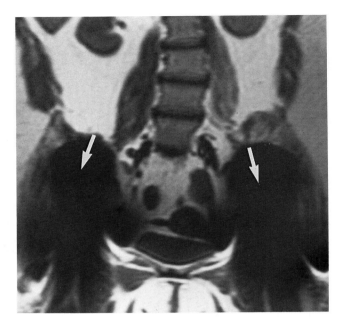

Figure 5-37
Low signal intensity artifact from bilateral total joint prosthesis *(arrows)*. T1-weighted coronal image; TR = 600 msec, TE = 20 msec.

Figure 5-38
Osteoid osteoma of the left femoral neck images with intermediate signal intensity circular nidus *(small arrow)*, low signal intensity cortical thickening *(curved arrow)*, and intermediate signal intensity effusion *(large arrow)*. T1-weighted axial image; TR = 600 msec, TE = 20 msec.

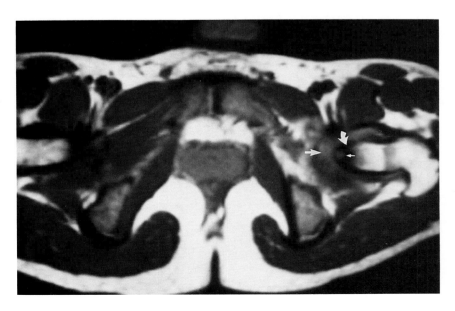

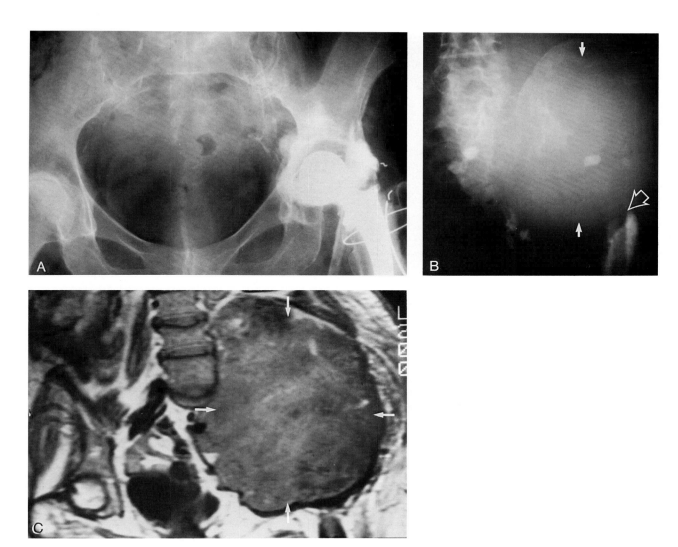

Figure 5-39

Aneurysmal bone cyst. *(A)* Initial AP radiograph showing left total hip prosthesis. *(B)* AP radiograph demonstrates progression of aggressive lytic destruction of the left pelvis *(closed arrows)* and proximal femur *(open arrow)* with a soft tissue density mass. *(C)* T1-weighted coronal image defining the extent of this well-marginated mass. TR = 500 msec, TE = 20 msec.

Figure continues on next page

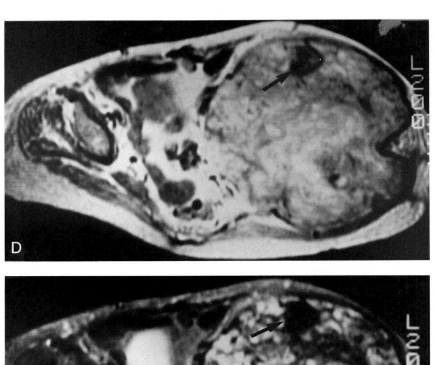

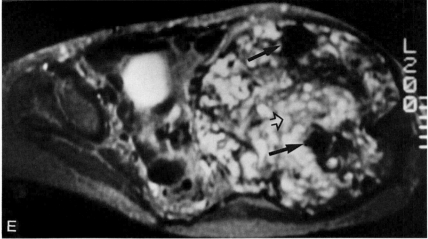

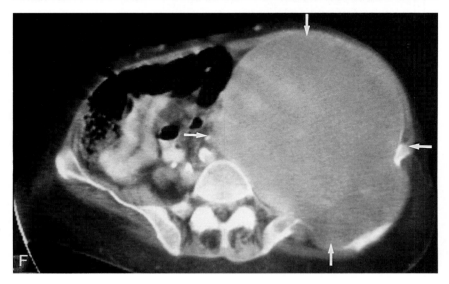

Figure 5-39 (continued)
Intermediate-weighted **(D)** and T2-weighted **(E)**
axial images show characteristic low signal intensity
hemosiderin deposits *(solid arrow)* mixed with high
signal intensity hemorrhagic elements *(open arrow)*.
TR = 2000 msec, TE = 20, 60 msec. **(F)**
Corresponding axial CT of the lesion *(arrows)* is
nonspecific for hemorrhagic constituents.

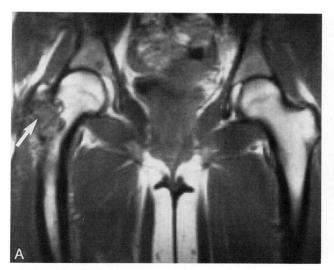

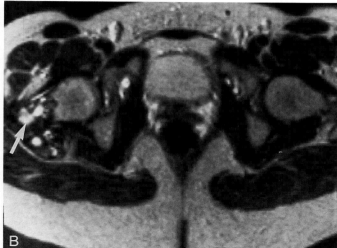

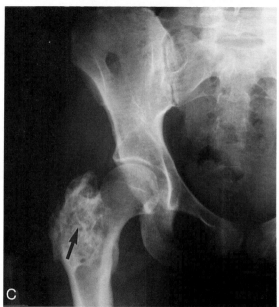

Figure 5-40

Recurrent chondroblastoma in an adult patient. **(A)** Lesion *(arrow)* images with low to intermediate signal intensity on T1-weighted coronal image. TR = 600 msec, TE = 20 msec. **(B)** Mixed inhomogeneity with high signal intensity chondroid components *(arrow)* is visualized on T2-weighted axial image. TR = 2000 msec, TE = 60 msec. **(C)** Conventional AP radiograph demonstrates greater trochanter location. Sclerotic appearance is the result of packing with bone chips *(arrow)*.

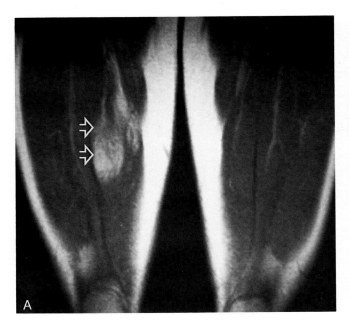

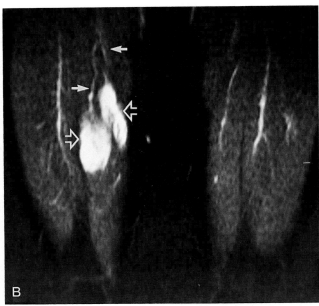

Figure 5-41

Hemangioma of the vastus medialis muscle. High signal intensity hemangioma *(open arrows)* is displayed on both T1-weighted *(A)* and STIR *(B)* images. The supplying vessels are identified with high signal intensity contrast on the STIR sequence *(closed arrows)*. The symmetry of vessel size with adjacent vasculature excludes fistula from the differential diagnosis. *(A)* TR = 600 msec, TE = 20 msec; *(B)* TR = 1400 msec, TI = 125 msec, TE = 40 msec.

Figure 5-42

Lipoma of the left thigh *(arrow)* is visualized with nulled or dark fat signal intensity on STIR sequence. TR = 1400 msec, TI = 125 msec, TE = 40 msec.

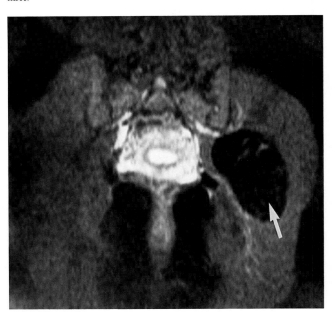

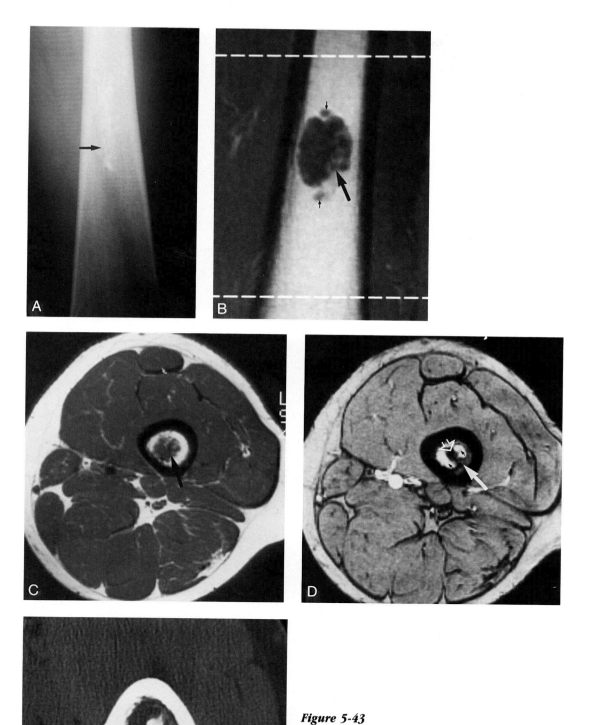

Figure 5-43

Enchondroma. *(A)* AP radiograph showing focus of calcification within distal femoral shaft. *(B)* T1-weighted coronal image displaying low signal intensity distal femoral enchondroma *(large arrow)* with two satellite lesions *(small arrows)*. TR = 600 msec, TE = 20 msec. On axial T1-weighted *(C)* and T2-weighted *(D)* images the enchondroma visualizes with low signal intensity *(large arrow)* and with high signal intensity *(small arrows)*, respectively. Cortical signal void is the result of calcification within the lesion *(open arrow)*. *(C)* TR = 600 msec, TE = 20 msec; *(D)* TR = 2000 msec, TE = 60 msec. *(E)* Corresponding axial CT confirms the presence of calcification *(open arrow)*.

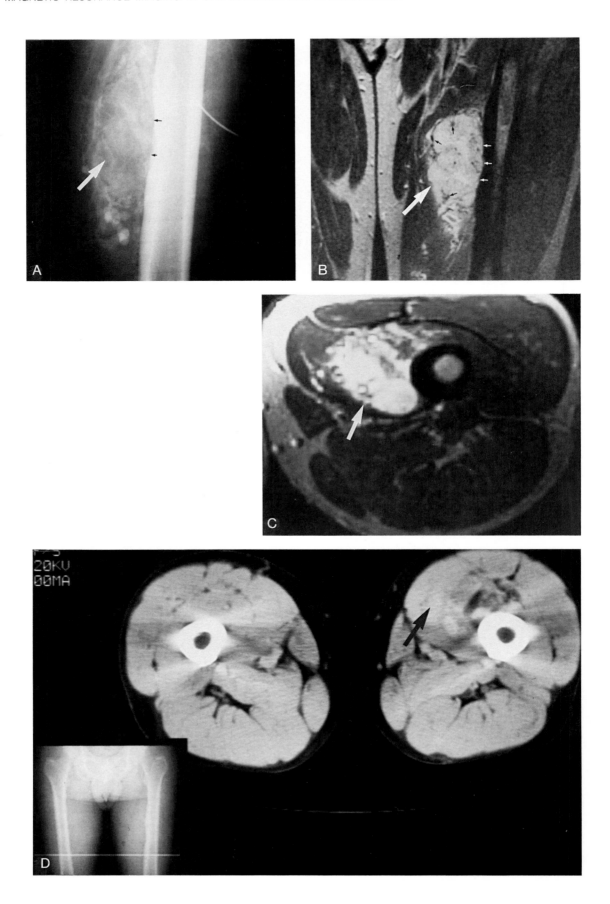

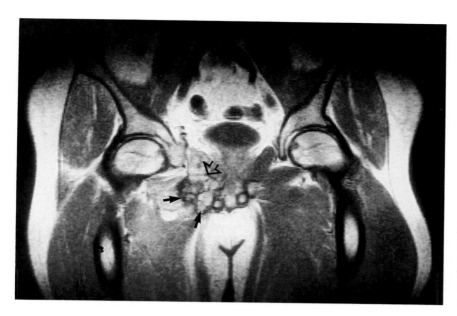

Figure 5-45

Multilobulated giant cell tumor *(closed arrows)* arising from the pubic ramis *(open arrow)*, images with nonuniform intermediate signal intensity on intermediate-weighted image. TR = 1500 msec, TE = 28 msec.

◄ **Figure 5-44**

Hemangiopericytoma of the vastus medialis and intermedius muscles. *(A)* Lesion demonstrates hypervascularity *(large arrow)* and erosion of the adjacent cortex *(small arrows)*. T2-weighted coronal *(B)* and axial *(C)* images demonstrating low signal intensity hypervascularity *(small black arrows)*, cortical erosion *(small white arrows)*, and bright signal intensity tumor *(large arrow)*. TR = 2000 msec, TE = 60 msec. *(D)* Corresponding axial CT identifying vague soft tissue mass *(arrow)*.

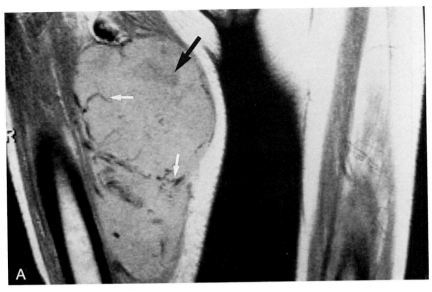

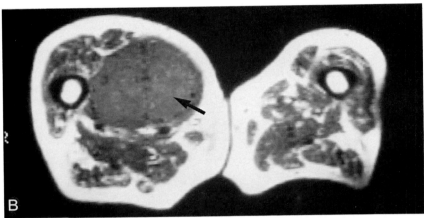

Figure 5-46

Malignant fibrous histiocytoma (MFH). *(A)* Large tumor mass *(black arrow)* involving the medial thigh compartment on an intermediate-weighted coronal image. Tumor hypervascularity is indicated *(white arrows)*. TR = 1800 msec, TE = 40 msec. T1-weighted *(B)* and T2-weighted *(C)* axial images of MFH lesion *(large arrow)* with low and high signal intensity, respectively. Areas of tumor inhomogeneity are apparent on T2-weighted image *(small arrows)*. *(B)* TR = 600 msec, TE = 20 msec; *(C)* TR = 2000 msec, TE = 60 msec.

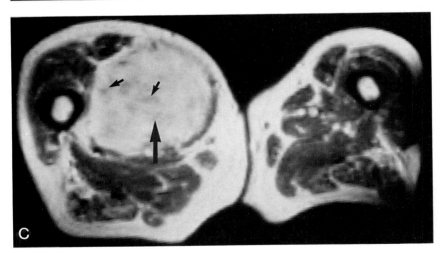

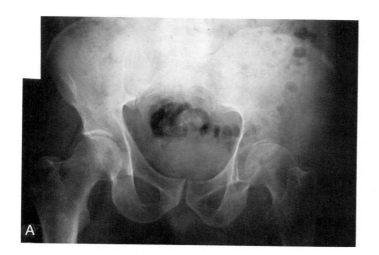

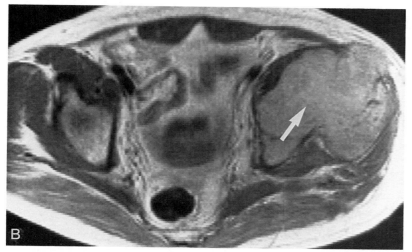

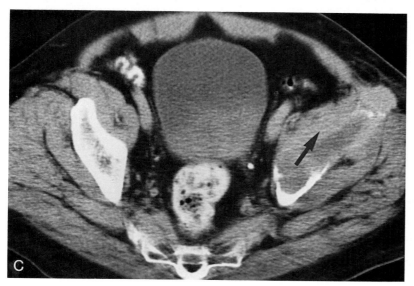

Figure 5-47

Plasmacytoma of the ilium. *(A)* Destruction of the left ilium as seen on AP radiograph of the pelvis. *(B)* T1-weighted axial MR imaging demonstrates intermediate signal intensity mass *(arrow)* with aggressive cortical transgression and soft tissue extension. TR = 600 msec, TE = 20 msec. *(C)* Axial CT identifies disrupted cortical bone *(arrow)*.

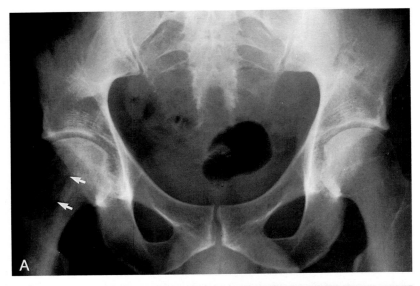

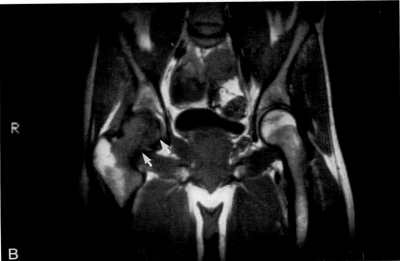

Figure 5-48

Metastatic melanoma. *(A)* Lesion seen as lytic area in lateral femoral neck *(arrows)* on AP radiograph. *(B)* T1-weighted coronal image shows nonspecific low signal intensity marrow replacement *(arrows)*. TR = 500 msec, TE = 30 msec.

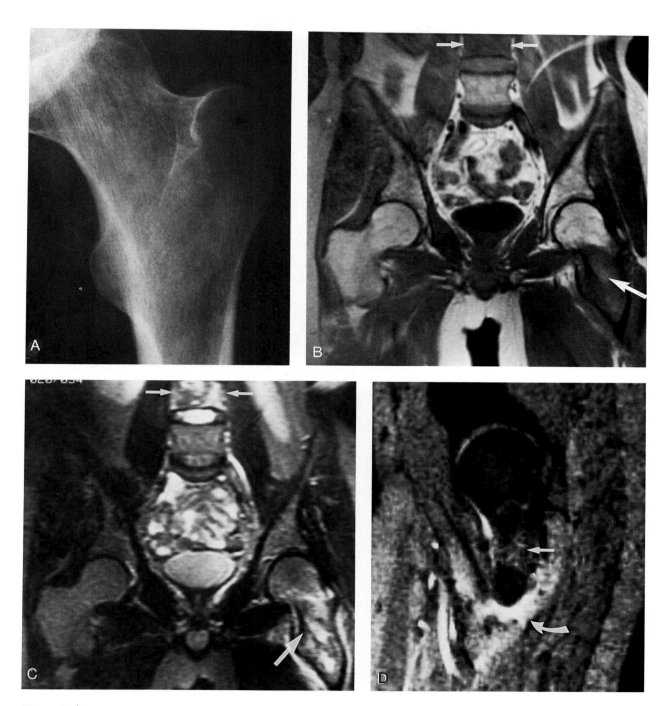

Figure 5-49

Metastatic lung carcinoma. *(A)* Negative AP radiograph. T1-weighted *(B)* and T2-weighted *(C)* images demonstrate low and high signal intensity, respectively, in L4 *(small arrows)* and proximal femur metastasis *(large arrow)*. *(B)* TR = 800 msec, TE = 20 msec; *(C)* TR = 2000 msec, TE = 60 msec. *(D)* Sagittal T2* gradient echo image displays high signal intensity metastatic deposit *(straight arrow)* and peritumoral edema *(curved arrow)*. TR = 400 msec, TE = 30 msec; flip angle = 30°.

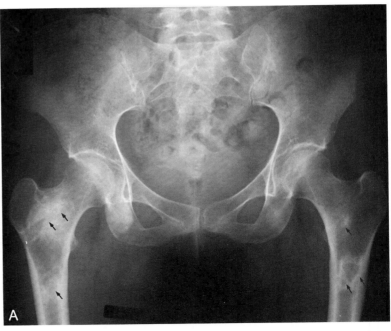

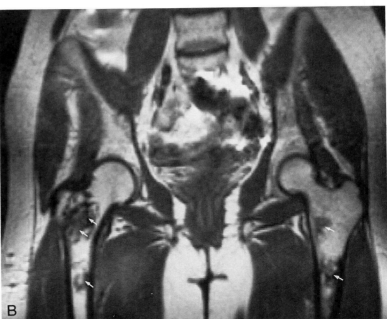

Figure 5-50

Metastatic medulloblastoma. *(A)* Mixed lytic and
sclerotic femoral lesions *(arrows)* are seen on AP
radiograph of the pelvis. *(B)* Corresponding T1-
weighted coronal image with metastatic deposits of
medulloblastoma *(arrows)* imaging with nonuniform
signal intensity (low to intermediate). TR = 500
msec, TE = 40 msec.

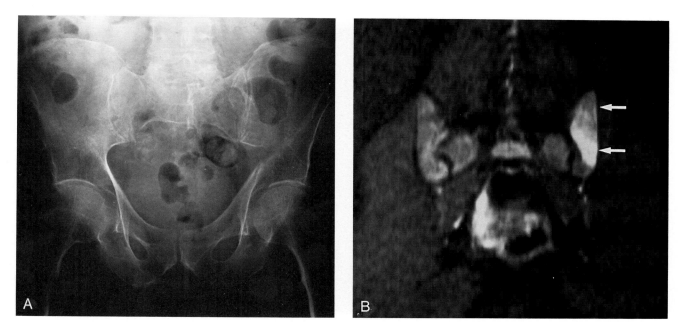

Figure 5-51

Lymphoma, focal pattern. *(A)* Negative AP radiograph. *(B)* High signal intensity lymphoma demonstrating asymmetric pattern of marrow involvement *(arrows)* in the posterior ilium on STIR sequence. TE = 1400 msec, TI = 125 msec, TR = 40 msec.

Figure 5-52

Lymphoma, nodular pattern. *(A)* Negative AP radiograph of the pelvis. *(B)* T1-weighted coronal image displays nonspecific low signal intensity proximal femurs *(large arrows)* and acetabulae *(small arrows)*. Fatty marrow of epiphysis and greater trochanter is spared. TR = 600 msec, TE = 20 msec. *(C)* STIR image demonstrates patchy nodularity of lymphomatous marrow involvement imaged with high signal intensity in the proximal femurs *(large white arrows)*, acetabulum *(small white arrows)*, and L4 vertebral body *(curved arrow)*. Spared yellow marrow of the greater trochanter and femoral epiphysis appears black. TR = 1400 msec, TI = 125 msec, TE = 40 msec.

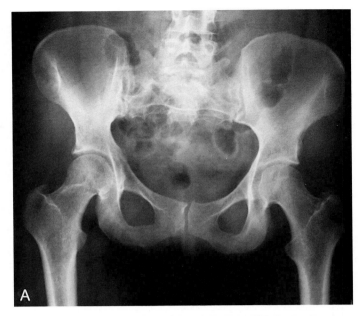

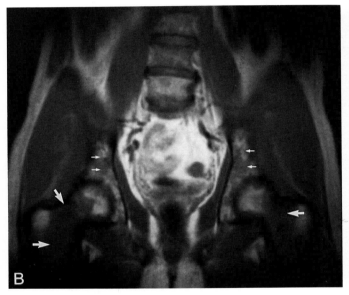

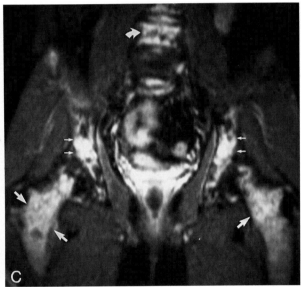

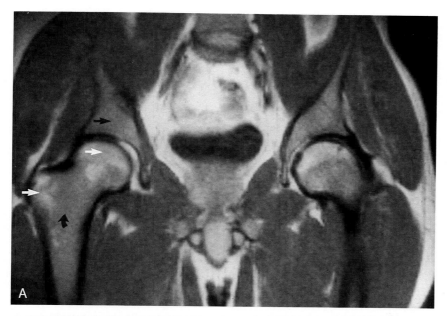

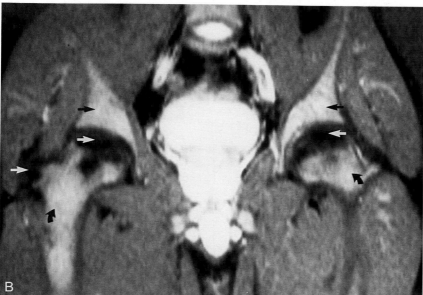

Figure 5-53

Diffuse marrow involvement with chronic myelogenous leukemia (CML) infiltrating regions of previous red marrow stores in the femurs *(curved arrows)* and acetabulum *(straight black arrows),* imaging with low signal intensity on T1-weighted image *(A)* and with high signal intensity on corresponding STIR image *(B).* Spared sites of yellow marrow (greater trochanter and femoral epiphysis) image with high signal intensity on T1-weighted image and with low signal intensity (nulled fat signal) on STIR sequence *(white arrows).* *(A)* TR = 600 msec, TE = 20 msec; *(B)* TR = 1400 msec, TI = 125 msec, TE = 40 msec.

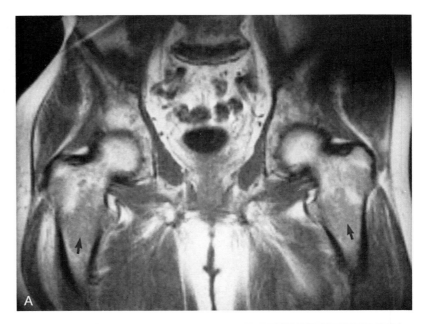

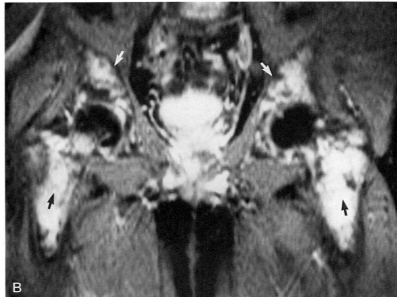

Figure 5-54

Hairy cell leukemia. Patchy pattern of marrow involvement mimicking the appearance of lymphoma. Leukemic infiltration images with low signal intensity *(black arrows)* on T1-weighted image *(A)* and with high signal intensity *(black and white arrows)* on STIR sequence *(B)*. *(A)* TR = 600 msec, TE = 20 msec; *(B)* TR = 1400 msec, TI = 125 msec, TE = 40 msec, respectively.

PERSPECTIVES ON MR IMAGING OF THE HIP

The hip is the focus of a variety of conditions in trauma, arthritis, and neoplasia. Early detection of these conditions may significantly alter patient morbidity and may direct proper treatment with either conservative or surgical intervention. Diagnosis and staging of osteonecrosis is more accurate with MR imaging than with conventional radiographs, CT, or bone scintigraphy. Femoral neck fractures can be identified and treated prior to their radiographic appearance, because of the excel-lent inherent contrast present in direct marrow imaging. The ability to visualize hyaline articular cartilage is invaluable in assessing the spectrum of hip disorders affecting pediatric patients. The hip is a common site for inflammatory and degenerative arthritides in which MR can provide information regarding the articular cartilage, joint capsule, and synovium structures not visualized with standard radiographic techniques. In the case of neoplasia, metastatic disease, and marrow disorders, MR has become a sensitive imaging modality for assessing the extent of disease and associated marrow infiltration.

REFERENCES

1. Fishman EK, et al: Multiplanar (MPR) imaging of the hip. RadioGraphics 6:7, 1986

2. Stoller DW, et al: Fast MR improves imaging for musculoskeletal system. Diagnostic Imaging February:98, 1988

3. Porter B, et al: Magnetic resonance imaging of bone marrow disorders. Radiol Clin North America June 1986

4. Porter BA, et al: Low-field STIR imaging of avascular necrosis, marrow edema, and infarction. Radiology 165P:83, 1987

5. Gillespy T III, et al: Magnetic resonance imaging of osteonecrosis. Radiol Clin North America 24:193, 1986

6. Berquist TH, Coventry MB: The pelvis and hips. In Berquist TH (ed): Imaging of Orthopedic Trauma and Surgery, pp 181–275. Philadelphia, WB Saunders, 1986

7. Mitchell DG, et al: Femoral head avascular necrosis: Correlation of MR imaging, radiographic staging, radionuclide imaging, and clinical findings. Radiology 162:709, 1987

8. Beltran J, et al: Femoral head avascular necrosis: MR imaging with clinical-pathologic and radionuclide correlation. Radiology 166:215, 1988

9. Mitchell MD, et al: Avascular necrosis of the hip: Comparison of MR, CT, and scintigraphy. AJR 147:67, 1986

10. Weissman BNW, Sledge CB: Orthopedic Radiology, chapter 8. Philadelphia, WB Saunders, 1986

11. Mankey M, et al: Comparison of MRI and bone scan in the early detection of osteonecrosis of the femoral head. Presented to the American Academy of Orthopaedic Surgeons, January 1987

12. Mitchell DG, et al: Chemical-shift MR imaging of the femoral head: An in vitro study of normal hips and hips with avascular necrosis. AJR 148:1159, 1987

13. Markisz JA, et al: Segmental patterns of avascular necrosis of the femoral heads: Early detection with MR imaging. Radiology 162:717, 1987

14. Lang P, et al: 2.0T MR imaging of the femoral head in avascular osteonecrosis: Histologic correlation (abstr). Sixth Annual Meeting and Exhibition of the Society of Magnetic Resonance in Medicine, New York City, August 17–21, 1987

15. Heuck A, et al: MR imaging in the evaluation of Legg-Perthes disease. Radiology 165P:83, 1987

16. Mitchell DG, et al: MRI of joint fluid in the normal and ischemic hip. AJR 146:1215, 1986

17. Burk DL Jr, et al: Acetabular fractures: Three-dimensional computed tomographic imaging and interactive surgical planning. CT 10:1, 1986

18. Fairclough J, et al: Bone scanning for suspected hip fractures. Radiology 164:886, 1987

19. Griffiths HJ, et al: Computed tomography in the management of acetabular fractures. Radiology 154:567, 1985

20. Stafford SA, et al: MRI in stress fracture. AJR 147:553, 1986

21. Ehman RL, Berquist TH: Magnetic resonance imaging of musculoskeletal trauma. Radiol Clin North America 24:291, 1986

22. Fisher MR, et al: Magnetic resonance imaging of the normal and pathologic musculoskeletal system. Magn Res Imag 4:491, 1986

23. Dooms GC, et al: MR imaging of intramuscular hemorrhage. JCAT 9:908, 1985

24. Szypryt P, et al: Synovial chondromatosis of the hip joint presenting as a pathological fracture. Br J Radiol 59:399, 1986

25. Stoller DW: MRI in juvenile (chronic) arthritis. Presented to Association of University Radiologists, Charleston, South Carolina, March 22–27, 1987

26. Brancaccio D, et al: Amyloid arthropathy in patients on regular dialysis: A newly discovered disease. Radiology 165P:335, 1987

27. Feldman F, et al: MR imaging of soft-tissue reactions to prostheses. Radiology 165P:84, 1987

28. Laakman RW, et al: MR imaging in patients with metallic implants. Radiology 157:711, 1985

29. Glass RBJ, et al: MR imaging of osteoid osteoma. JCAT 10:1065, 1986

30. Resnick D, Niwayama, G: Diagnosis of Bone and Joint Disorders, 2nd ed, vol 6, chapter 91. Philadelphia, WB Saunders, 1988

31. Beltran J, et al: Aneurysmal bone cysts: MR imaging at 1.5T. Radiology 158:689, 1986

32. Kaplan PA, Williams SM: Mucocutaneous and peripheral soft-tissue hemangiomas: MR imaging. Radiology 163:163, 1987

33. Petasnick JP, et al: Soft-tissue masses of the locomotor system: Comparison of MR imaging with CT. Radiology 160:125, 1986

34. Brady TJ, et al: NMR imaging of forearms in healthy volunteers and patients with giant-cell tumors of bone. Radiology 144:549, 1982

35. Olson D, et al: Magnetic resonance imaging of the bone marrow in patients with leukemia, aplastic anemia, and lymphoma. Investigative Radiology July 1986

36. Porter B, et al: MR may become routine for imaging bone marrow. Diagnostic Imaging February 1987

37. Thompson J, et al: Magnetic resonance imaging of bone marrow in hairy cell leukemia: Correlation with clinical response to α-Interferon. Leukemia April 1987

David W. Stoller
John V. Crues III

Chapter 6   THE SHOULDER

Conventional radiographic evaluation of the shoulder is limited to display of osseous changes and calcifications without direct visualization of the rotator cuff and glenohumeral capsular mechanism. More invasive techniques, such as single and double contrast arthrography, permit assessment of the rotator cuff by the identification of the abnormal passage of contrast material into the subacromial-subdeltoid bursa.[1] Even with arthrography, however, superficial or substance tears that do not involve the deep surface of the rotator cuff cannot be identified. The glenoid labrum and capsule can be visualized with computed arthrotomography or CAT, which involves the intraarticular injection of air and contrast material.[2–4] Recently, ultrasonography has been used to visualize areas of increased echogenicity in the rotator cuff.[5–7] Athough the accuracy rate of sonography approaches 90% (similar to conventional arthrography), this technique is operator-dependent and individual tendons cannot be differentiated on sonograms.

Magnetic resonance (MR) imaging of the shoulder offers the advantages of noninvasive direct imaging of the rotator cuff muscles and tendons and of the glenohumeral joint in axial, coronal-oblique, and sagittal planes.[8–13] With its excellent soft tissue and bony discrimination, MR has shown potential in characterizing the spectrum of changes seen in the shoulder impingement syndrome.[14,15] Arthritis, infection, and neoplastic disorders involving shoulder anatomy have also been identified and evaluated with MR.[16]

IMAGING PROTOCOLS FOR THE SHOULDER

Advances in MR imaging of the shoulder have not kept pace with other musculoskeletal areas, in part because of poor surface coil designs and applications. The shoulder girdle presents unique problems in acquiring high-resolution images obtained at small fields of view (FOVs) from a larger anatomic region. Early surface coils were placed posterior to the shoulder and did not provide uniform signal intensity or penetration. New sleeve-shaped surface coils, which conform to the shoulder, permit better signal-to-noise and uniform depth penetration of both the rotator cuff and of the glenohumeral joint (Fig. 6-1). Off axis image capability is required to eliminate the necessity of positioning the shoulder in the center of the magnet.

Aliasing or wrap around artifact is often the limiting factor in image quality when using FOVs of less than 20 cm. Software advances have eliminated phase wrap by allowing the acquisition of data in a 512 × 512 matrix format. Another recent approach uses a transmit coil, separate from the body coil, to selectively excite protons in the limited area of anatomic interest (the transmit coil avoids the aliasing back of information outside the chosen FOV).

High-resolution shoulder imaging is achieved using a dedicated sleeve surface coil, a 256 × 256 acquisition matrix, 16 to 18-cm FOV, two excitations (NEX), and 5-mm slice thickness. Routine protocols for evaluating the rotator cuff and the glenoid labrum begin with an axial plane localizer. Coronal images, obliqued between 25° and 35°, are acquired parallel to the supraspinatus muscle as determined on axial images through the superior shoulder. Images in the coronal-oblique plane are generated with a TR of 1500 msec and a TE of 20 and 60 to 80 msec. The patient's arm is positioned in external rotation to facilitate elongation of the supraspinatus muscle. The glenoid labrum is evaluated with either 3-mm or 5-mm T1-weighted axial images, acquired at a TR of 600 msec and a TE of 20 msec. Sagittal images, optional in rotator cuff examinations, provide another plane in which to evaluate the conjoined insertion of the supraspinatus and intraspinatus tendons. Images, covering the extent of the supraspinatus muscle and tendon in the sagittal direction, are acquired with a TR of 600 msec and a TE of 20 msec.

Evaluation of shoulder neoplasms requires T1- and T2-weighted images in the axial plane to delineate margins; marrow extension; and relationships to adjacent soft tissue, muscle, and neurovascular structures. In extensive lesions or defects, the body coil can be used for a larger FOV and for comparison with the opposite shoulder.

NORMAL MR ANATOMY OF THE SHOULDER

Axial Images

On superior axial images the normal oblique course of the supraspinatus muscle is visualized with intermediate signal intensity (Fig. 6-2). The supraspinatus tendon, from its insertion on the capsule and greater tuberosity (posterior to the bicipital groove) to the supraspinatus fossa of the scapula, is visualized with low signal intensity. Marrow fat of high signal intensity is present in the acromion, localized laterally and parallel to the supraspinatus. At the level of the superior coracoid process,

Figure 6-2
Superior axial image through the shoulder demonstrating intact supraspinatus muscle *(large white arrows)* and low signal intensity tendon *(small white arrows)*. Humeral head *(open black arrow)* and acromion *(flagged arrow)* are identified. T1-weighted image; TR = 600 msec, TE = 20 msec.

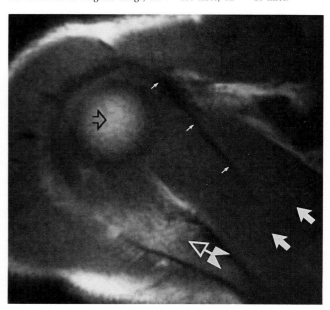

Figure 6-1
Circular sleeve design for dedicated shoulder extremity coil.

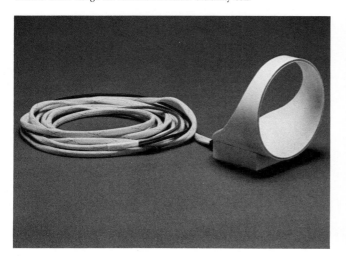

the long axis of the infraspinatus takes origin from the posteroinferior surface of the scapula, crosses the glenohumeral joint posterior to the supraspinatus, and inserts on the lateral aspect of the greater tuberosity. As it approaches the greater tuberosity posterolaterally, the low signal intensity infraspinatus tendon merges with the low signal intensity cortex of the humerus. The spine of the scapula separates the supraspinatus and infraspinatus muscles. The teres minor is visualized posterolateral to the infraspinatus, originating from the axillary border of the scapula to insert on the inferior facet of the greater tuberosity. In cross section, the tendon of the long head of the biceps is seen as a low signal intensity structure within the bicipital groove, sometimes associated with a small amount of high signal intensity fat. At the level of the glenohumeral articulation, inferior to the coracoid, the dark, low spin density fibrocartilaginous labrum is demonstrated (Fig. 6-3). The anterior and posterior labrum should have well-defined triangular shapes. With internal rotation, the anterior labrum is reported to be larger than the posterior. Glenohumeral articular cartilage follows the concave shape of the glenoid cavity and visualizes with intermediate signal intensity. Anterolateral to the glenoid, the subscapularis muscle arises from the subscapular fossa to insert on the lesser tuberosity. The low signal intensity subscapularis tendon can be identified anterior to the apex of the anterior glenoid labrum. The collapsed subacromial-subdeltoid bursa is identified posteriorly, between the infraspinatus and deltoid muscles, and images with the high signal intensity of associated fat.

Coronal Images

In rotator cuff evaluations, the supraspinatus tendon anatomy is best displayed on coronal planar images (Fig. 6-4). On anterior and midcoronal-oblique images, the supraspinatus muscle and its central tendon are visualized in continuity. The low spin density supraspinatus tendon is defined at its insertion on the greater tuberosity. The collapsed subacromial-subdeltoid bursa, interposed between the supraspinatus tendon and the acromion, is surrounded by high signal intensity fat. On anterior coronal images, the subscapularis muscle fibers and multitendinous fibers can be identified converging on the lesser tuberosity. The acromioclavicular joint and coracoclavicular ligaments are also demonstrated on coronal sections. On midcoronal images the belly of the supraspinatus extends laterally to the glenoid before its central tendon emerges to blend with the rotator cuff. On mid- to posterior coronal sections there is a subtle transition between the supraspinatus and conjoined insertion of the infraspinatus tendons. The supraspinatus muscle then assumes a thick elliptical shape, and the

Figure 6-3
Axial image through the glenohumeral joint identifying infraspinatus muscle *(open white arrow)*, infraspinatus tendon *(curved white arrow)*, deltoid muscle *(open black arrow)*, subdeltoid bursa *(straight black arrow)*, biceps tendon *(curved black arrow)*, and fibrocartilage glenoid labrum *(small white arrows)*. T1-weighted image; TR = 600 msec, TE = 20 msec.

Figure 6-4
Intact intermediate signal intensity supraspinatus muscle *(open arrows)* and low signal intensity supraspinatus tendon *(solid arrows)* displayed on T1-weighted coronal image. TR = 800 msec, TE = 20 msec.

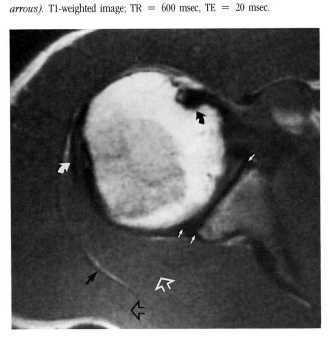

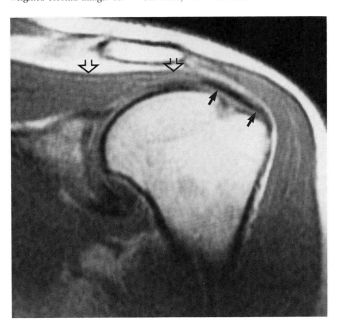

tendon seen lateral to this is from the infraspinatus. On these sections the infraspinatus tendon may be mistaken for the supraspinatus tendon that is now out of the plane of section. Humeral head articular cartilage, intermediate in signal intensity, is interposed between the low signal intensity supraspinatus tendon (superiorly) and cortex (inferiorly).

Sagittal Images

The muscle groups of the deltoid, supraspinatus, infraspinatus, teres minor, teres major, subscapularis, and coracobrachialis are defined on sagittal plane MR images (Fig. 6-5). On mid- and lateral sagittal images the supraspinatus and infraspinatus conjoined cuff tendons are visualized between the acromion and superior articular surface of the humeral head. They image with low signal intensity. The tendon visualized on the anterior half of the sagittal image is that of the supraspinatus, whereas the tendon that arches over the posterior half of the humeral head represents the infraspinatous component. The coracoacromial ligament is seen as a low signal intensity band that arches over the anterior aspect of the rotator cuff, connecting the acromion and coracoid. Medial sagittal sections display the clavicle and acromioclavicular joint in profile. The oblique-transverse oriented physis is also delineated on sagittal images. Marrow inhomogeneity, seen frequently as red to yellow marrow conversion, may not be complete distal to the physis in the metadiaphyseal region. The low signal intensity glenoid labrum is also defined on sagittal images that transect the glenohumeral joint.

THE ROTATOR CUFF AND SHOULDER IMPINGEMENT SYNDROME

The rotator cuff is composed of the supraspinatus, infraspinatus, teres minor, and subscapularis muscles and tendons that fuse with and reinforce the fibrous capsule of the shoulder, providing strength and stability to the joint. Degenerative changes, which develop at the attachment of the tendinous fibers of the rotator cuff, are most prominent in the hypovascular critical zone or in the area near the insertion of the supraspinatus.[15,17,18] The supraspinatus tendon, anatomically confined by bone on both its superior and inferior surfaces, is at risk for injury. Bursal inflammation and tendinitis, promoted by this confinement, may lead to advancing degeneration and precipitation of a tear. Ossification of the rigid coracoacromial ligament (which forms the anterior acromial arch) may contribute to the formation of an acromial spur, further narrowing the subacromial space. This critical area of tendon disintegration is the site of initiation of most tears of the rotator cuff.

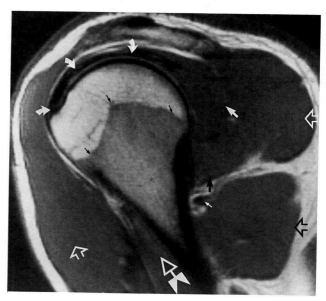

Figure 6-5

Sagittal image identifying low signal intensity supraspinatus tendon *(curved white arrows)*, deltoid muscle *(open white arrow)*, infraspinatus muscle *(large white arrow)*, teres minor *(large black arrow)*, teres major *(open black arrow)*, corachobrachialis *(flagged arrow)*, posterior humeral circumflex artery *(small white arrow)*, and normal physeal division between yellow marrow in the epiphysis and red marrow in the metaphysis *(small black arrows)*. T1-weighted image; TR = 600 msec, TE = 20 msec.

Shoulder Impingement Syndrome

The pathogenesis of rotator cuff tears is thought to involve the *shoulder impingement syndrome.*[15,17–20] There is some controversy as to whether impingement precedes the development of rotator cuff lesions[17,20] or whether primary degeneration of the cuff results in inflammation and secondary impingement. The latter may be more common in professional athletes who place the rotator cuff under repetitive stress.

Neer has developed a three-tier clinical staging system for shoulder impingement that helps to establish indications for surgical treatment of rotator cuff lesions.[15,17,18,20] In this system the pretear impingement lesion represents one end of the spectrum that can culminate in the development of a complete rotator cuff tear. In stage 1 lesions there is edema and hemorrhage within the rotator cuff, and the shoulder responds to conservative management. Stage 2 is characterized by fibrosis and tendinitis. Thickening of the subacromial soft tissues and partial tears may be present in this stage. While most stage 2 lesions respond to conservative management, symptoms (recurrent pain) beyond 6 to 12 months usually indicate the necessity for surgical treatment (an open anterior acromioplasty or arthroscopic decompression of the subacromial space). In stage 3 there is a complete rupture or tear of the rotator cuff that requires an open repair to restore both structure and function.

The spectrum of MR changes in shoulder impingement has also been characterized and documented.[15] Spurs or callus of the inferior margins of the acromion and acromioclavicular joint, hypertrophy of the acromioclavicular joint capsule, and displacement (inferior) of the acromion relative to the distal clavicle have all been identified on MR images (Fig. 6-6). Impingement is classified into three types based on coronal MR images. Type 1 is characterized by the presence of subacromial bursitis which images as thickening of the normally high signal intensity subacromial-subdeltoid bursal line. On T1-weighted images this thickening may visualize with intermediate signal intensity relative to fat

Figure 6-6

Impingement syndrome. A spectrum of minimal *(A)*, mild *(B)*, moderate *(C)*, and severe *(D)* impingement of the supraspinatus muscle/tendon is visualized with callus-osteophyte formation about the acromioclavicular joint *(large curved arrow)*. Reactive edema in the area of tendinitis *(small curved arrow)* is shown with severe impingement *(D)*. Old avulsion *(small arrows)* of greater tuberosity is shown in *(A)*.

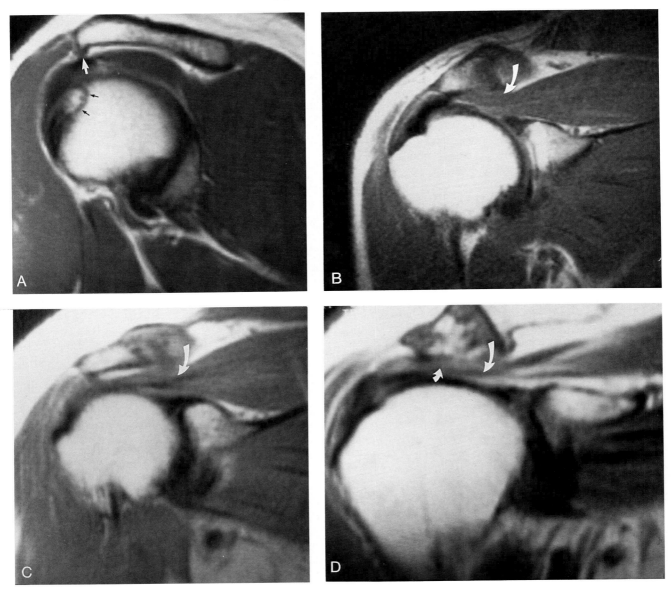

associated with the synovial lining. Signal intensity in the supraspinatus muscle and tendon remains unchanged, intermediate and low, respectively.

In type 2 impingement, signal intensity of the supraspinatus tendon is high on T1-weighted images (Fig. 6-7). Increased or bright signal intensity of the tendon on T2-weighted images represents a type 2b change. Type 3 impingement is characterized by the addition of supraspinatus muscle retraction, with complete disruption of the rotator cuff. Complete tears have been confirmed in type 2 and type 3 lesions. High signal intensity visualized within the supraspinatus tendon on T2-weighted images is thus considered pathognomonic for a cuff tear.

In our experience, either low or high signal intensity, depending on the absence or presence of marrow fat, may be found in subacromial and acromioclavicular spurs. High signal intensity can be demonstrated in areas of the supraspinatus tendon compressed by hypertrophic bone. Further studies are needed to document the importance of the impingement syndrome and to correlate MR findings with the clinical pathogenesis proposed by Neer.

Rotator Cuff Tears

Rotator cuff tears are classified as partial or complete Fig. 6-8).[17,18] Only complete or full thickness tears allow direct communication between the subacromial bursa and the glenohumeral joint (Fig. 6-9). MR has demonstrated potential in identifying rotator cuff tears prior to radiographic detection.[21,22] In a series of 25 patients with either known or suspected rotator cuff tears, MR studies revealed signs consistent with a tear in 20 of 22 patients, with tears confirmed by arthrography or surgery.[22] A tear was judged to be complete if discontinuity of the cuff could be identified (Fig. 6-10).

The coronal plane is the most sensitive for identifying rotator cuff lesions. Rarely is a tear detected only on sagittal planar images, and we studied one patient with a rotator cuff disruption, with complete tearing of the supraspinatus muscle and tendon, which was most accurately displayed on axial planar images (Fig. 6-11). In this patient a posterolateral Hill-Sachs compression fracture was seen, in association with the full-thickness cuff tear.

On T2-weighted images most tears demonstrate increased signal intensity, and partial tears usually exhibit signal characteristics similar to those described for full thickness or complete tears. Complete absence of the rotator cuff also indicates tendinous disruption. T2-weighted images are important in demonstrating areas of bright signal in fluid, granulation tissue, or hypertrophied synovium, all of which have low to intermediate signal intensity on relative T1-weighted images. In contradistinction to arthrographic findings, on MR images

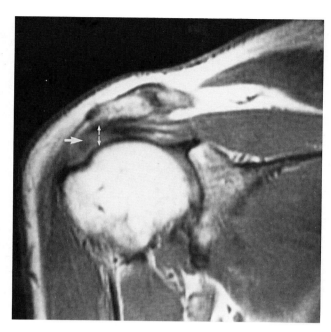

Figure 6-7

Subacromial impingement with decreased subacromial space *(small vertical arrows)* and increased signal intensity in underlying supraspinatus tendon *(large horizontal arrow).* T1-weighted coronal image; TR = 1000 msec, TE = 20 msec.

joint effusions associated with complete rotator cuff tears are not usually seen extending into the subacromial-subdeltoid bursa, superior and lateral to the greater tuberosity.

Secondary signs imaged in rotator cuff tears include supraspinatus muscle atrophy and retraction of the musculotendinous junction medial to the glenoid on coronal-oblique images (Fig. 6-12).[15] A wavy contour may be visualized in torn tendinous fibers. Chronic tears may be more difficult to diagnose if no increased signal intensity is observed on T2-weighted images.

MR imaging has also been used preliminarily to evaluate postoperative *rotator cuff repairs.* Following the theory that impingement leads to tears of the rotator cuff, the procedure of choice should involve an acromioplasty, subacromial decompression, and assessment of the acromioclavicular joint with claviculoplasty.[17] The acromioplasty is required to gain exposure and to repair the torn cuff. Since the supraspinatus frequently tears at its insertion on the greater tuberosity, primary repairs are fixed directly to bone. Only in the presence of extensive acromioclavicular degeneration is a Mumford procedure (resection of the lateral clavicle) performed (Fig. 6-13). Nonabsorbable sutures are used when reattaching the tendon to a raw (bleeding) bone surface. Drill holes in the acromion may provide additional fixation in repairing the deltoid reflected during surgery.

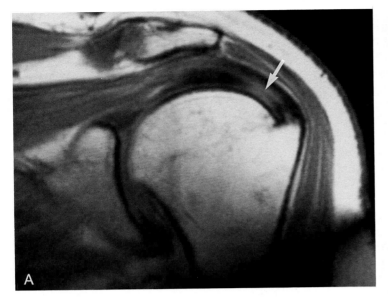

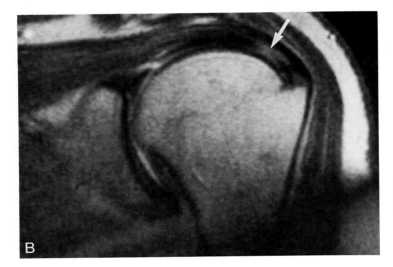

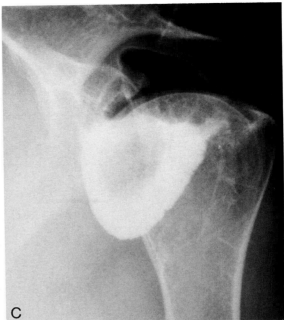

Figure 6-8
Partial rotator cuff tear with tendinitis. Intermediate signal intensity supraspinatus edema *(arrow)* in partial tendon tear is identified on intermediate *(A)* and T2-weighted *(B)* spin echo sequence. TR = 1500 msec, TE = 20, 70 msec. *(C)* Rotator cuff lesion was missed on corresponding double contrast arthrogram (AP view).

Acromial or clavicular resections are satisfactorily displayed on coronal plane images. Drill holes or suture sites are visualized as foci of low signal intensity. T2-weighted images are useful in identifying fluid collec-tions and tears at sites of reattachment (Fig. 6-14). In general, the same criteria used to diagnose tears in the native rotator cuff are used for postsurgical supraspina-tus repairs.

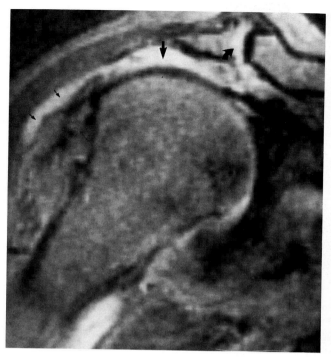

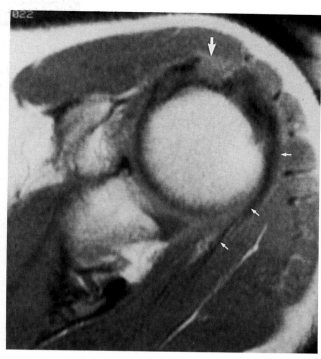

Figure 6-9

Rotator cuff tear with high signal intensity in subacromial-subdeltoid bursa *(straight arrow)* seen tracking lateral and inferior to greater tuberosity *(small arrows)*. Acromioclavicular joint fluid is identified *(curved arrow)*. T2-weighted coronal image; TR = 2000 msec, TE = 60 msec.

Figure 6-10

Infraspinatus tendon tear *(large arrow)* is displayed as an area of intermediate signal intensity on T1-weighted axial image. Intact low signal intensity is identified posterolaterally *(small arrows)*. TR = 600 msec, TE = 20 msec.

Figure 6-11

Rotator cuff tear *(large white arrow)* and Hill-Sachs fracture *(black arrows)* are displayed on superior axial image through the shoulder. Disrupted low signal intensity supraspinatus tendon *(small white arrows)* and intermediate signal intensity joint effusion *(curved white arrow)* are identified. TR = 1500 msec, TE = 40 msec.

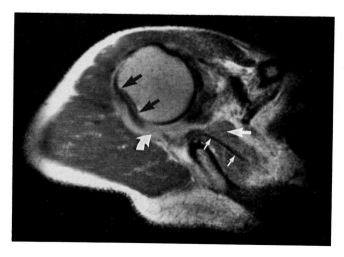

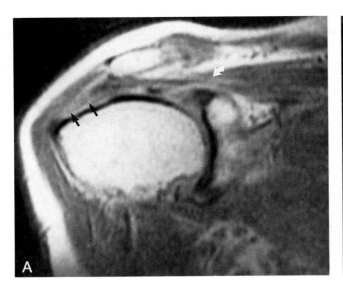

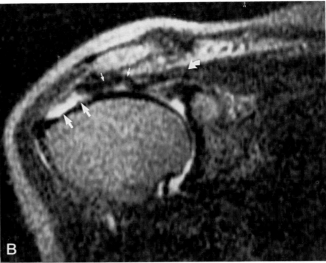

Figure 6-12

Rotator cuff tear. Supraspinatus tendon tear is visualized with intermediate signal intensity *(black arrows)* on proton density (1st echo) weighted image *(A),* and with high signal intensity edema *(large white arrows)* on T2-weighted image *(B).* Retracted supraspinatus muscle *(curved arrow)* and irregular unattached supraspinatus tendon are identified *(small straight arrows in **B**).* TR = 1500 msec, TE = 20, 70 msec.

Figure 6-13

Postsurgical rotator cuff tear. Widened acromioclavicular joint with osteotomy of lateral clavicle *(straight arrow)* and recurrent tear of the supraspinatus *(curved arrow)* are shown on intermediate *(A)* and T2-weighted *(B)* coronal images. TR = 1500 msec, TE = 20, 70 msec.

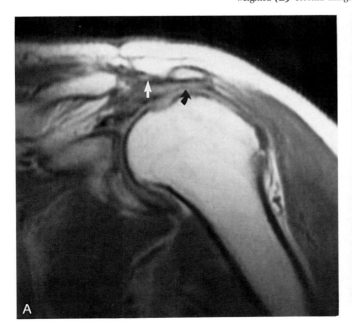

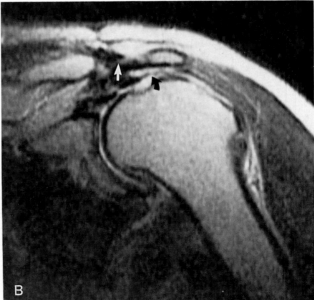

THE GLENOHUMERAL JOINT

The stability of the glenohumeral joint depends on support provided by the rotator cuff, the glenohumeral ligaments, and the fibrocartilaginous glenoid labrum.[23–26] Glenohumeral joint subluxations and dislocations may be associated with Hill-Sachs compression fractures, tears or detachments of the capsular mechanism and la-

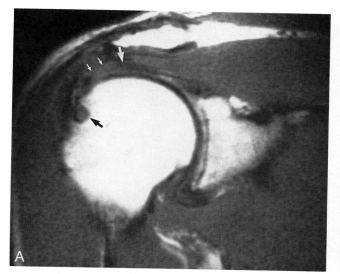

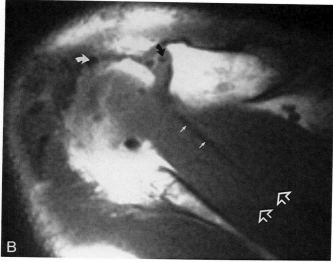

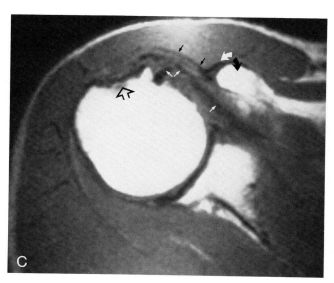

Figure 6-14

(A) Torn rotator cuff repair. Coronal image with increased signal intensity *(small white arrows)* at site of previous primary supraspinatus repair. The transition to normal low signal intensity tendon is indicated *(large white arrow)*. Degenerative cystic change *(black arrow)* is seen in the region of the greater tuberosity. TR = 600 msec, TE = 20 msec. ***(B)*** Superior axial view demonstrating supraspinatus muscle *(double open arrow)*, supraspinatus tendon *(double small straight arrows)*, and low signal intensity suture artifacts anterolaterally *(curved white arrow)* and at osteotomy site *(curved black arrow)*. TR = 600 msec, TE = 20 msec. ***(C)*** Axial image at the level of the coracoid process *(curved black arrow)* showing the overlying low signal intensity tendon of the coracobrachialis-biceps attachment *(curved white arrow)*, distended anterior joint capsule *(small black arrows)*, subscapularis tendon *(small white arrows)*, and postsurgical humeral head defect near site of cuff insertion *(open black arrow)*. TR = 600 msec, TE = 20 msec.

brum, and a large or redundant subscapularis bursa. Computed tomography (CT) air contrast arthrography has been successfully used to identify labral, capsular, and glenohumeral ligament tears in patients with anterior, posterior, or multidirectional instabilities.[2,3,27] Initial MR experience has shown that areas of increased signal intensity within the anterior or posterior labrum correspond to imbibed contrast material seen in CT air contrast arthrography studies.

MR imaging protocol to evaluate the glenoid labrum includes T1-weighted axial images through the glenohumeral joint, using either 3-mm or 5-mm thick sections without an interslice gap. The intact fibrocartilaginous glenoid labrum is low in signal intensity on T1- and T2-weighted images.[10] Large tears and detachments may image with a diffuse increase in signal intensity, whereas discrete tears maintain linear morphology (Fig. 6-15). In two of our patients, anterior labral tears were identified on MR images and later confirmed with CAT and surgery (Fig. 6-16). MR is also sensitive to abnormal labral outlines, identifying regions of blunting or stripping from the underlying bone.

In a series of 35 patients with histories of subluxation or dislocations, axial MR images demonstrated abnormal attenuation or tears of the glenoid labrum in 100% of cases (Fig. 6-17).[28] Intermediate signal intensity in the subscapularis tendon was associated with anterior capsular trauma. Larger, controlled comparisons among MR, CT arthrography, and arthroscopy are needed before MR can replace traditional radiographic evaluation of the glenohumeral joint and capsular mechanism.

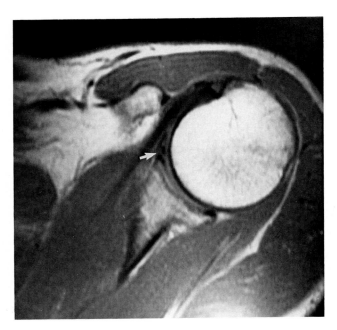

Figure 6-15
Tear of the anterior glenoid labrum visualized as a linear area of high signal intensity *(arrow)* on T1-weighted axial image. TR = 600 msec, TE = 20 msec.

GENERAL PATHOLOGIC CONDITIONS IN THE SHOULDER

Calcific Tendinitis

Calcification in the rotator cuff most commonly occurs in the supraspinatus tendon.[29] These deposits of hydroxyapatite are seen in profile on conventional radiographs with external rotation of the shoulder. Calcifications *(calcium hydroxyapatite crystal deposition)* are thought to form in degenerative muscles or tendons. Although the focus of calcification may remain silent, rupture into the subacromial bursa or adjacent tendon can result in adhesive periarthritis with an acute and painful inflammatory reaction. We have imaged one patient with a low signal intensity calcium deposit localized on coronal MR images of the supraspinatus tendon (Fig. 6-18). No adjacent inflammatory reaction was observed within the critical zone of the supraspinatus.

Arthritis

Primary degenerative osteoarthritis of the glenohumeral joint is not common.[30] Cartilage narrowing, hypertrophic bone, subchondral cysts, and associated soft tissue abnormalities of the rotator cuff or biceps tendon may be associated with this condition (Figs. 6-19 and

Figure 6-16
Labral tear. *(A)* Air contrast CT demonstrating anterior labral tear *(arrow)*. *(B)* Corresponding T1-weighted axial image showing increased signal intensity in labral tear *(white arrows)*. TR = 600 msec, TE = 20 msec.

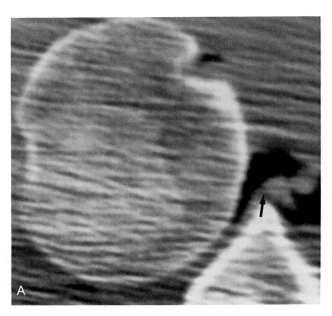

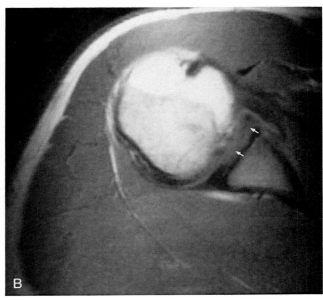

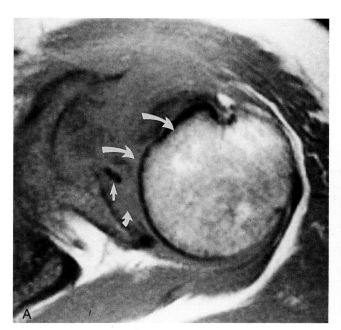
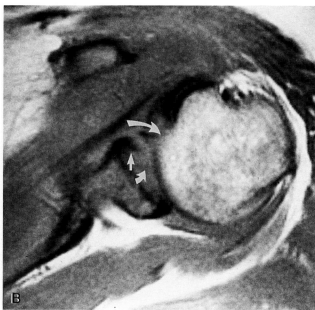

Figure 6-17

(A–B) Posterior subluxation of the humeral head *(large curved arrows)*, glenolabral detachment *(straight arrow)*, and joint effusion *(small curved arrow)* are imaged at the level of the glenohumeral joint in a patient with rheumatoid arthritis. T1-weighted axial images; TR = 600 msec, TE = 20 msec.

Figure 6-18

Calcific tendinitis. *(A)* Calcific density is identified in the region of the greater tuberosity *(arrow)* on AP radiograph. *(B)* On T1-weighted coronal image calcification images with low signal intensity focus *(arrow)* in the supraspinatus-infraspinatus conjoined insertion. TR = 600 msec, TE = 20 msec.

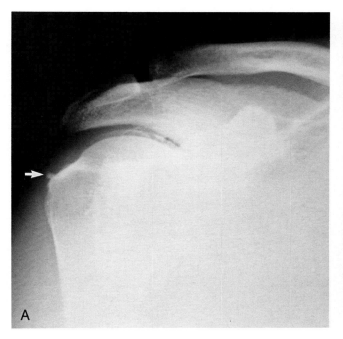
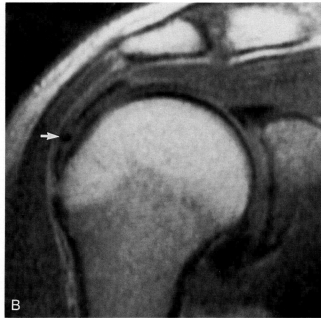

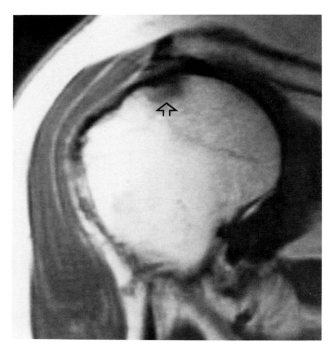

Figure 6-19
Low signal intensity degenerative sclerosis in the superior humeral head *(open arrow)*. T1-weighted coronal image; TR = 600 msec, TE = 20 msec.

6-20). *Secondary osteoarthritis* is seen in younger patients, with an underlying defect in the articular cartilage or humeral head as the initial event in development of joint incongruity. In *rheumatoid disease* of the shoulder, pathologic findings include synovitis and synovial proliferation with destruction of the capsule, rotator cuff, biceps tendon, articular cartilage, and subchondral bone.

Our experience with arthritides about the shoulder is limited. We have observed thinning of the glenohumeral articular cartilage seen in association with labral abnormalities. In a rheumatoid patient, subcortical cysts and low signal intensity sclerosis about the greater tuberosity were imaged. In a series of five rheumatoid patients, MR findings included joint effusions, muscular atrophy, rotator cuff rupture, and synovial cyst formation.[10]

Biceps Tenosynovitis

Bicipital tenosynovitis or inflammation of the biceps tendon synovial sheath can be the result of trauma (e.g., cuff tear), calcific deposition, or infection. The biceps tendon is optimally visualized on axial planar images through the glenohumeral joint. Increased fluid in the biceps sheath, nonspecific for infection, images with low signal intensity on T1-weighted images and with high signal intensity on T2-weighted images (Figs. 6-21 and

Figure 6-20
Degenerative humeral head cyst *(curved arrow)* with low signal intensity on intermediate-weighted axial image *(A),* and with high signal intensity on T2-weighted axial image *(B).* Anterior labral tear is identified *(small arrow).* TR = 1500 msec, TE = 20, 70 msec.

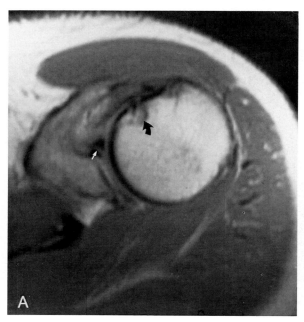

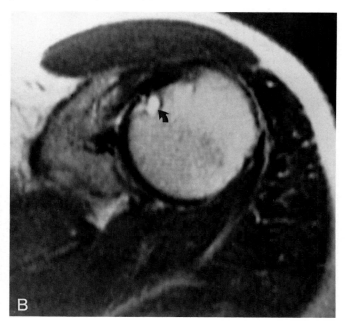

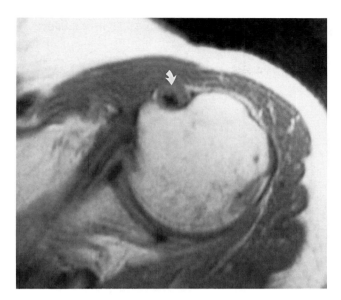

Figure 6-21
Bicipital tendon sheath fluid *(curved arrow)* is visualized as a thickened ring of intermediate signal intensity on T1-weighted axial image. TR = 800 msec, TE = 20 msec.

6-22).[31] Comparison with the opposite shoulder may be useful in assessing the significance of tendon inflammation and associated fluid.

Infection

We have performed MR studies in two cases of staphylococcal *osteomyelitis* involving the shoulder. In one patient, infection was limited to the glenohumeral joint. An extensive joint effusion (purulent debris) was seen and had crossed the rotator cuff into the subacromial-subdeltoid bursa. Subchondral bone involvement, visualized as a low signal intensity focus on T1-weighted images that demonstrated increased signal intensity on T2-weighted images, led to the MR diagnosis (Fig. 6-23). There was additional irregularity and attentuation of overlying articular cartilage and cortex.

A second patient developed an unusual form of multifocal sclerosing osteomyelitis involving the humeral diaphysis. On T2-weighted images proliferative bone and sequestra were visualized with low signal intensity, and adjacent marrow with bright signal intensity.

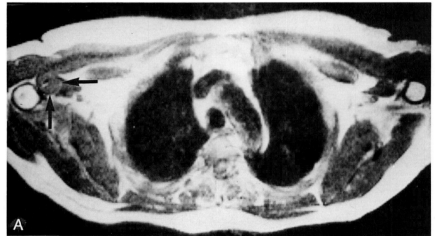

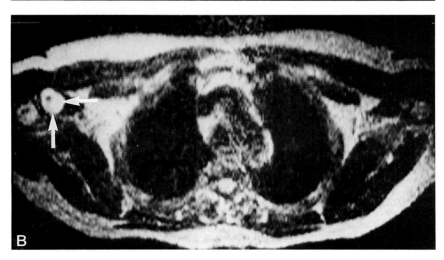

Figure 6-22
Bicipital tenosynovitis shown as low signal intensity thickening *(black arrows)* of the bicipital tendon sheath on T1-weighted axial image *(A)* and as high signal intensity *(white arrows)* on T2-weighted axial images *(B)*. *(A)* TR = 1000 msec, TE = 40 msec; *(B)* TR = 2000 msec, TE = 60 msec.

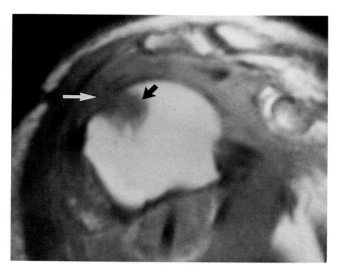

Figure 6-23
Osteomyelitis (staphylococcal) of the right humeral head images as a focus of intermediate signal intensity transgressing cortical and trabecular bone *(black arrow)*. Purulent fluid in the glenohumeral joint and subacromial-subdeltoid bursa obscures rotator cuff insertion *(white arrow)*. T1-weighted image; TR = 1000 msec, TE = 20 msec.

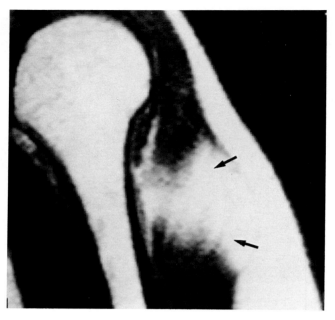

Figure 6-24
High signal intensity lipoma *(arrows)* infiltrating deltoid muscle laterally on T1-weighted coronal image. TR = 500 msec, TE = 31 msec.

Neoplasia

Although there are no tumors specific to the shoulder, there are several MR imaging characteristics of neoplastic disease targeting the shoulder girdle that represents both flat (scapula) and long bone (humerus) structure.[16]

Benign Lesions

Lipomas have the MR signal characteristic of fat and image with bright signal intensity on T1- and T2-weighted images (Fig. 6-24).[32] Deep lipomas occurring in the extremities commonly involve either the shoulder or the thigh. Although intramuscular lipomas are well-defined lesions, we have imaged several that have ill-defined borders and which demonstrate infiltration into adjacent muscle tissue.

Chondroblastomas involve the humerus in 20% of cases, with a 90% involvement of the proximal epiphysis.[33] Low to intermediate signal intensity is observed on T1-weighted images, with increased signal inhomogeneity in uncalcified chondroid tissue on T2-weighted images (Fig. 6-25).

Osteochondromas are metaphyseal tumors frequently involving the long bones—in 20% of cases, the humerus.[33] Scapular exostoses are reported to have an occurrence rate of 4% and usually involve the anterior surface. Osteochondromas involving flat bones may present with a more cauliflowerlike, expansile configuration. On MR examination of osteochondroma of the coracoid in a 14-year-old athlete, the lesion was defined in all planes and associated soft tissue mass was excluded (Fig. 6-26). Athough bony detail was greater on corresponding CT, T2* gradient echo sequences were useful in defining the thickness of the high signal intensity cartilage cap, which may be as thick as 3 cm in adolescents and less than 1 cm in adults.

Malignant Lesions

The tubular bones of the appendicular skeleton are a common site of involvement for *osteosarcoma,* and the humerus is affected in up to 15% of cases.[33] As in other locations, lesions image with low to intermediate signal intensity on T1-weighted images and with bright signal intensity on T2-weighted images.[34] On MR examination of an aggressive, dedifferentiated osteosarcoma involving the proximal humerus of a 24-year-old patient, a necrotic, hemorrhagic fluid-fluid level was imaged within the more distal marrow cavity, a unique feature not detected by corresponding CT (Fig. 6-27). Since these tumors usually occur in children and young adults, they are discussed in more detail in Chapter 2.

Fibrosarcoma is a rare malignant tumor with a fibrous proliferative matrix devoid of cartilage, osteoid, or bone. Fibrosarcoma of bone has a poorer prognosis than primary soft tissue fibrosarcoma.[33] MR imaging characteristics include low signal intensity on T1-weighted images, as a function of histologic differentiation, and uniform high signal intensity on T2-weighted

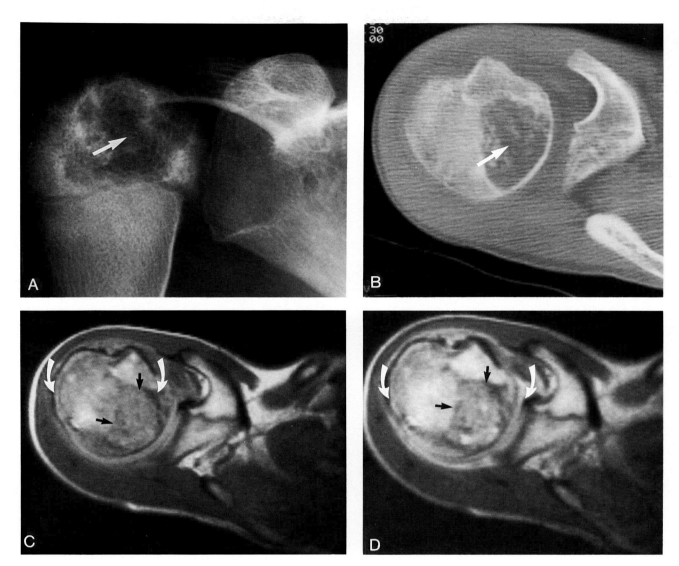

Figure 6-25

Chondroblastoma of the humeral epiphysis is identified as a lytic defect *(arrow)* on AP radiograph *(A)* and axial CT scan *(B)*. Humeral head *(curved white arrows)* cartilage tumor *(straight black arrows)* is visualized as low to intermediate signal intensity on first echo *(C)* and as an inhomogeneous area of mixed signal intensity on second echo *(D)* of T2-weighted sequence. TR = 1500 msec, TE = 20, 60 msec.

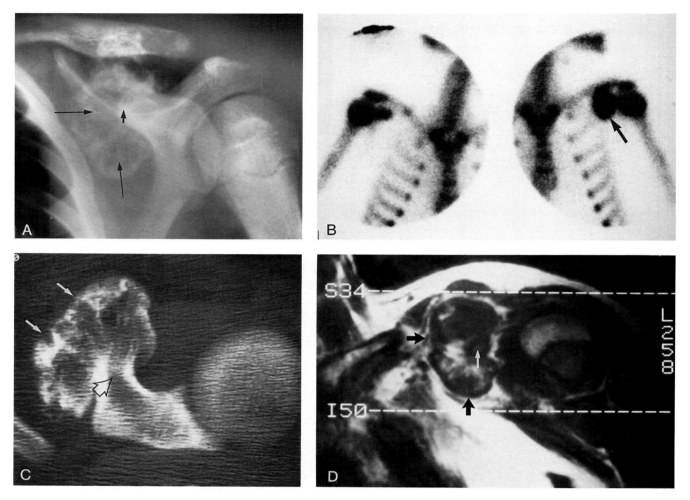

Figure 6-26

Benign osteochondroma. *(A)* Cauliflowerlike bony excrescence *(long arrows)* arising from the coracoid process *(short arrow)* on AP radiograph. *(B)* Increased uptake of bone tracer in region of left coracoid on nuclear scintigraphy *(arrow)*. *(C)* Enlarged cap *(white arrows)* continuous with cortex and spongiosa of adjacent bone *(open arrow)* on axial CT. *(D)* Low signal intensity mass *(black arrows)* emanating from low spin density coracoid *(white arrow)* on T1-weighted coronal image. The cartilage cap is difficult to distinguish from cortex without a T2-weighted pulse sequence.
TR = 600 msec, TE = 20 msec.

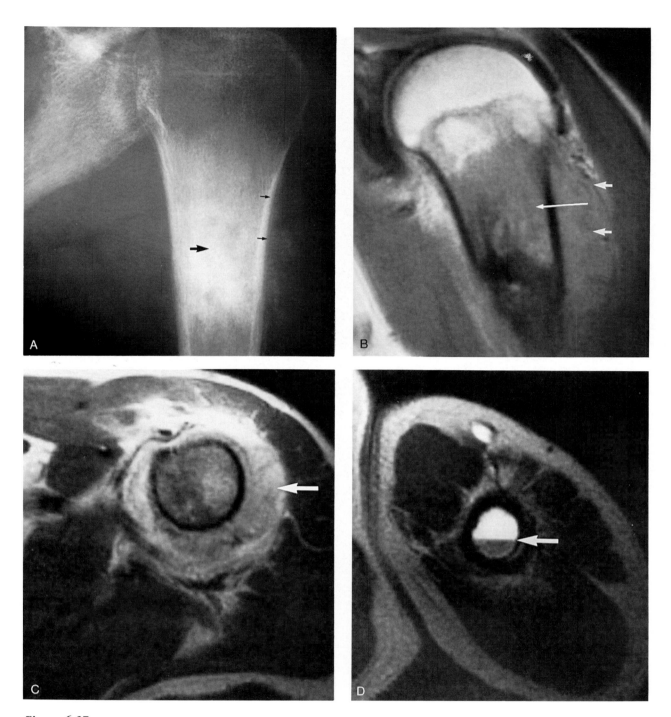

Figure 6-27

Dedifferentiated osteosarcoma involving the proximal humerus. **(A)** AP radiograph with sclerosis *(large arrow)* and aggressive periosteal reaction *(small arrows)*. **(B)** Corresponding T1-weighted coronal image demonstrating soft tissue mass *(short arrows)* and marrow involvement *(long arrow)*. TR = 600 msec, TE = 20 msec. T2-weighted axial images display increased intensity in circumferential soft-tissue component *(arrow)* proximally **(C)** and fluid-fluid level *(arrow)* in area of marrow necrosis distally **(D)**. TR = 2000 msec, TE = 60 msec.

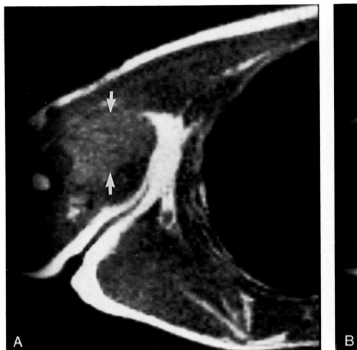 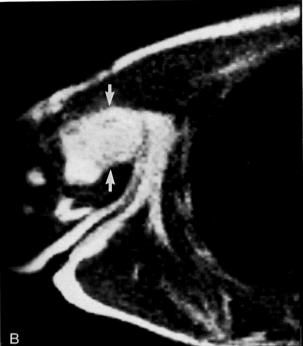

Figure 6-28

Upper arm soft tissue fibrosarcoma *(arrows)* involving the biceps brachii muscle group medially. Tumor visualizes with low signal intensity on T1-weighted axial image **(A)** and with high signal intensity on T2-weighted axial image **(B). (A)** TR = 500 msec, TE = 28 msec; **(B)** TR = 1500 msec, TE = 56 msec.

images (Fig. 6-28). In one case of soft tissue fibrosarcoma involving the upper arm, we were able to identify the lesion without evidence of cortical transgression. The fibrosarcomas that occur in children are different from their adult counterparts. In children tumor occurrence is usually within the first 2 years of life, and the prognosis is more favorable.

PERSPECTIVE ON MR IMAGING OF THE SHOULDER

By providing detailed imaging and identification of the rotator cuff, glenoid, and capsular mechanism of the shoulder, MR offers a noninvasive alternative to conventional radiographic and arthrographic imaging techniques. Individual tendons can be identified on MR images, in contrast to sonograms of the shoulder. Plain film radiography and arthrography may not be sensitive to the spectrum of changes described in the various stages of impingement and rotator cuff pathology. As further documentation becomes available from prospective, controlled studies, MR imaging of the rotator cuff

and labrum will become more routine. With superior contrast resolution and discrimination, MR is particularly well suited for assessing neoplastic disease about the shoulder and upper arm.

REFERENCES

1. Mink JH, Harris E, Rappaport M: Rotator cuff tears: Evaluation using double-contrast shoulder arthrography. Radiology, 157:621, 1985
2. Rafii M, et al: Athlete shoulder injuries: CT arthrographic findings. Radiology, 162:559, 1987
3. Rafii M, et al: CT arthrography of capsular structures of the shoulder. AJR, 146:361
4. Resnik CS: The shoulder. In Scott WW Jr, Magid D, Fishman EK (eds): Contemporary Issues in Computed Tomography—Computed Tomography of the Musculoskeletal System, pp 139–154. New York, Churchill Livingstone, 1987
5. Middleton WE, et al: Sonographic detection of rotator cuff tears. AJR 144:349, 1985
6. Crass JR, Craig EV, Feinberg SB: Sonography of the postoperative rotator cuff. AJR 146:561, 1986

7. Mack LA, et al: US evaluation of the rotator cuff. Radiology, 157:205, 1985

8. Middleton WD, et al: High-resolution MR imaging of the normal rotator cuff. AJR, 148:559, 1987

9. Middleton WD, et al: High resolution surface coil magnetic resonance imaging of the joints: Anatomic correlation. RadioGraphics, 7:645, 1987

10. Kieft GJ, et al: Magnetic resonance imaging of glenohumeral joint diseases. Skeletal Radiol, 16:285, 1987

11. Huber DJ, et al: MR imaging of the normal shoulder. Radiology, 158:405, 1986

12. Seeger LL, et al: MR imaging of the normal shoulder: Anatomic correlation. AJR, 148:83, 1987

13. Kieft GJ, et al: Normal shoulder: MR imaging. Radiology, 159:741, 1986

14. Hardy DC, Vogler JB III, White RH: The shoulder impingement syndrome: Prevalence of radiographic findings and correlation with response to therapy. AJR, 147:557, 1986

15. Seeger LL, et al: Shoulder impingement syndrome: MR findings in 53 shoulders. AJR, 150:343, 1988

16. Zlatkin MB, et al: MR imaging of the shoulder: Spectrum of abnormalities in 65 patients and correlation with arthrography and surgery. Radiology, 165P:148, 1987

17. Brems J: Rotator cuff tear: Evaluation and treatment. Orthopedics, 11:69, 1988

18. Ellman H: Shoulder arthroscopy: Current indications and techniques. Orthopedics, 11:45, 1988

19. Kieft GJ, et al: Rotator cuff impingement syndrome: MR imaging. Radiology, 166:211, 1988

20. Neer CS: Anterior acromioplasty for the chronic impingement syndrome in the shoulder: A preliminary report. J Bone Joint Surg, 54A:41, 1972

21. Kneeland JB, et al: Rotator cuff tears: Preliminary applications of high-resolution MR imaging with counter rotating current loop-gap resonators. Radiology, 160:695, 1986

22. Kneeland JB, et al: MR imaging of the shoulder: Diagnosis of rotator cuff tears. AJR, 149:333, 1987

23. Goss TP: Anterior glenohumeral instability. Orthopedics, 11:87, 1988

24. Hawkins RJ, McCormack RG: Posterior shoulder instability. Orthopedics, 11:101, 1988

25. Arendt EA: Multidirectional shoulder instability. Orthopedics, 11:113, 1988

26. Zlatkin MB, et al: Cross-sectional imaging of the capsular mechanism of the glenohumeral joint. AJR, 150:151, 1988

27. Singson RD, Feldman F, Bigliani L: CT arthrographic patterns in recurrent glenohumeral instability. AJR, 149:749, 1987

28. Seeger LL, et al: MR imaging of shoulder instability. Radiology, 165P:148, 1987

29. Resnick D, Niwayama, G: Diagnosis of Bone and Joint Disorders, 2nd ed, chapter 49. Philadelphia, WB Saunders, 1988

30. Kerr R, et al: Osteoarthritis of the glenohumeral joint: A radiologic-pathologic study. AJR, 144:967, 1985

31. Beltran J, et al: Tendons: high-field-strength, surface coil MR imaging. Radiology, 162:735, 1987

32. Petasnick JP, et al: Soft-tissue masses of the locomotor system: Comparison of MR imaging with CT. Radiology, 160:125, 1986

33. Resnick D, Niwayama G: Diagnosis of Bone and Joint Disorders, 2nd ed, vol 6, chapter 91. Philadelphia, WB Saunders, 1988

34. Sundaram M, McGuire MH, Herbold DR: Magnetic resonance imaging of osteosarcoma. Skeletal Radiol, 16:23, 1987

David W. Stoller

Chapter 7 THE HAND, WRIST, AND ELBOW

Interest in the wrist and its pathology has grown enormously in recent years. An increasing number of papers has been devoted to this topic at annual meetings of the American Society for Surgery of the Hand, and an entire conference on "wrist instability" was held in 1986. Many specific ligamentous injuries, which lead to a myriad of instability patterns, have been described, and the diagnosis of "wrist sprain" is now considered too general and of little practical use.

Conventional radiographic evaluation of the hand, wrist, and elbow joints is restricted primarily to dem-

onstrating osseous structures. When the pathologic process can be localized, select views, such as the scaphoid and carpal tunnel view, may provide additional information. Arthrography, an invasive technique, has been used to evaluate articular cartilage, synovium, ligamentous integrity, and the status of the triangular fibrocartilage in patients with posttraumatic wrist pain.[1-3] Elbow arthrography has been performed to evaluate loose bodies, articular cartilage, and synovium.[4] Computed tomography (CT) has limited application in the study of the carpal tunnel and of nonbony structures about the hand

and wrist, and cannot optimally resolve subtle differences in closely related soft tissue attenuation values. Ultrasound has been used to study the gross motion of tendons in the carpal tunnel during flexion and extension.[5] Fluoroscopic or cine CT study of wrist biomechanics may give indirect evidence of pathology in tendons, ligaments, and cartilage, without direct visualization of these structures.

With a surface coil, magnetic resonance (MR) imaging can provide the high spatial and contrast resolution of both soft tissue and osseous components needed for evaluation of the small and complex anatomy in the articulations of the forearm (hand, wrist, and elbow).[6–11] MR can provide high-resolution images of muscles, ligaments, tendons, tendon sheaths, vessels, nerves, marrow, and cortical bone at small fields of view (FOVs) with uniform depth penetration. Thin section, nonorthogonal (multiplanar) images permit direct anatomic and pathologic discrimination in axial, coronal, sagittal, and oblique planes, without the delayed reconstructions or reformatting necessary for CT. In the wrist and hand, MR has shown application in the study of avascular necrosis; trauma (fracture); ligament, tendon, and cartilage abnormalities; carpal tunnel syndrome; arthritis; infection; and neoplasia.

IMAGING PROTOCOLS FOR THE HAND, WRIST, AND ELBOW

The hand, wrist, and elbow are imaged using a dedicated surface or extremity coil to optimize signal-to-noise in obtaining high spatial resolution images (0.31 × 0.31 pixels to 0.47 × 0.47 pixels; Fig. 7-1). T1-weighted images, obtained routinely in the axial and coronal planes and optimally in the sagittal plane, are acquired with a repetition time (TR) of 600 msec and an echo time (TE) of 20 to 25 msec. Thin (5 mm) slices at a 256 × 256 acquisition matrix are preferred. At an 8 to 10-cm FOV, two signal averages (NEX) provide excellent signal-to-noise ratios (SNRs) while larger FOVs (12 to 16 cm) can be acquired with only one NEX. A larger FOV is useful when greater anatomic coverage is required.

If T2-weighted sequences are needed, they are acquired using the orthogonal plane, best suited to display the area of pathologic interest. Spin echo T2-weighted images are generated with a TR of 1500 to 2000 msec and a TE of 20 and 60 to 80 msec. Gradient echo effective T2- (T2*)-weighted fast scan images can be substituted for conventional spin echo T2-weighted images. These scans are obtained using a TR of 400 msec, a TE of 30 msec, and theta flip angle of 30° (< 90°).

Patient positioning for studies of the hand, wrist, and elbow depends on the design of the surface coil used. The patient is either prone, with the arm outstretched and supinated, or is supine, with the upper extremity supinated at the patient's side. The axial sequence is acquired first and is used to localize landmarks for the coronal and sagittal images.

When high spatial resolution (and therefore a smaller FOV) is required, comparison with the contralateral extremity is performed in separate acquisitions. If only gross anatomic pathology needs to be visualized, a larger FOV will suffice and both hands can be placed in the same coil.

NORMAL MR ANATOMY OF THE HAND, WRIST, AND ELBOW

Hand and Wrist

Axial Images

In the axial plane, the flexor digitorum superficialis and profundus muscles are visualized as tubular structures, of low signal intensity that invest the synovial sheaths and image with intermediate signal intensity (Fig. 7-2). The thin flexor retinaculum, spanning the palmar border of the carpal tunnel, images with low signal intensity (Fig. 7-3). Its distal attachments to the hook of the hamate and tubercle of the trapezium are more reliably defined than the proximal attachments to the tubercles of the pisiform and scaphoid. Dorsally, the low spin density extensor tendons are visualized deep to the extensor retinaculum. On proximal sections, the flexor pollicis longus can be identified deep to the median nerve. Distally it is flanked by the adductor pollicis medially and by the thenar muscles laterally toward the

Figure 7-1

Circular extremity coil for use in imaging the hand, wrist, or elbow.

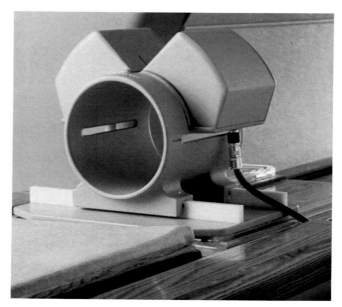

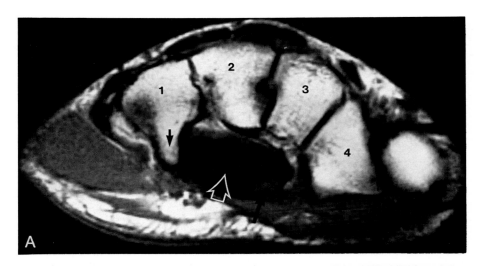

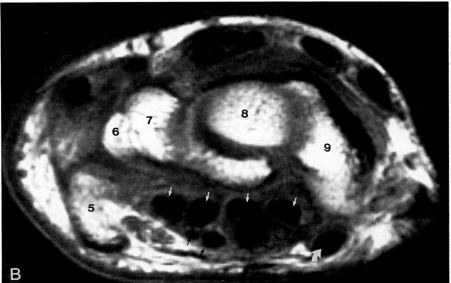

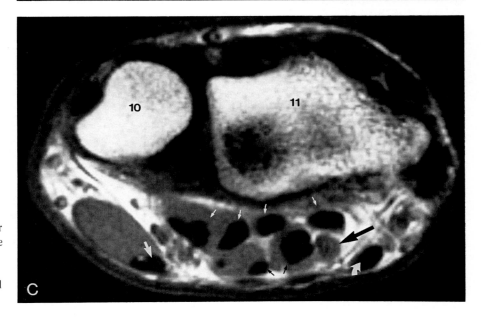

Figure 7-2

Axial anatomy of the wrist: Hamate *(1)*, capitate *(2)*, trapezoid *(3)*, trapezium *(4)*, pisiform *(5)*, triquetrium *(6)*, lunate *(7)*, scaphoid *(8)*, styloid process of radius *(9)*, ulna *(10)*, radius *(11)*. Flexor tendons *(open arrow)*, median nerve *(large black arrow)*, hook of hamate *(medium black arrow)*, flexor digitorum profundus tendons *(small white arrows)*, flexor digitorum superficialis tendons *(small black arrows)*, flexor carpi ulnaris tendon *(large white arrow)*, and flexor carpi radialis tendon *(curved white arrow)* are identified. T1-weighted images; TR = 600 msec, TE = 20 msec. *(A)* At distal carpal row. *(B)* At proximal carpal row. *(C)* At distal radial-ulna.

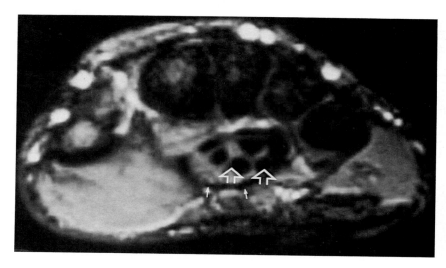

Figure 7-3

Low-spin density flexor tendons *(open arrows)* image deep to the flexor retinaculum *(small arrows)* on T2* gradient recall axial image. TR = 400 msec, TE = 30 msec; flip angle = 30°.

thumb. The two central tendons of the superficial flexor group are located superiorly within the carpal tunnel, before fanning out to their insertions on the middle phalanx. Definition of the four separate tendons of the

Figure 7-4

Sagittal image identifying low signal intensity flexor digitorum superficialis *(small white arrow)* and flexor digitorum profundus *(large white arrow)* tendons in profile. Capitate *(1)*, lunate *(2)*, distal radius *(3)*. TR = 600 msec, TE = 20 msec.

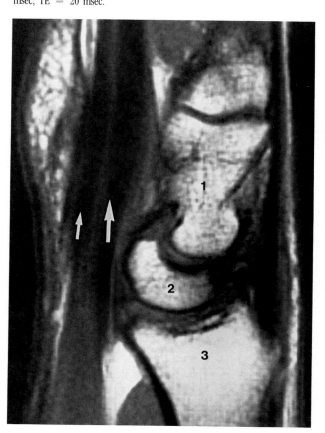

flexor profundus group is possible on axial planar images. In axial sections through the distal carpal tunnel, the lumbrical muscle origins are seen deep to the flexor tendons and image with intermediate signal intensity. The median nerve can be identified in the superficial radial aspect of the carpal tunnel, imaging with intermediate signal intensity. In axial images through the midmetacarpals, the flexor tendons are seen anterior to the ventral interosseii muscles, whereas the dorsal interosseii are identified lying between the metacarpal bones.

Blood vessels image with low signal intensity, except in venous structures demonstrating even echo rephasing or paradoxical enhancement secondary to slow flow. By using gradient echo techniques, both arterial and venous structures can be imaged with high signal intensity.

Sagittal Images

The sagittal imaging plane has not been used extensively for MR evaluations of the wrist (Fig. 7-4). In the hand and digits, however, parasagittal sections display the separate insertions of the flexor digitorum superficialis tendons on the middle phalanx and the profundus tendons on the distal phalanx. Abnormalities of metacarpal or phalangeal joint alignment, as well as capsular anatomy, can be assessed on sagittal plane images.

Coronal Images

Coronal plane images are important in understanding the relationship between cartilage and ligamentous structures of the wrist. On coronal images the triangular fibrocartilage is visualized as a curvilinear "bow-tie" band of low, homogeneous signal intensity (Fig. 7-5). The band extends horizontally to the base of the ulnar styloid process from the ulnar surface of the distal radius. Differentiation of the triangular fibrocartilage from the adjacent meniscus, which often prevents communication between the radiocarpal and the pisiform-triquetral compartments, may not be possible.

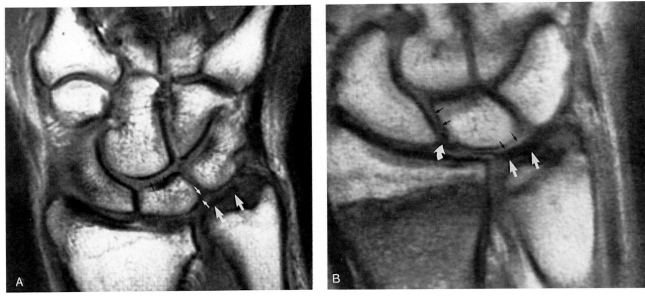

Figure 7-5
Coronal images of normal wrists demonstrating intact low signal intensity triangular fibrocartilage *(large white arrows)* and intermediate signal intensity hyaline articular cartilage of the carpal bones *(black arrows)*. Scapholunate *(curved white arrow)* and lunatotriquetral *(small white arrows)* interosseous ligaments are identified. T1-weighted images; TR = 600 msec, TE = 20 msec. *(A)* 10-cm FOV. *(B)* 8-cm FOV.

Figure 7-6
Volar coronal anatomy. *(A)* Normal anatomy of low signal intensity flexor tendon *(large arrow)* and intermediate signal intensity palmar aponeurosis *(small arrows)* distal to carpal tunnel. T1-weighted coronal image; TR = 600 msec, TE = 20 msec. *(B)* Low signal intensity flexor tendons *(small white arrows)* passing through carpal tunnel. Trapezium *(large white arrow)* and pisiform *(black arrow)* are visualized. T1-weighted image; TR = 600 msec, TE = 20 msec.

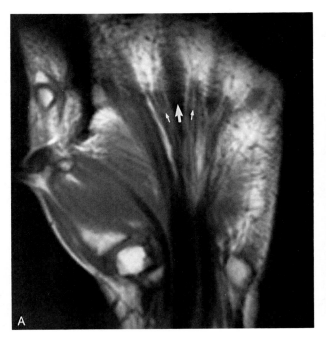

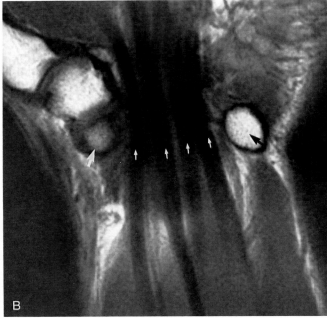

The inferior radioulnar joint, demarcated from the radiocarpal compartment by the triangular fibrocartilage, is well defined in the coronal plane. The scapholunate interosseous ligament images with low signal intensity and, in our experience, has been identified intact in over 50% of T1-weighted coronal images of the wrist. The lunatotriquetral ligament has been less satisfactorily imaged in the coronal plane. On T2-weighted images, conventional spin echo or gradient echo, the interosseous ligaments image with low signal intensity and are contrasted with the high intensity signal of surrounding fluid.

On images of the volar aspect of the wrist, the low signal intensity bands of the flexor digitorum tendons are seen en face, passing through the carpal tunnel between the hook of the hamate and the trapezium (Fig. 7-6). The intermediate signal of the median nerve may also be discerned in this plane of section. The cartilage surfaces of the carpal bones image with intermediate signal intensity and may be seen between the proximal and distal carpal rows on high resolution images by using a small (8 to 12-cm) FOV.

Detailed venous anatomy can be traced on superficial coronal images on either volar or dorsal surfaces of the hand (Fig. 7-7). The dorsal interosseii muscles are demonstrated between the metacarpal shafts.

Anatomic Variants

In the wrist, the lumbrical muscles, which are attached to the profundus tendons, may appear contiguous with both the superficialis and profundus groups.[12] Partial flexion of the digits can pull the proximal lumbricals into the carpal tunnel and may mimic synovial thickening on axial images. A persistent median artery and aberrant course of the medial nerve have also been observed on MR images through the wrist. Partial voluming effects may simulate inhomogeneities or defects in the triangular fibrocartilage and scapholunate ligament.

Elbow

Axial Images

Axial scans best display the anatomic relationship of the superior radioulnar joint (Fig. 7-8) and elbow joint proper (Fig. 7-9). The radial nerve, of intermediate signal intensity, is interposed between the brachioradialis muscle and the brachialis muscle medially. The ulnar

Figure 7-7
Venous signal enhancement *(arrows)* in basilic tributary on T2* gradient echo coronal image. TR = 400 msec, TE = 30 msec; flip angle = 30°.

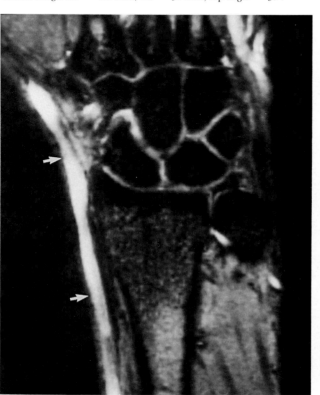

Figure 7-8
Proximal radiolunar joint. Low signal intensity bands of the annular ligament are visualized encircling the radial head *(white arrows)*. Radioulnar joint hyaline cartilage demonstrates intermediate signal intensity *(small black arrows)*. Radial head *(large straight arrow)* and ulna *(curved arrow)* are identified. T1-weighted axial image; TR = 600 msec, TE = 20 msec.

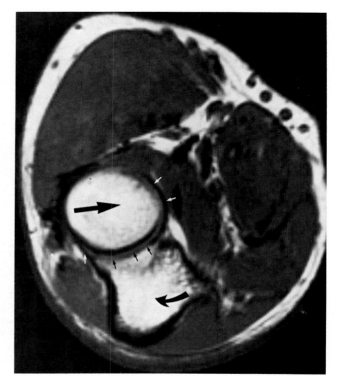

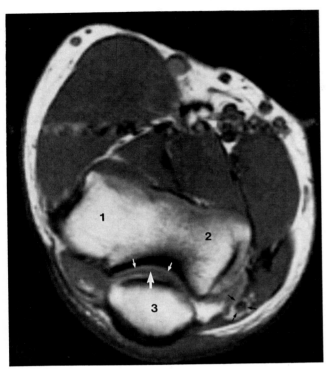

Figure 7-9

Normal anatomy of the elbow joint *(large white arrow)* with intermediate signal intensity hyaline articular cartilage *(small white arrows)*. The ulnar nerve *(small black arrows)* is seen posterolaterally. Capitellum *(1)*, trochlea *(2)*, olecranon *(3)*. T1-weighted axial image; TR = 600 msec, TE = 20 msec.

nerve is of similar signal intensity, and is identified posteromedial to the semilunar incisura (posterior to the medial epicondyle). The radial head should be positioned within the concave semilunar notch of the ulna. The thin, annular ligament, which secures the head of the radius and images with low signal intensity, can be differentiated from adjacent articular cartilage of the radial head, which images with intermediate signal intensity.

The brachialis as well as the biceps muscles, tendon, and aponeurosis are optimally imaged on axial sections. The lateral and medial muscle groups can be separated on paraaxial images through the elbow joint. The brachial artery is visualized as an area of signal void medial to the biceps and superficial to the brachialis muscles. Just distal to the elbow joint, the brachial artery can be seen to divide into radial and ulnar branches.

Sagittal Images

Two of the three joints of the elbow—the trochlear-ulnar and the capitellar-radial articulations—are defined on medial and lateral sagittal images, respectively (Fig. 7-10). The conjoined insertion of the triceps muscle is visualized with low signal intensity at its attachment to the posterosuperior surface of the olecranon. The anconeus muscle, which extends from the medial epicondyle to the posterolateral olecranon, can be visualized on either sagittal or axial images. The biceps and brachialis muscle groups are visualized in long axis on sagittal images. The biceps tendon (superior to the muscle proper) is particularly well delineated on sagittal images. The anterior and posterior fat pads are identified

Figure 7-10

Normal parasagittal anatomy of the elbow: olecranon apophysis (cartilage; *1)*, coronal process *(2)*, trochlea (cartilage; *3)*, anterior fat pad *(4)*, posterior fat pad *(5)*, biceps *(6)*, proximal radius *(7)*. Biceps tendon *(white arrows)* and triceps tendon *(black arrows)* are identified.

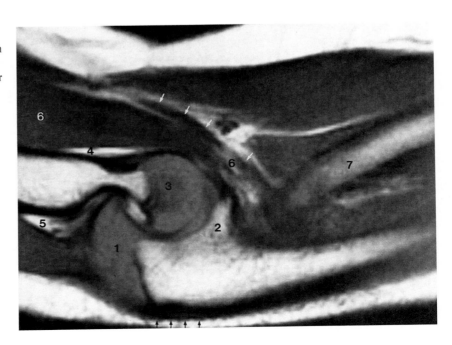

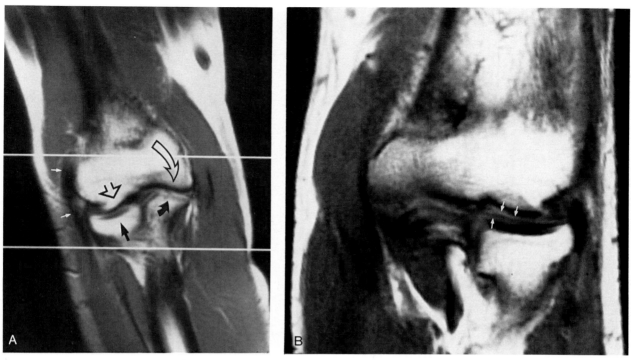

Figure 7-11
Coronal anatomy. **(A)** Normal coronal anatomy identifying capitellum *(straight open arrow)*, trochlea *(curved open arrow)*, radial head *(solid straight arrow)*, coranoid process *(solid curved arrow)*, and low signal intensity lateral collateral ligament *(small white arrows)*. T1-weighted image; TR = 800 msec, TE = 20 msec. **(B)** Intermediate signal intensity hyaline articular cartilage on radial head *(single arrow)* and opposing capitellum *(double arrows)*.

as high signal intensity bands, proximal to the trochlea, in the coronoid and olecranon fossae, respectively. The hyaline articular cartilage of the radial head-capitellum articulation and the trochlear-olecranon joints is displayed with intermediate signal intensity on sagittal images through the elbow. In the immature skeleton, cartilage thickness is especially prominent in the unfused apophysis.

Coronal Images

The trochlear-ulnar and capitellar-radial head joints can be visualized on the same coronal image through the elbow (Fig. 7-11). Articular cartilage of intermediate signal intensity and medial and lateral collateral ligaments of low signal intensity are also well defined in the coronal plane. The anatomy of the radial head and the physeal plates or scars is also shown in this plane of section. The pronator teres and extensor carpi radialis muscles flank the medial and lateral articulations of the elbow, respectively. Posteriorly, the olecranon fossa may be visualized bordered by a semicircular region of low signal intensity. On midjoint coronal images, the biceps and supinator muscles are identified inferior to the capitellum and radial head. The ulnar nerve, as it courses posterior and distal to the medial epicondyle of the humerus, images with intermediate signal intensity and can be differentiated from the adjacent flexor carpi ulnaris muscle by the high signal intensity of encasing perineural fat.

Anatomic Variants

In the elbow, anatomic structures may be more discernable when imaged in varying degrees of elbow flexion.[10,11] A transverse line of low to intermediate signal intensity in the articular surface of the radial head represents a partial volume artifact, and not a fracture. This can be confirmed by imaging of the contralateral elbow.

PATHOLOGY IN THE HAND, WRIST, AND ELBOW

Avascular Necrosis

Avascular necrosis (AVN) in the wrist primarily affects the scaphoid bone in posttraumatic cases and the lunate bone in Kienböck's disease (lunatomalacia).[9,13] Most

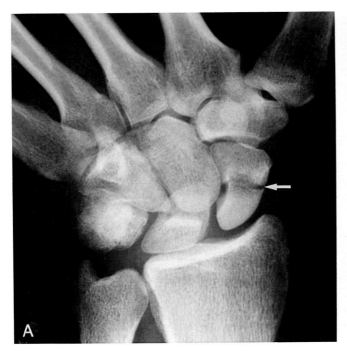
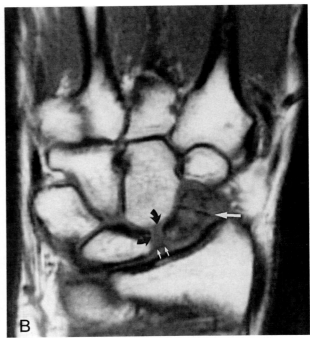

Figure 7-12

Scaphoid fracture *(arrow)* with avascular necrosis (AVN). *(A)* AP radiograph with scaphoid wrist fracture. No sclerosis is demonstrated in proximal or distal fragments. *(B)* Corresponding T1-weighted coronal image with low signal intensity necrotic marrow in both proximal and distal scaphoid poles. Low signal intensity scapholunate ligament *(small white arrows)* and fluid in widened scapholunate space *(curved arrows)* are indicated. TR = 600 msec, TE = 20 msec.

scaphoid fractures of the proximal one third, and up to 33% of fractures of the middle one third ("waist" fractures), are associated with AVN (Fig. 7-12). Nondisplaced fractures may be missed on conventional radiographs, and detection of sclerosis at the fracture site may not be apparent on plain films for as long as 2 weeks after the initial insult. Kienböck's disease of the lunate, especially in the early stages of vascular compromise, is also particularly difficult to detect by standard radiologic methods. The changes of sclerosis, resorption, and collapse, as demonstrated by plain radiographs, represent an advanced stage of the disease.

The application of MR imaging to the detection and evaluation of avascular necrosis in the wrist is facilitated by the normally bright signal generated from the yellow marrow of the carpal bones. Abnormal areas of decreased marrow signal intensity can be associated with AVN. MR has been reported to be as sensitive as bone scintigraphy in the detection of AVN, and to possess even greater specificity in diagnosis.[14,15] Using a short TR/TE sequence, MR sensitivity rates for the detection of decreased marrow signal associated with AVN are 87.5%. With the addition of T2-weighted sequences, specificity is reported to be 100%. In contrast, specificity for bone scintigraphy may be as low as 18.2%.

Early MR detection of both AVN of the scaphoid and in Kienböck's disease has been documented in cases with negative radiographs. Although nuclear scintigraphy may be a satisfactory screening tool, the poor specificity and limited spatial resolution provided may not be sufficient for early detection and precise anatomic localization of disease.

The most common imaging pattern in AVN of the scaphoid is low signal intensity in the proximal pole on both T1- and T2-weighted images. In cases of diffuse necrosis, low signal intensity marrow may not be restricted to the proximal pole of the scaphoid. In addition, in the literature and in our own experience, early cases of AVN have been identified that show evidence of T2 prolongation, usually secondary to associated marrow edema or associated fluid (Fig. 7-13). On heavily T2-weighted sequences, therefore, high-signal intensity will sometimes be seen.

It is possible that early marrow edema (which images with low signal intensity on T1-weighted sequences) may be confused with AVN in a patient who has sustained traumatic fracture. With marrow edema, however, a diffuse increase in signal intensity should be evident on T2-weighted sequences; a pattern not reported with AVN in the literature to date.

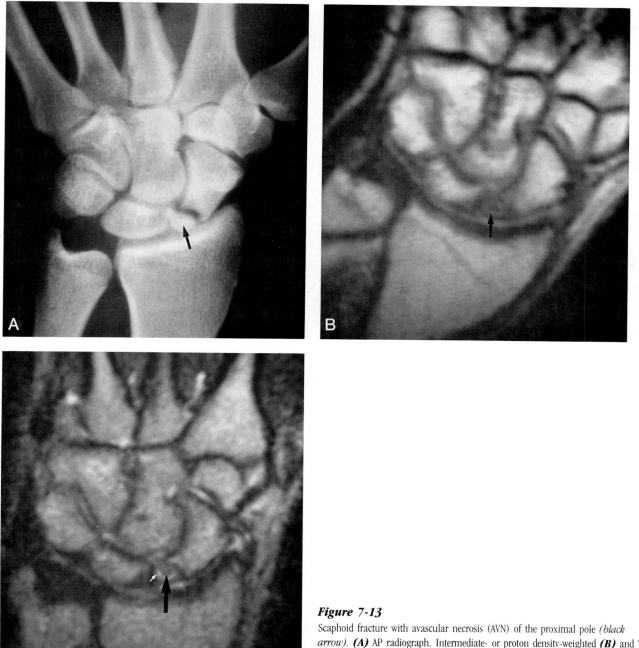

Figure 7-13
Scaphoid fracture with avascular necrosis (AVN) of the proximal pole *(black arrow)*. *(A)* AP radiograph. Intermediate- or proton density-weighted *(B)* and T2-weighted *(C)* images. Necrotic segment remains low in signal intensity on T2-weighted image except for peripheral rim of edema *(small white arrow)*. TR = 1500 msec, TE = 20, 60 msec.

In three of the five cases of Kienböck's disease we have studied, disruption of the scapholunate ligament could be identified on both T1- and T2-weighted images (Fig. 7-14).

Our experience with AVN in the elbow is restricted to a single case of Panner's disease in the capitellum of the humerus. Although radiographs appeared normal, MR images revealed abnormal, low signal intensity marrow.

Nonscaphoid Fracture about the Wrist

Nonscaphoid fractures about the wrist have not been associated with significant marrow edema. In a case report

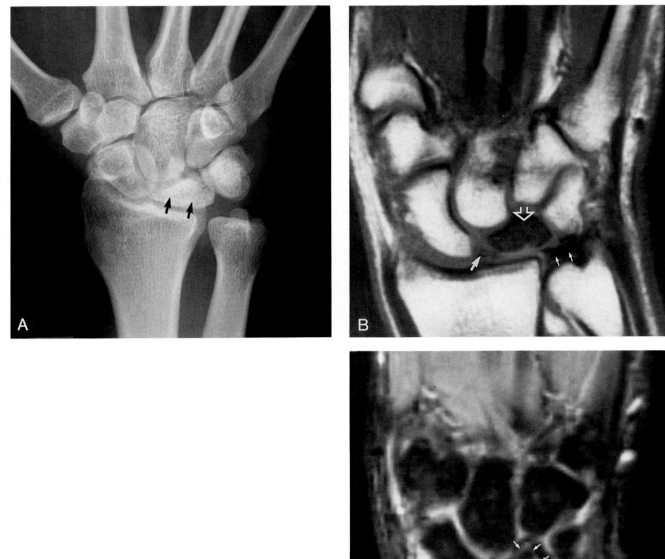

Figure 7-14

Kienböck disease. *(A)* AP radiograph displaying sclerosis and collapse of lunate *(arrow)*, associated with negative ulnar variance. *(B)* Corresponding T1-weighted coronal image identifying low-signal intensity necrotic lunate *(open arrow)* and disrupted scapholunate ligament *(large white arrow)*. Intact triangular fibrocartilage is identified *(small white arrows)*. TR = 600 msec, TE = 20 msec. *(C)* T2* gradient echo coronal image demonstrating free fragment *(large solid arrow)* and edema *(small arrows)* associated with necrotic lunate *(open arrow)*.

of a subacute fracture of the hamate with negative radiography and positive bone scintigraphy, the fracture fragment was detected on MR as a linear area of low signal intensity with preservation of high signal intensity marrow fat in the fractured segment. In a chronic fracture of the distal radius with intraarticular extension, the low signal intensity site of cortical and trabecular disruption—corresponding to linear sclerosis on conventional radiography—was clearly delineated on MR. Frac-

tures of the radiocarpal joint have been associated with linear areas of intermediate signal intensity in ruptured radioulnar ligaments.

Carpal Tunnel Syndrome

Impairment of motor or sensory function of the median nerve as it transgresses the carpal tunnel (carpal tunnel syndrome) may be caused by fractures and dislocations about the wrist, intraneural hemorrhage, infection, infiltrative disease, and various soft tissue injuries. Distal radial fractures may also contribute to the development of an acute carpal tunnel syndrome. If the neuropraxia does not respond to a course of conservative immobilization, surgical exploration may be necessary.

Early detection of the cause of carpal tunnel syndrome requires soft tissue discrimination not possible with standard radiographs or CT. Axial and coronal MR imaging of the wrist, however, has shown potential for evaluating patients with clinical presentations of median nerve deficits (Fig. 7-15).[12,15] In a series of six patients with carpal tunnel syndrome, MR studies of three showed diffuse swelling of the median nerve, whereas the remaining three showed segmental enlargement at

the level of the pisiform bone. In a case of postpartum carpal tunnel syndrome, there was increased signal intensity demonstrated on T2-weighted images through the median nerve. In two patients, fibrous proliferation (imaging with low signal intensity) surrounding the median nerve and thickened synovial tendon sheaths were identified.

Up to two thirds of patients with carpal tunnel syndrome have bilateral involvement, rendering comparison with the contralateral wrist for normal anatomy misleading. A persistent median artery has been postulated to predispose to carpal tunnel syndrome, and in one patient with signs of median nerve compression, a benign tumor of the wrist—a fibrolipoma—was noted. The relatively rare finding of thinning of the median

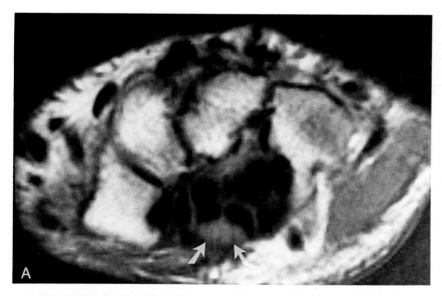

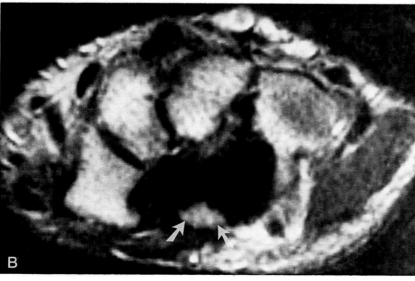

Figure 7-15

Carpal tunnel syndrome. Enlarged and edematous median nerve *(arrows)* is visualized as intermediate signal intensity on intermediate-weighted *(A)* and high signal intensity on T2-weighted *(B)* images. Axial images: TR = 1500 msec, TE = 20, 80 msec.

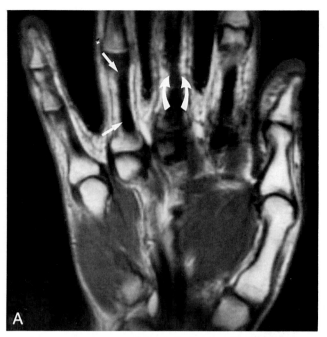

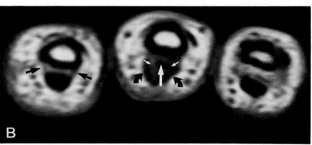

Figure 7-16

Intact flexor tendon repair. **(A)** Attentuated low signal intensity flexor tendon at site of primary surgical repair *(curved arrows)*. Normal contour of uninvolved flexor tendon is shown for comparison *(straight arrows)*. T1-weighted cornal image; TR = 600 msec, TE = 20 msec. **(B)** Corresponding axial image demonstrating central low signal intensity flexor digitorum profundus *(large white arrow)* and the dividing tendons of the flexor digitorum superflicialis *(curved black arrows)*. Fibrous thickening of the tendon sheaths is imaged with intermediate signal intensity *(small white arrows)*. Intact digital fibrous sheaths forming the osseofibrous canal are shown supporting the flexor tendons *(straight black arrows)*. TR = 600 msec, TE = 20 msec.

nerve in patients with symptoms of carpal tunnel syndrome may be related to a more chronic or advanced stage of the disorder. Enlargement or swelling of the median nerve proximal to the carpal tunnel, referred to as a "pseudoneuroma," has also been documented with MR. This condition may actually be associated with constriction of the median nerve distal to the point of swelling, within the carpal tunnel. Edematous changes, which image with high signal intensity on T2-weighted images, have also been documented in the median nerve of patients with carpal tunnel syndrome. Chronic induration

after transverse carpal ligament release visualizes on MR as an area of neural constriction.

The ability to display the cross-sectional anatomy of the median nerve and adjacent structures on axial sections, and to trace the flexor tendons on coronal plane images, makes MR valuable in characterizing normal anatomy and pathology in the carpal tunnel. Attempts have been made to use MR in the measurement of the diameter and in the area of affected portions of the median nerve, although clinical application needs further documentation.

Subluxations and Disorders of Tendons, Triangular Fibrocartilage, and Interosseous Ligaments

One of the more interesting applications of MR imaging in the wrist and hand is the assessment of tendinous anatomy.[16] In two cases of primary flexor tendon repair studied with MR, we have identified and confirmed continuity of collagen fibers (Fig. 7-16). In a documented case of flexor tendon laceration, tendon disruption (complete discontinuity) was differentiated from scarring (intrasheath high signal intensity) using MR imaging.[15] Normal adjacent tendons with structurally intact pulley mechanisms could be confirmed preoperatively. In a patient with lateral epicondylitis (tennis elbow), partial tearing of the origin of the extensor tendon on the lateral epicondyle of the distal humerus is visualized with increased signal intensity, representing edema, on T2-weighted images (Fig. 7-17).

To date, there have been no reports in the literature comparing the accuracy of arthrography, MR, and arthroscopy in identifying triangular fibrocartilage tears. The ability to reliably image the triangular fibrocartilage complex with MR has, however, been documented. T1-weighted coronal images appear to be sufficient to detect areas of intermediate or increased signal intensity (associated with pathology) within this normally low spin density structure. In preliminary studies, we have identified torn triangular fibrocartilages in four patients with posttraumatic injury to the wrist, with surgical confirmation in two of these cases (Figs. 7-18 and 7-19). In a patient with psoriatic arthritis involving the wrist, complete disruption of the triangular fibrocartilage was identified.

The anatomy of the interosseous scapholunate ligament has been demonstrated with MR studies in normal volunteers and in patients with Kienböck's disease. Disruption of the scapholunate ligament in Kienböck's disease is visualized as an abnormal wavy contour along the low signal intensity ligaments. In a posttraumatic scapholunate dissociation, a frayed attachment of the scapholunate ligament was identified at its scaphoid insertion (see Fig. 7-19). On T2-weighted images, small amounts of fluid in the wrist may help to identify other

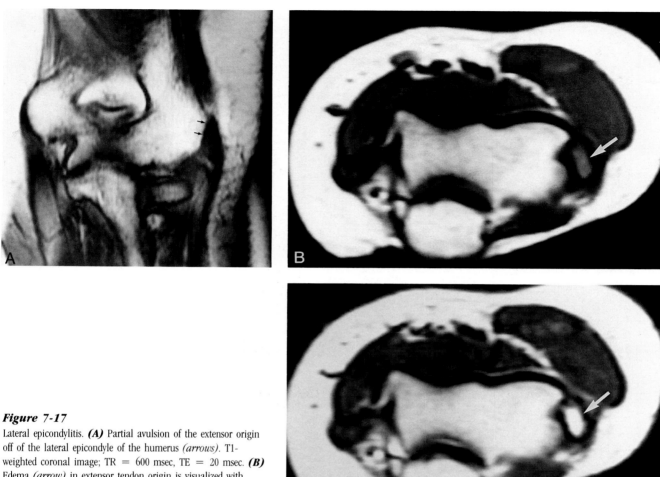

Figure 7-17

Lateral epicondylitis. **(A)** Partial avulsion of the extensor origin off of the lateral epicondyle of the humerus *(arrows)*. T1-weighted coronal image; TR = 600 msec, TE = 20 msec. **(B)** Edema *(arrow)* in extensor tendon origin is visualized with intermediate signal intensity on intermediate- or balanced-weighted images **(B)** and with high signal intensity on T2-weighted images **(C)**. TR = 1500 msec, TE = 20, 70 msec.

interosseous ligaments, such as the lunatotriquetral ligament. In these cases, the high intensity signal of fluid is reflected off the low spin density (and low signal intensity) ligaments.

In cases of joint subluxations, axial MR images have proven very useful in demonstrating dorsal subluxation of the radius of both arthritic and traumatic origin (Fig. 7-20). Normally, the radius is positioned within the concavity of the ulnar semilunar notch. Chronic posterolateral subluxation of the radial head was visualized in the elbow joint of a two year-old child with a lax collateral ligament and capsule (Fig. 7-21). Nonossified epiphyseal cartilage, not evident on conventional radiographs, was identified on MR studies.

Arthritis

Conventional radiography has been the cornerstone of the evaluation and followup of arthritides involving the hand, wrist, and elbow. The superior soft tissue discrim-

ination of MR imaging, however, has proven useful in evaluating patients in both the initial and advanced stages of arthritis. MR imaging achieves noninvasive, accurate delineation of hyaline articular cartilage (Fig. 7-22), ligaments, tendons, and synovium as distinct from cortical bone. Alterations in joint morphology or structure are identified with MR studies before changes can be seen on standard radiographs. Although MR should neither replace radiography nor be used in every patient receiving rheumatologic evaluation, it can, in selected cases, offer the clinician specific information that may modify the patient's diagnosis or treatment.

Rheumatoid Arthritis

To date, the number of patients with adult or juvenile onset rheumatoid arthritis who have received MR evaluation studies in the hand and wrist is limited.[15,17] In patients with chronic rheumatoid disease, the findings of subluxations and erosions affecting the phalanges, carpals, metacarpals, and ulnar styloid are documented

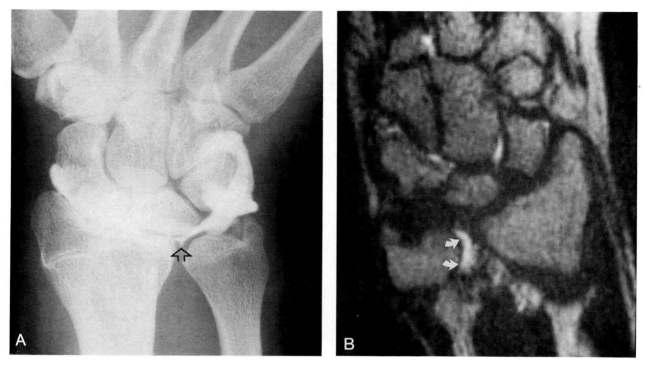

Figure 7-18
Triangular fibrocartilage tear. **(A)** AP view of wrist arthrogram demonstrating partial tear in the triangular fibrocartilage *(open arrow)*. **(B)** Corresponding T2-weighted coronal image with high signal intensity effusion *(curved arrows)* in the inferior radioulnar compartment. TR = 2000 msec, TE = 60 msec.

Figure 7-19
Scapholunate dissociation. **(A)** Scapholunate dissociation *(open arrow)* with a positive Terry Thomas sign (scapholunate diastasis) is seen on AP radiograph. **(B)** Corresponding T1-weighted coronal image showing absence of the scapholunate ligament *(open arrow)* and disrupted triangular fibrocartilage *(small solid white arrows)*. Attachment of triangular fibrocartilage can be followed to the ulnar styloid *(larger solid white arrow)*. TR = 600 msec, TE = 20 msec.

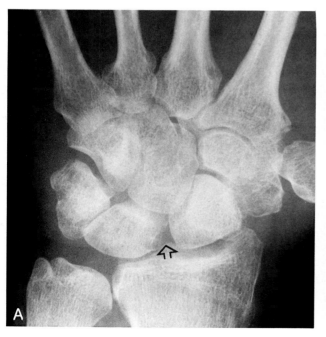

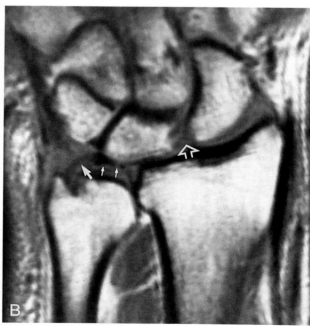

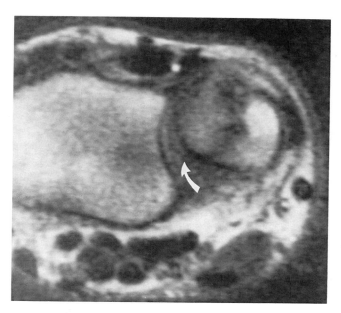

Figure 7-20

Posttraumatic dorsal subluxation of the ulna *(curved arrow)* on T1-weighted axial image. TR = 600 msec, TE = 20 msec.

with both MR and plain film radiography (Fig. 7-23). The changes are more pronounced on MR images. Alterations in soft tissue anatomy and the development of pannus around carpal and interphalangeal joints are displayed only on MR. Because they prolong tissue T1 and T2 relaxation times, both acute inflammation with edema and joint effusion image with low signal intensity on T1-weighted images and with high signal intensity on T2-weighted images. Inflammatory edema may also extend into the subcutaneous tissues where it is visualized with high signal intensity on T2-weighted images. In contrast, chronically inflamed tissue has been reported to remain low in signal intensity on both T1- and T2-weighted images. In our experience, with more advanced rheumatoid disease, pannus formation images with low to intermediate signal intensity on both T1- and T2-weighted images, whereas areas of adjacent fluid collection demonstrate increased signal intensity on T2-weighted acquisitions. Although the signal intensity of localized edematous or inflammatory tissue may be similar to synovial fluid, noninflammatory effusions in the wrist have not, when imaged on T2-weighted sequences, been observed to display an irregular pattern or focal distribution at multiple sites.

Cystic carpal erosions are better delineated on MR images than on corresponding AP radiographs. In a series of four patients with rheumatoid arthritis with wrist involvement, destruction of cartilage and joint arthrosis was distinctly visualized on T1-weighted images. Marrow changes (subchondral sclerosis), present on both sides of the joint or carpal articulation, helped to differentiate arthrosis from intermedullary edema.

In four patients with juvenile rheumatoid arthritis with wrist involvement, early fluid collections along tendon sheaths, subarticular erosions, and cysts, as well as attenuated intercarpal articular cartilage were detected on MR images but were not appreciated on conventional radiographs. Subluxations and areas of bone destruction were equally evident on MR images and on plain films.[18]

MR has the potential to become an important adjunct in the diagnosis and monitoring of patients with rheumatoid disease. Further studies with larger patient populations and comparison with conventional radiographic studies are required before standardized indications can be implemented in rheumatoid patients. MR may also prove to be valuable in monitoring a patient's response to drug therapy, including remitative agents such as methotrexate or gold in juvenile and adult rheumatoid disease.

Other Arthritides

In evaluating nonrheumatoid arthritic disease, we have had the opportunity to evaluate patients with psoriatic arthritis, Lyme disease, intraosseous sarcoid, hemophilia, calcium pyrophosphate deposition disease, and the more commonly found osteoarthritis.

In *psoriatic arthritis,* destruction of the triangular fibrocartilage with pancompartmental joint space narrowing, erosions, scapholunate ligament disruption, and subchondral low signal intensity (sclerosis) in the carpus have been detected with MR studies (Fig. 7-24). Synovitis of the flexor carpi radialis tendon, inferior radioulnar compartmental fluid, intermediate signal intensity inflammatory tissue, and dorsal subluxation of the distal ulna were identified on T1- and T2-weighted axial images (Fig. 7-25). The integrity of an artificial Silastic interphalangeal joint replacement was assessed on coronal images and imaged with low signal intensity without artifact. The site of fusion, in the interphalangeal articulation of the thumb, was degraded by residual metallic artifact, despite prior surgical removal of fixation pins. In a patient presenting with diffuse soft tissue swelling of a single digit secondary to psoriatic arthritis, MR was successful in excluding the diagnosis of osteomyelitis of the bone.

MR studies of *Lyme arthritis* of the wrist were performed in a patient with negative conventional radiographs (Fig. 7-26). Two separate pockets of fluid collection, characterized by high signal intensity on T2-weighted images, were detected on MR images. A scalloped contour of the fluid interface was demonstrated adjacent to inflamed synovium. No joint deformities or cartilaginous erosions were detected.

The hand is a predominant site in patients affected with the relatively rare disorder *skeletal sarcoidosis.* In one case studied, conventional radiographs demonstrated lytic changes, characteristic of sarcoid, in both the middle and distal phalanges (Fig. 7-27). Although MR images did not provide any additional diagnostic in-

Text continues on p. 302

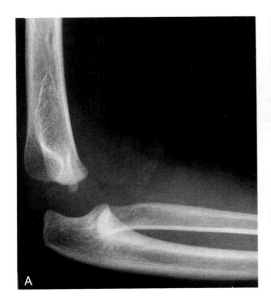

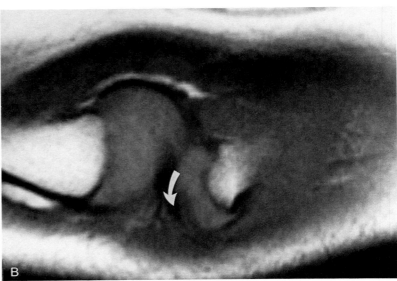

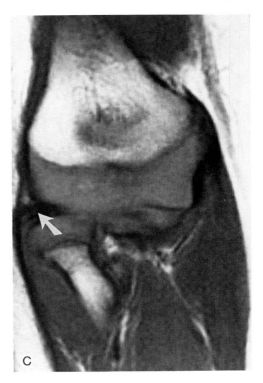

Figure 7-21

Elbow subluxation. **(A)** Lateral radiograph of the elbow without alignment of the radial shaft and capitellar ossific center. Corresponding T1-weighted MR images demonstrating posterior subluxation *(curved arrow)* of the radial head on sagittal image **(B)** and lateral subluxation *(straight arrow)* on coronal image **(C).** Epiphyseal cartilage of the distal humerus and radial head image with intermediate signal intensity. TR = 600 msec, TE = 20 msec.

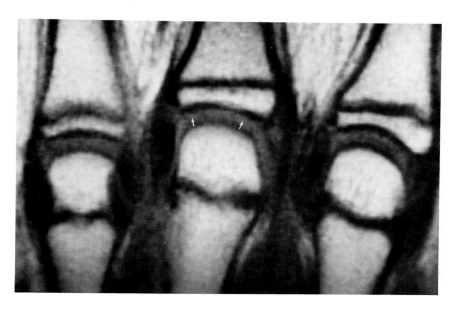

Figure 7-22
Metacarpophalangeal joint hyaline articular cartilage *(arrows)* of normal thickness demonstrates intermediate signal intensity in this T1-weighted coronal image. TR = 800 msec, TE = 20 msec.

Figure 7-23
Rheumatoid arthritis. *(A)* AP radiograph of the hand of an adult with rheumatoid arthritis demonstrating carpal erosions, collapse, subluxation, and marginal erosive changes. *(B)* Corresponding T1-weighted coronal image identifies capitate erosion *(small black arrows)*, low signal intensity fluid and pannus about the ulnar styloid *(small white arrow)*, and radiocarpal compartment *(curved arrow)*. Scaphoid and lunate are difficult to identify because they also image with low signal intensity. TR = 600 msec, TE = 20 msec.

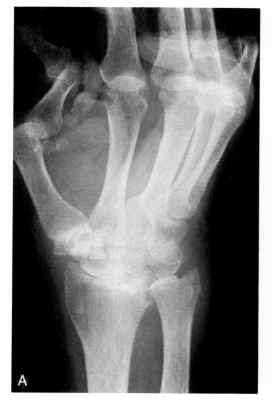

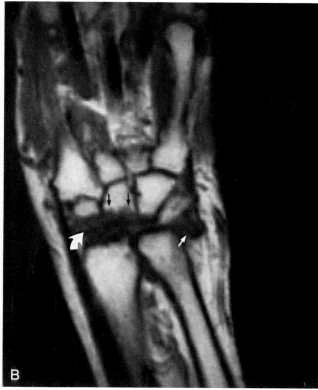

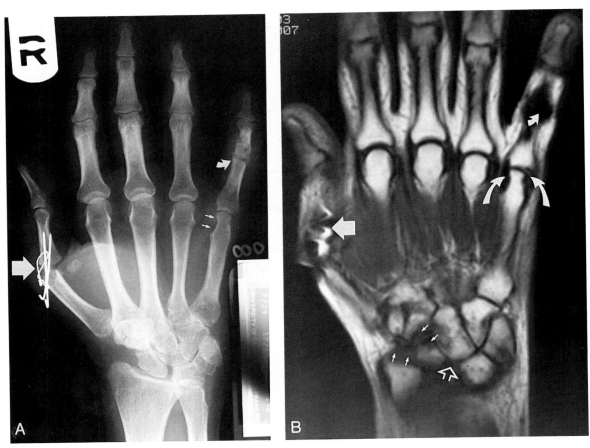

Figure 7-24

Psoriatic arthritis. **(A)** AP radiograph of the first metacarpophalangeal joint postfusion for subluxation *(large arrow)*. Fifth metacarpal head erosions *(small arrows)* and proximal interphalangeal joint Silastic implant *(curved arrow)* are shown. Diffuse carpal joint space narrowing is evident. **(B)** Corresponding T1-weighted coronal MR image demonstrating first metacarpophalangeal metallic artifact *(large solid arrow)*, low signal intensity Silastic joint *(small curved arrow)*, proximal interphalangeal joint erosions and fibrous tissue *(large curved arrows)*, scapholunate dissociation *(open arrow)*, and subchondral sclerosis of the scaphoid *(small arrows)*. TR = 600 msec, TE = 20 msec.

formation, the extent of soft tissue granulomatous proliferation in the cystic defects and areas of cortical destruction were more accurately demonstrated on coronal and axial MR images (Fig. 7-28). The noncaseating, granulomatous tissue in sarcoid images with low to intermediate signal intensity on T1-weighted sequences and with high signal intensity on T2-weighted images.

In an adult *hemophiliac* presenting with a mass on the volar aspect of his wrist, acute hemorrhage into the soft tissues was imaged with a fluid-fluid level present. Higher signal intensity serum was observed layering above hemorrhagic sediment.

We have imaged one patient with *calcium pyrophosphate deposition disease.* On T1-weighted images, areas of intraarticular calcification were not satisfactorily demonstrated when compared to high-quality magnification radiographs. T2-weighting and photography at high contrast settings may prove useful in identifying areas of calcified crystalline deposits, but these have yet to be assessed.

In degenerative *osteoarthrosis* of the wrist, MR has provided information regarding the thickness of the hyaline articular cartilage, the integrity of the triangular cartilage, and associated effusions not identified on plain

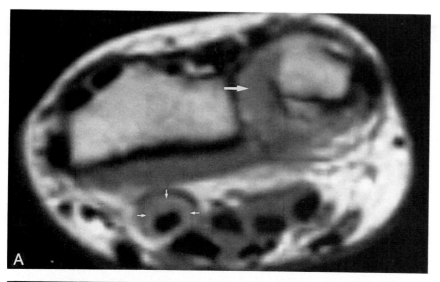

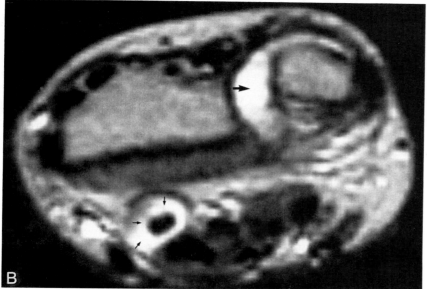

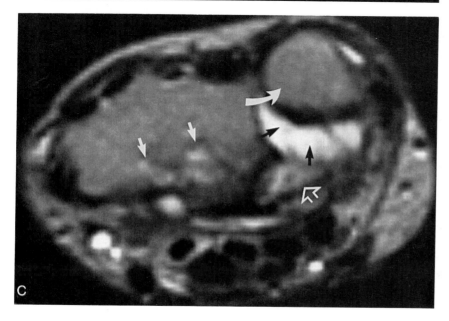

Figure 7-25

Wrist of patient with psoriatic arthritis. Axial images depicting tenosynovitis of a deep flexor tendon *(small arrows)* and fluid collecting in the radioulnar space *(large arrow)* as low signal intensity on T1-weighted images *(A)* and as high signal intensity on T2-weighted images *(B)*. *(A)* TR = 600 msec, TE = 20 msec; *(B)* TR = 2000 msec, TE = 80 msec. *(C)* Distal axial T2-weighted image of the wrist demonstrates dorsal radial subluxation *(curved arrow)* with associated joint effusion *(black arrows)* and intermediate intensity synovial hypertrophy *(open arrow)*. Erosions of the distal radius are identified *(white arrows)*. TR = 2000 msec, TE = 80 msec.

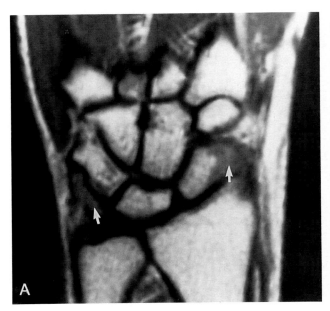 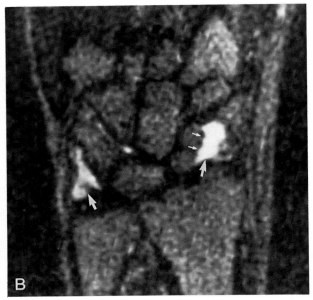

Figure 7-26

Synovitis of the wrist with focal fluid pockets *(large arrows)* images with low signal intensity on T1-weighted coronal image *(A)* and with high signal intensity on T2-weighted coronal image *(B)*. Irregular or corrugated contour of the fluid represents contact with inflamed synovium *(small arrows)*. *(A)* TR = 1000 msec, TE = 20 msec; *(B)* TR = 2000 msec, TE = 80 msec.

film examinations. Subchondral sclerosis of the first carpometacarpal and trapezioscaphoid space are visualized as intramedullary areas of low signal intensity on both surfaces of the joint. Subchondral cysts (Fig. 7-29) and intraarticular fragments (Fig. 7-30) of the elbow, not detected on radiographs, have been identified on corresponding MR images.

Experience with MR in arthritis of the hand, wrist, and elbow is preliminary, and documentation of clinical applications is still ongoing. However, the ability to characterize synovial processes, ligaments, and tendinous structures offers a potential advantage over plain film radiography.

Other Abnormalities of the Synovium

In addition to the changes seen in arthritis, other abnormalities of the synovium—synovial cysts or ganglions, tenosynovitis, and capsular synovitis—have been characterized on MR images of the hand, wrist, and elbow.[15]

Cystic swellings overlying a joint or tendon sheath are referred to as *ganglions,* and are thought to be secondary to protrusions of synovial tissue. On MR images, ganglions generate uniformly low signal intensity on T1-weighted images and high signal intensity on T2-weighted images (Fig. 7-31). Fibrous septations may cause loculation of the ganglion. Even without infiltra-

tion or edema of adjacent tissues, these lesions are well demarcated on MR. Intercarpal communication of a ganglion is more frequent than communication with the radiocarpal joint. Here the role of MR is to identify the joint or tendon of origin and to exclude other soft tissue masses, such as neoplasms, when an accurate preoperative clinical assessment is difficult and wrist arthrography is not satisfactory. We have identified ganglions in the wrist associated with the flexor carpi radialis tendon and the dorsal extensor surface. The narrow tail associated with the ganglion frequently can be traced on MR images (Fig. 7-32). Similarly, a large juxtaarticular ganglion was demonstrated in the elbow joint, with the same T1 and T2 prolongation seen in cysts about the wrist (Fig. 7-33).

Tenosynovitis and *capsular synovitis* may be associated, as part of the spectrum of rheumatoid disease, or they may exist as isolated conditions with a traumatic or infectious etiology. Thickening, swelling, or fluid associated with an irritated synovial tendon sheath may be demonstrated on MR images (Fig. 7-34). An edematous sheath images with a rim of increased signal intensity on T2-weighted images. We have seen examples of both flexor and extensor tenosynovitis without history of infection. Capsular distention may be evident in the small interphalangeal or metacarpal joints when small amounts of synovial fluid accumulate (Fig. 7-35).

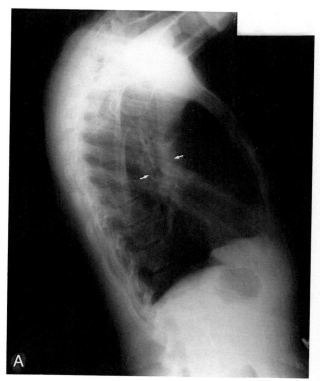

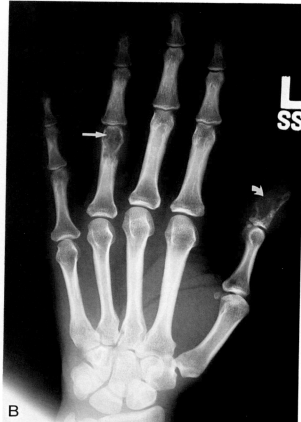

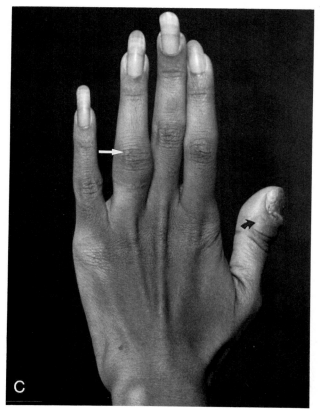

***Figure* 7-27**
Skeletal sarcoid. **(A)** Hilar lymphadenopathy *(arrows)* on lateral chest
radiograph. **(B)** Lytic lesions of sarcoid demonstrated in the proximal phalanx
of the fourth digit *(straight arrow)* and in the distal phalanx of the thumb
(curved arrow). **(C)** Photograph depicting soft tissue swelling of the fourth
proximal interphalangeal joint *(straight arrow)*. Characteristic nail changes and
swelling are shown in the thumb *(curved arrow)*.

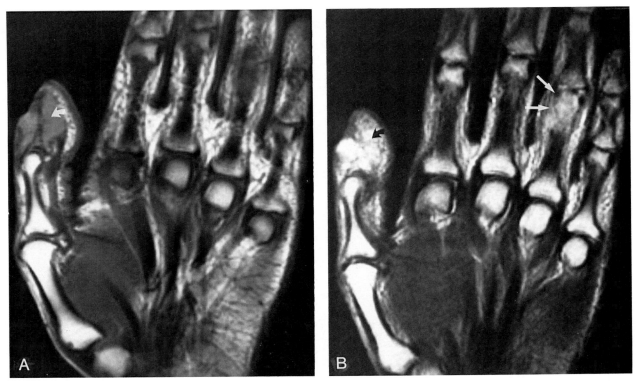

Figure 7-28
Skeletal sarcoid on MR (see also corresponding radiographs in Figure 7-27. **(A)** Intermediate signal intensity soft tissue mass and cortical destruction *(curved arrow)* are shown on T1-weighted coronal image. TR = 600 msec, TE = 20 msec. **(B)** High signal intensity is demonstrated in granulomatous tissue in the distal phalanx of the thumb *(curved arrow)* and proximal phalanx *(straight arrows)* of the ring finger on T2-weighted coronal image. TR = 2000 msec, TE = 60 msec.

Neoplasms

Benign Lesions

The spectrum of vascular lesions is well depicted by MR (Figs. 7-36, 7-37, 7-38). *Arteriovenous malformations* (AVM) about the wrist and elbow visualize with signal void, secondary to fast blood flow, through a serpiginous tangle of vessels.[15] In cases of capillary AVM, however, increased signal intensity is seen in areas of slow blood flow (Fig. 7-39). In a postoperative recurrence of intraosseous hemangioma, the lesion demonstrated nonspecific low intensity signal on T1-weighted images and increased intensity on T2-weighted images (Fig. 7-40).

Fibrolipomas, consisting of both fibrous connective tissue and fatty elements, demonstrate heterogeneous signal characteristics. In one patient, with a fibrolipoma involving the carpal tunnel, T1-weighted sequences depicted thin, fibrous bands of low signal intensity within a fatty mass of high signal intensity.[9] *Simple lipomas* image with uniform, high signal intensity on T1-weighted images and with intermediate signal intensity on T2-weighted images (Fig. 7-41).

Plexiform neurofibromas involving nerves of the upper extremity, near the wrist and elbow, appear on MR as fusiform enlargements tracking along the course of the involved nerve.[19] In our experience, these have demonstrated uniform, increased signal intensity, most pronounced on T2-weighted sequences, with low to intermediate signal intensity on T1-weighted sequences.

MR images of *giant cell tumor* of the distal radius are characterized by the presence of an eccentric, expansile subarticular lesion demonstrating low and intermediate signal intensity on T1- and T2-weighted images, respectively.[20]

Enchondromas involving the digits of a patient with multiple enchondromatosis (Ollier's disease) demonstrated expansion of the cortex and signal inhomogeneity on both T1- and T2-weighted images. However, these are not reliable criteria for suspecting malignant degeneration in the more aggressive lesions (Fig. 7-42).

Malignant Lesions

In a number of instances MR has demonstrated its usefulness in the assessment of malignant lesions about the hand, wrist, and elbow. In one instance of postbiopsy

Text continues on p. 316

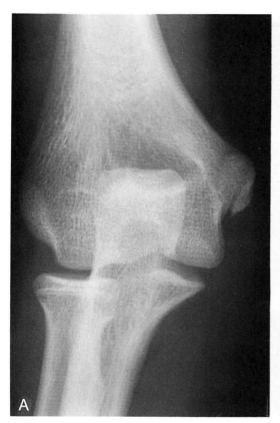

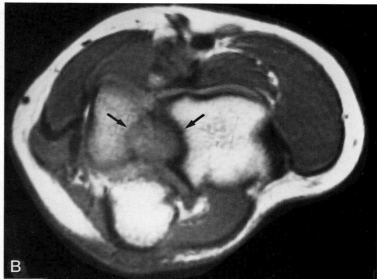

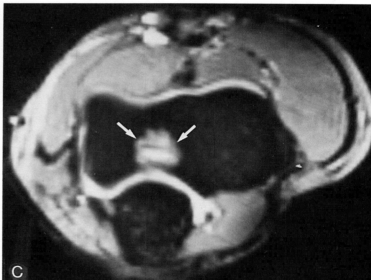

Figure 7-29

Traumatic subarticular cyst *(arrows)* between the trochlea and capitellum of the distal humerus in a 12-year-old gymnast. *(A)* Normal radiographic evaluation. *(B)* Viscous synovial fluid contents generate low signal intensity on T1-weighted image. TR = 600 msec, TE = 20 msec. *(C)* Increased signal intensity is seen on T2* gradient echo image. TR = 400 msec, TE = 30 msec; flip angle = 30°.

Figure 7-30

Low signal intensity free fragment *(straight arrow)* surrounded by high signal intensity fluid *(curved arrow)* in the elbow joint on T2* gradient echo axial images.

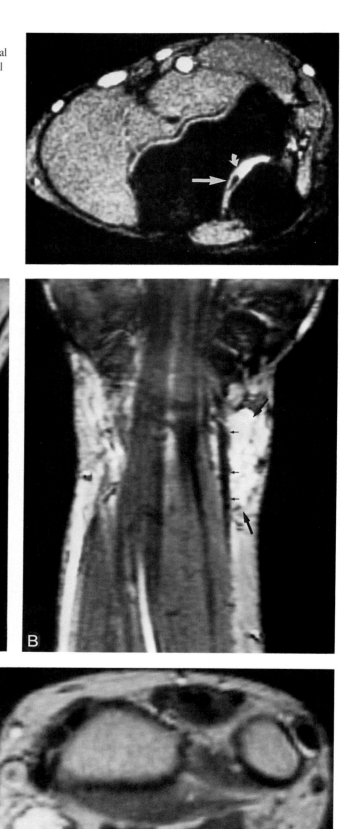

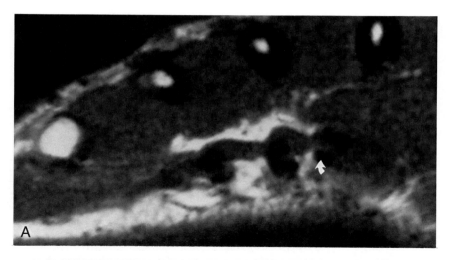

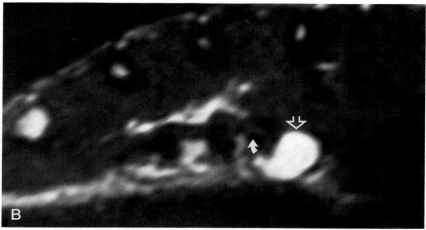

Figure 7-32

Flexor tendon ganglion *(open arrow)* is not visualized on T1-weighted axial image *(A),* but is defined with high signal intensity on heavily T2-weighted axial image *(B).* Involved tendon images with low signal intensity *(curved arrow).* *(A)* TR = 800 msec, TE = 20 msec; *(B)* TR = 2000 msec, TE = 60 msec.

◀ ***Figure 7-31***

Wrist ganglion. Synovial ganglion *(large arrows)* associated with flexor carpi radialis tendon *(small arrows)* on T1-weighted *(A)* and T2* gradient echo *(B)* coronal images, and on T1-weighted *(C)* and T2-weighted *(D)* axial images. The relationship of the cyst *(curved arrow)* to flexor tendon *(straight arrow)* is displayed on the axial image. Mucinous synovial contents demonstrate low signal intensity on T1-weighted images and high signal intensity on T2-weighted images. *(A)* TR = 600 msec, TE = 20 msec; *(B)* TR = 400 msec, TE = 30 msec, flip angle = 30°; *(C)* TR = 600 msec, TE = 20 msec; *(D)* TR = 2000 msec, TE = 60 msec.

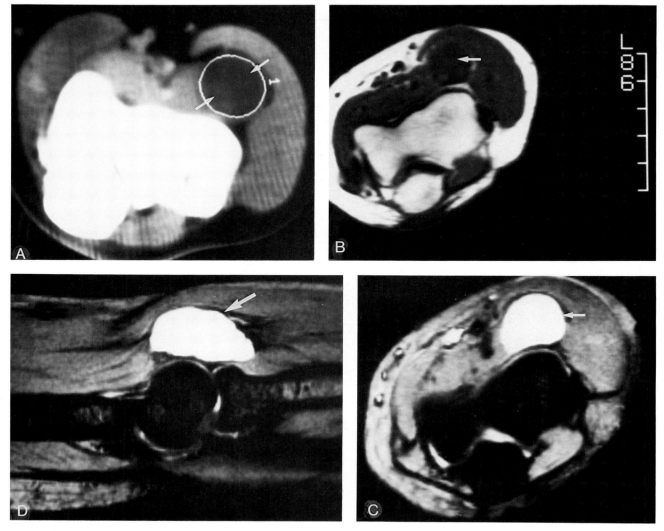

Figure 7-33

Juxstaarticular synovial cyst about the elbow. *(A)* CT demonstrates cyst as low attenuation lesion deep to the brachioradialis *(white arrows)*. *(B)* Corresponding T1-weighted axial image showing cyst *(arrow)* isointense with adjacent muscle tissue. T2* gradient echo axial *(C)* and sagittal *(D)* images demonstrating cyst with uniform high signal intensity *(white arrow)*. TR = 400 msec, TE = 80 msec; flip angle = 30°.

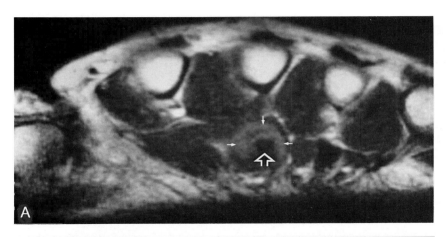

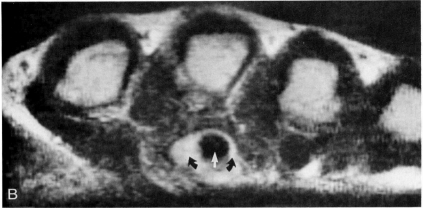

Figure 7-34
Peritendinous edema in flexor tendon tenosynovitis.
Edema images with low signal intensity *(small
arrows)* on intermediate- or proton density-weighted
image *(A)* and with high signal intensity *(curved
arrows)* on T2-weighted axial image *(B)*. Flexor
tendon is visualized with low signal intensity
(central arrow). TR = 1500 msec, TE = 20, 60
msec.

Figure 7-35
Synovitis. *(A)* Capsular synovitis with bowing of overlying extensor tendon in the first metacarpal
phalangeal joint *(large and small arrows)*. *(B)* Normal contralateral metacarpal phalangeal joint shown
(arrow). T1-weighted coronal image; TR = 800 msec, TE = 20 msec.

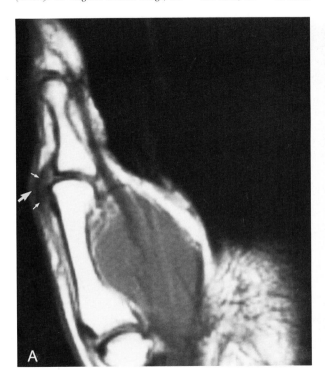

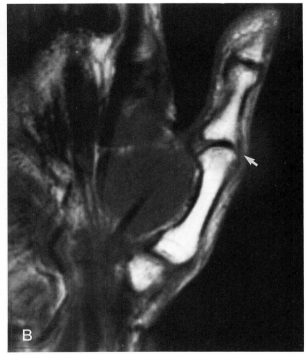

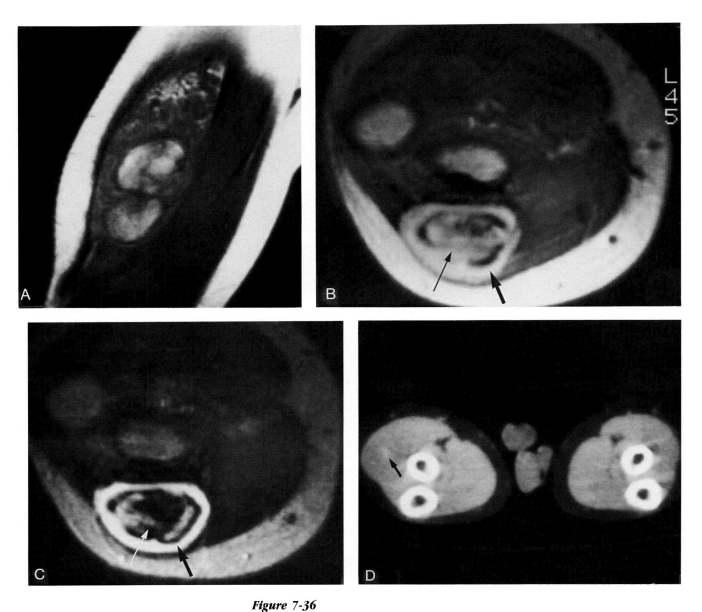

Figure 7-36

Hemorrhagic hemangioma. **(A)** Hemorrhagic intramuscular hemangioma images with high signal intensity elements on T1-weighted coronal image through the forearm. TR = 800 msec, TE = 20 msec. **(B)** Corresponding T1-weighted axial image demonstrating high signal intensity central portion *(long thin arrow)* and surrounding high signal intensity peripheral ring *(short thick arrow).* TR = 800 msec, TE = 20 msec. **(C)** With T2-weighting the central hematoma *(white arrow)* becomes less intense (T2 shortening effect), whereas the outer core of more chronic blood and clot is visualized with bright signal intensity *(black arrow).* TR = 2000 msec, TE = 80 msec. **(D)** Axial CT scan demonstrates nonspecific soft tissue mass with focal area of high attenuation *(arrow).*

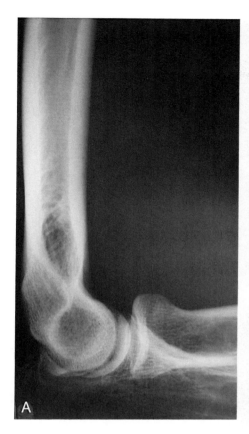

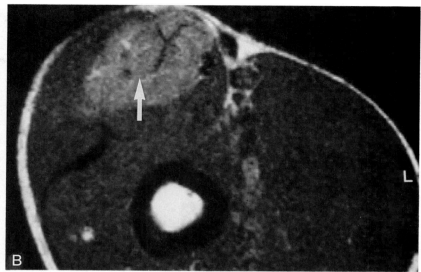

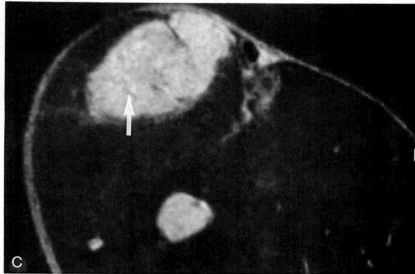

Figure 7-37

Hemangioma. *(A)* Normal lateral radiograph of the distal humerus and elbow. Intermediate signal intensity soft tissue hemangioma deep to the biceps brachii *(arrow)* on T1-weighted image *(B)* increasing in signal intensity on T2-weighted sequence *(arrow; C)*. *(B)* TR = 800 msec, TE = msec; *(C)* TR = 2000 msec, TE = 80 msec.

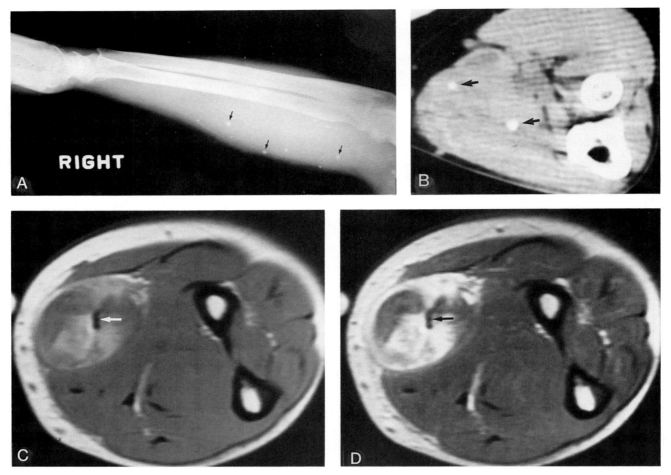

Figure 7-38

Hemangioma involving the forearm. *(A)* Lateral radiograph of a volar soft tissue hemangioma with phleboliths identified *(arrows)*. *(B)* Axial CT demonstrates punctate calcifications and indistinct soft tissue mass within pronator teres and flexor digitorum superficialis *(arrows)*. Intermediate-weighted *(C)* and T2-weighted *(D)* axial images demonstrate a progressive increase in signal intensity. Central vessel with signal void is indicated *(arrow)*. TR = 2000 msec, TE = 20, 80 msec.

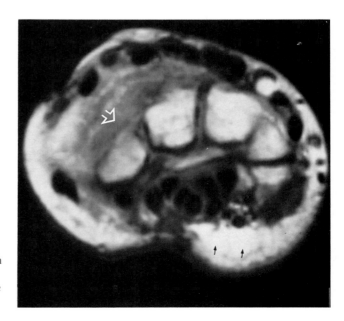

Figure 7-39

Postoperative recurrent capillary hemangioma *(black arrows)* is seen as a high signal intensity soft tissue mass on T1-weighted axil image through the carpal tunnel. Postoperative fibrosis is visualized as intermediate signal intensity *(open arrow)*. TR = 800 msec, TE = 20 msec.

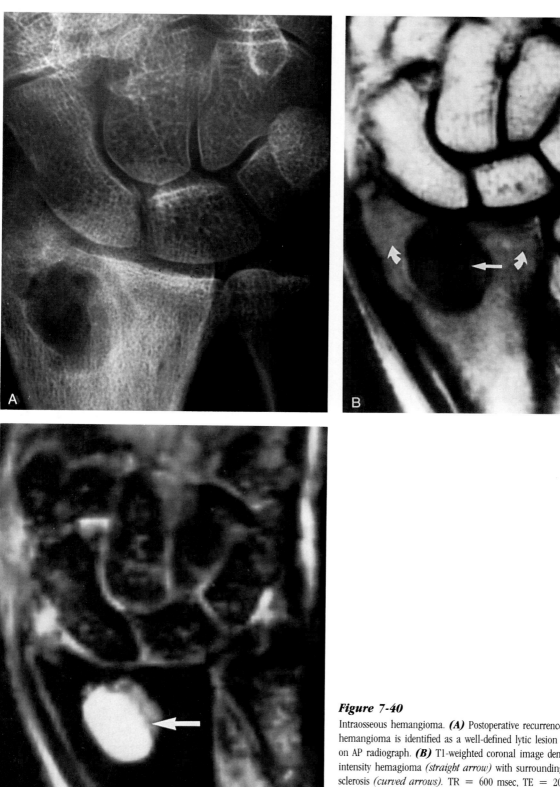

Figure 7-40

Intraosseous hemangioma. *(A)* Postoperative recurrence of an intraosseous hemangioma is identified as a well-defined lytic lesion with reactive sclerosis on AP radiograph. *(B)* T1-weighted coronal image demonstrating low signal intensity hemagioma *(straight arrow)* with surrounding low signal intensity sclerosis *(curved arrows)*. TR = 600 msec, TE = 20 msec. *(C)* Corresponding T2* gradient echo image revealing uniform high signal intensity within the subarticular lesion *(arrow)*. TR = 400 msec, TE = 30 msec; flip angle = 30°.

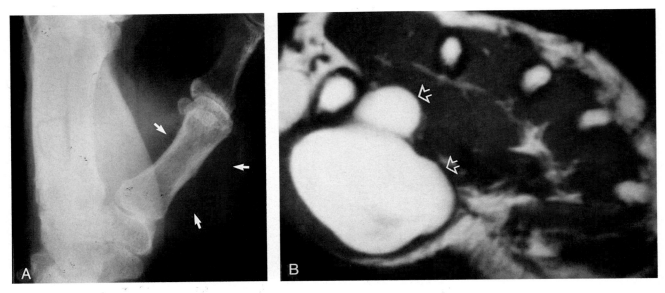

Figure 7-41

Lipoma. **(A)** Low-density soft tissue mass of thenar eminence *(arrows)* on lateral radiograph. **(B)** Corresponding T1-weighted axial image showing multilobulated lipoma with subcutaneous and marrow fat signal intensity *(arrows)*. TR = 600 msec, TE = 20 msec.

synovial sarcoma, arising within the first web space of the hand, MR—although demonstrating in this case intermediate signal intensity on T2-weighted images in contrast to significantly increased signal intensity in other cases of appendicular synovial sarcoma—clearly showed the extent and distribution of involvement by the neoplasm (Fig. 7-43).[21]

In a case of Ollier's disease affecting the distal radial shaft, the malignant degeneration of an enchondroma to *chondrosarcoma* was indicated by: the MR appearance of a dominant lesion with higher intensity signal than adjacent enchondromas; periosteal elevation; a soft tissue mass; and frank cortical bone destruction. These criteria are not documented, however, and correlation with clinical symptoms such as pain and interval changes in imaging characteristics may need to be considered when making a diagnosis.

MR was found to be superior to CT for demonstration of the soft tissue components of a myxomatous tumor of the proximal radius and for identification of an undifferentiated sarcoma about the elbow (Figs. 7-44 and 7-45). In the latter, areas of necrosis with fluid-fluid levels separate from adjacent tumor and neurovascular structures were clearly depicted on MR images.

Short TI inversion recovery (STIR) imaging sequences are valuable in the assessment of marrow malignancy, because the normally high intensity signal of fat is nulled.[22,23] Using STIR in a case of *Ewing sarcoma* infiltrating a metacarpal, areas of involvement were easily identified as regions of high intensity signal replacing the low intensity signal (nulled fat signal) of normal marrow (Fig. 7-46).

MR, with superior soft tissue contrast and marrow imaging capabilities, shows great potential for multiplanar tumor imaging about the upper extremity in both pre- and postoperative assessments.

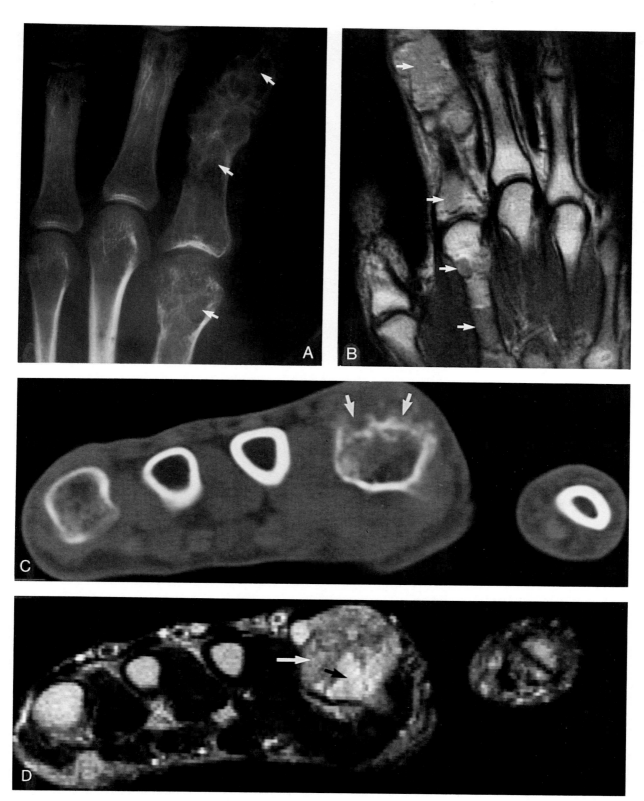

Figure 7-42

Ollier's disease. AP radiograph *(A)* and T1-weighted coronal image *(B)* identifying multiple enchondromatous foci *(arrows)* in the second ray. TR = 1000 msec, TE = 40 msec. *(C)* Corresponding axial CT demonstrating cortical irregularity *(arrows)*. *(D)* Increased signal intensity is appreciated in cartilaginous foci *(black arrow)* within the affected digit *(white arrow)* on axial spin echo T2-weighted sequence. TR = 2000 msec, TE = 80 msec.

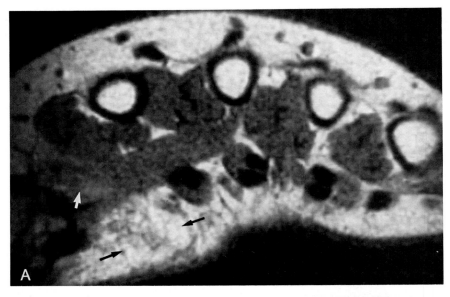

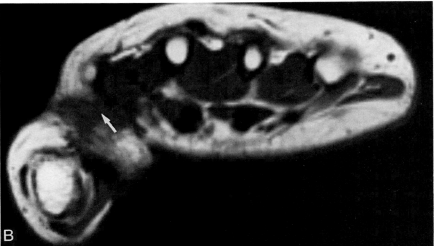

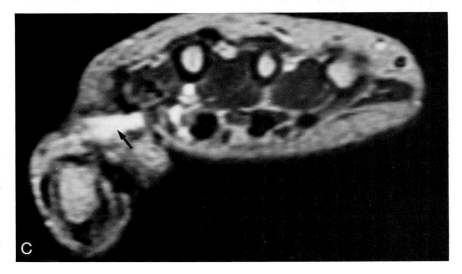

Figure 7-43

Synovial sarcoma. *(A)* Postbiopsy synovial sarcoma *(white arrow)* of the first web space (intermediate signal intensity) with inhomogeneity of overlying subcutaneous fat *(black arrows)*. T1-weighted axial image; TR = 800 msec, TE = 20 msec. Subsequent postoperative images demonstrating fluid collection *(arrow)* after removal of second ray; low signal intensity on T1-weighted axial image *(B)*, and high signal intensity on T2-weighted axial image *(C)*. *(B)* TR = 800 msec, TE = 20 msec; *(C)* TR = 2000 msec, TE = 60 msec.

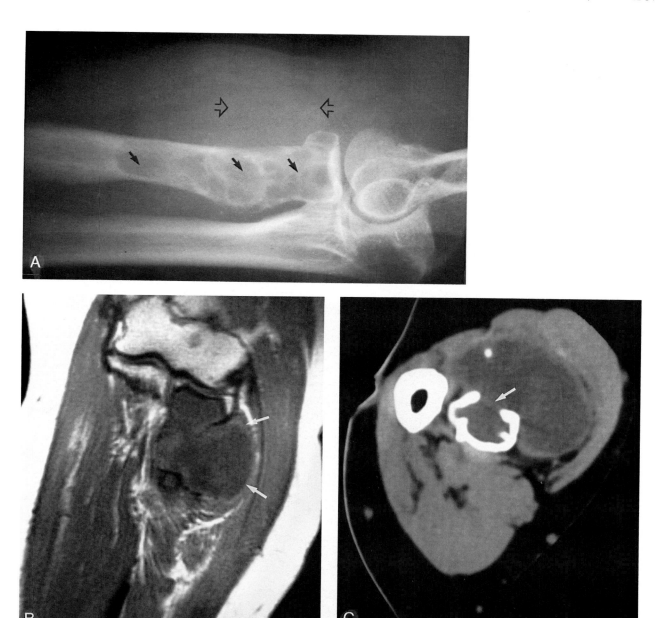

Figure 7-44

Myxoid tumor of the proximal radius. **(A)** Lateral radiograph demonstrating aggressive lytic lesions *(solid arrows)* and associated soft tissue mass *(open arrows)*. **(B)** T1-weighted coronal image depicting low to intermediate signal intensity tumor with cortical breakthrough and soft tissue mass. TR = 600 msec, TE = 20 msec. **(C)** Axial CT displaying bone detail in cortical breakthrough *(arrows)*.

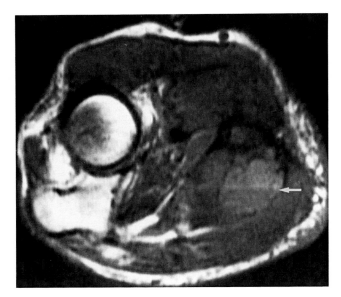

Figure 7-45

Undifferentiated sarcoma. Fluid-fluid level in necrotic component of
undifferentiated sarcoma *(arrow)* treated with chemotherapy and radiation.
T1-weighted axial image; TR = 600 msec, TE = 20 msec.

PERSPECTIVE ON MR IMAGING OF THE HAND, WRIST, AND ELBOW

MR imaging is still in the early stages of its development as a diagnostic tool, and it is not always possible to correlate MR findings with clinical signs and symptoms. For example, clinical correlation with MR findings in difficult diagnostic entities such as injuries of the distal radioulnar joint, the triangular fibrocartilage complex, and the intercarpal ligaments is not yet available.

Nonetheless, MR offers exquisite multiplanar depiction of the complex anatomy about the hand, wrist, and elbow not available in conventional imaging techniques. In AVN of the scaphoid and lunate bones, and for fractures about the wrist, MR provides precise anatomic localization and depiction of the extent of involvement. Patient's with Kienböck's disease may benefit greatly from earlier diagnosis and initiation of followup of AVN. Axial images obtained by MR show great potential in the diagnosis of pathology involving the carpal tunnel. Similarly, MR holds diagnostic potential in the assessment of pathology within the complex tendons, cartilages, and interosseous ligaments of the upper extremity.

Figure 7-46

Ewing sarcoma of the metacarpal in a patient undergoing radiation therapy. *(A)* Conventional T1-weighted sagittal image. TR = 900 msec, TE = 40 msec. *(B)* STIR image demonstrates high signal intensity contrast *(arrows)* in infiltrated bone marrow. Normal marrow is black. TR = 400 msec, TI = 125 msec, TE = 40 msec.

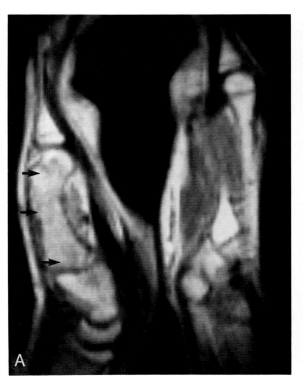

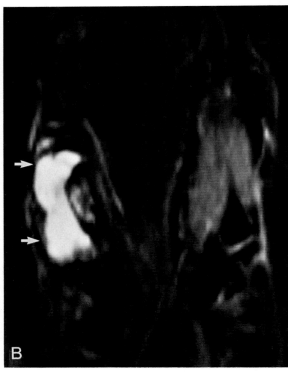

Although still in the preliminary stages, MR imaging of arthritides may ultimately prove useful in the early detection and monitoring of arthritic conditions. Excellent soft tissue differentiation and anatomic depiction afforded by MR images provide important information in synovial and neoplastic pathologies, demonstrating morphology, tissue of origin, extent, and distribution of involvement.

As comparisons among arthrography, fluoroscopy, MR imaging, and arthrotomy become available, MR imaging will assume its proper place in the diagnostic workup and may supercede many or all of these other tests.

REFERENCES

1. Manaster BJ: Digital wrist arthrography: Precision in determining the site of radiocarpal-midcarpal communication. AJR, 147:563, 1986

2. Braunstein EM, et al: Fluoroscopic and arthrographic evaluation of carpal instability. AJR, 144:1259, 1985

3. Tirman RM, et al: Midcarpal wrist arthrography for detection of tears of the scapholunate and lunatotriquetral ligaments. AJR, 144:107, 1985

4. Singson RD, et al: Elbow joint: Assessment with double-contrast CT arthrography. Radiology 160:167, 1986

5. DeFlaviis L, et al: High-resolution ultrasonography of wrist ganglia. JCU, 15:17, 1987

6. Weiss KL, et al: High-field strength surface-coil imaging of the hand and wrist, Part I: Normal anatomy. Radiology, 160:143, 1986

7. Baker LL, et al: High-resolution magnetic resonance imaging of the wrist: Normal anatomy. Skeletal Radiol, 16:128, 1987

8. Middleton WD, et al: High resolution surface coil magnetic resonance imaging of the joints: Anatomic correlation. RadioGraphics, 7:645, 1987

9. Koenig H, et al: Wrist: Preliminary report on high-resolution MR imaging. Radiology, 160:463, 1986

10. Mark S, et al: High resolution MR imaging of peripheral joints using a quadratus coil at 0.35T. ROFO, 146:397, 1987

11. Fisher MR, et al: MR imaging using specialized coils. Radiology, 157:443, 1985

12. Middleton WD, et al: MR imaging of the carpal tunnel: Normal anatomy and preliminary findings in the carpal tunnel syndrome. AJR, 148:307, 1987

13. Ruby LK, et al: Natural history of scaphoid nonunion. Radiology, 156:856, 1985

14. Reinus WR, et al: Carpal avascular necrosis: MR imaging. Radiology, 160:689, 1986

15. Weiss KL, et al: High-field MR surface-coil imaging of the hand and wrist, Part II: Pathologic correlations and clinical relevance. Radiology, 160:147, 1986

16. Baker LL, et al: High-resolution magnetic resonance imaging of the wrist: Normal anatomy. Skeletal Radiol, 16:128, 1987

17. Yulish BS, et al: Juvenile rheumatoid arthritis: Assessment with MR imaging. Radiology, 165:149, 1987

18. Stoller DW, et al: MRI in juvenile rheumatoid (chronic) arthritis. Presented to the Association of University Radiologists, Charleston, South Carolina, March 22–27, 1987

19. Levine E, et al: Malignant nerve-sheath neoplasms in neurofibromatosis: Distinction from benign tumors by using imaging techniques. AJR, 149:1059, 1987

20. Brady TJ, et al: NMR imaging of forearms in healthy volunteers and patients with giant-cell tumors of bone. Radiology, 144:549, 1982

21. Sundaram M, et al: Magnetic resonance imaging of lesions of synovial origin. Skeletal Radiol, 15:133, 1986

22. Olson D, et al: Magnetic resonance imaging of the bone marrow in patients with leukemia, aplastic anemia and lymphoma. Investigative Radiology, June, 1986

23. Porter B, et al: MR may become routine for imaging bone marrow. Diagnostic Imaging, February, 1987

David W. Stoller
Harry K. Genant
Philipp Lang

Chapter 8   THE SPINE

OUTLINE

Accurate diagnosis and evaluation of the cervical, thoracic, and lumbar spines are necessary in the specialties of orthopedics, rheumatology, neurology, and neurosurgery. At best, standard radiographs of the spine provide a limited interpretation of nonosseous events occurring in the discs, cord, cerebrospinal fluid (CSF), and ligaments (structures not directly visualized on plain film studies). Myelography, an invasive procedure, indirectly evaluates the disc by visualizing the contour of the thecal sac and nerve root sleeves. Computed tomography (CT) is useful in delineating bone detail, and direct axial scans of the spine provide soft tissue discrimination of the disc, nerve roots, and thecal sac.[1-5]

Sagittal, coronal, or oblique views, however, cannot be directly acquired, and require reformations. Although CT is excellent for assessing postoperative pseudoarthrosis, fibrosis and scarring may be difficult to differentiate from disc material, especially in the absence of contrast enhancement. Magnetic resonance (MR) imaging complements CT and myelography in the routine evaluation of the spine for degenerative disc disease, trauma, infection, neoplasia, and intrinsic cord disease.[6-31]

With MR imaging, the separate components of the disc, including the nucleus pulposus and anulus fibrosus, can be distinguished and assessed in early degenerative disc disease. The disc-thecal sac interface is defined without administration of a contrast agent; the structure of the cord is visualized in contrast with surrounding CSF; and the dura and supporting ligaments of the spine are demonstrated in either sagittal or axial images. MR has the unique advantage of direct marrow imaging in the study of patients with marrow infiltrative diseases, metastasis, infection, or reactive endplate changes.[32–35] MR imaging of the spine has advanced in parallel with the development of improved surface coils and software. Oblique imaging, cardiac gating, and gradient echo and short TI inversion recovery (STIR) sequences have all been used to maximize the information obtained from MR images. Improved signal-to-noise and excellent spatial and contrast resolution have made it possible to define spinal anatomy in direct sagittal, oblique, and axial planes with MR images obtained from circular and rectangular surface coils (Fig. 8-1).

IMAGING PROTOCOLS FOR THE CERVICAL SPINE

The cervical spine is studied with a custom-designed posterior or anterior cervical spine coil. With anterior placement, greater respiratory artifact may be introduced because of closer proximity to the trachea.

In the *sagittal imaging plane,* T1-weighted images are obtained with a TR of 600 msec and a TE of 20 msec. Thin (5 mm) sections, with or without an interslice gap (1 mm), are acquired with a 16- to 20-cm field of view (FOV), a 256 × 256 acquisition matrix, and four signal averages or excitations (NEX). T2-weighted contrast in the sagittal plane is achieved using effective T2 or T2* gradient echo images that minimize pulsation artifacts from CSF and cause flow related enhancement of signal intensity. Gradient echo or refocused images can be generated using a TR of 400 msec, TE of 15 msec, and a flip angle of 30°. With long acquisition times (long TR/TE) CSF flow-related artifacts are more common, but can be reduced by gating the acquisition to the cardiac cycle using an electrograph (ECG) or pulse trigger.[13,36]

Axial images are generated with T2* gradient echo sequences similar to those used in the sagittal plane. Conventional T1-weighted images, if obtained, should be acquired with flow compensation to minimize vascular and CSF flow artifacts. Conventional T2-weighted images in the axial plane have poor signal-to-noise and are degraded by motion artifact unless some form of cardiac gating is employed.

NORMAL MR ANATOMY OF THE CERVICAL SPINE

Sagittal Images

T1-Weighted Images
On T1-weighted sagittal images of the cervical spine the yellow or fatty marrow of the vertebral bodies is visualized as bright signal intensity (Fig. 8-2). The fibrocartilaginous cervical discs are intermediate in signal intensity, and CSF, which is of low signal intensity, is imaged in contrast with the higher signal intensity of the cord.

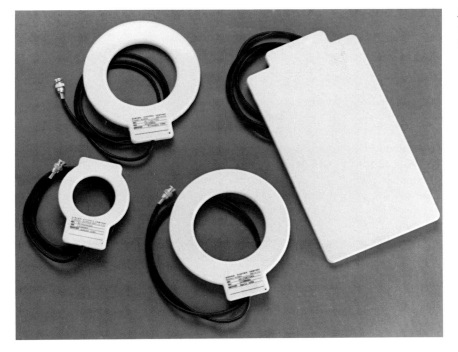

Figure 8-1
Circular and rectangular planar surface coils for the thoracic and lumbar spine.

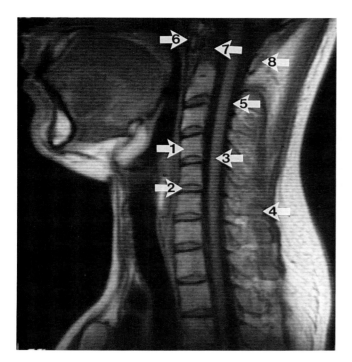

Figure 8-2

Midsagittal anatomy of cervical spine: bright marrow signal intensity vertebral body *(1)*, intermediate signal intensity disc *(2)*, spinal cord *(3)*, spinous process *(4)*, low signal intensity CSF *(5)*, anterior arch of first cervical vertebra *(6)*, odontoid *(7)*, posterior arch of C1 *(8)*. T1-weighted sagittal image; TR = 600 msec, TE = 20 msec.

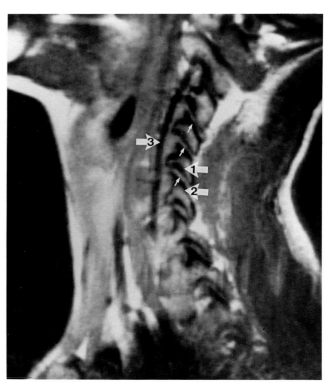

Figure 8-3

Parasagittal anatomy of cervical spine at level of the facet joints: superior articular facet *(1)*, inferior articular facet *(2)*, vertebral artery *(3)*. Intermediate signal intensity facet cartilage *(small white arrows)* is identified. T1-weighted parasagittal image; TR = 600 msec, TE = 20 msec.

Differentiation of posterior cortical bone, longitudinal ligaments, and CSF is difficult, because all generate low signal intensity on short TR/TE sequences. The dorsal and ventral roots in the neural foramina are identified on peripheral sagittal images. They image with intermediate signal intensity and are surrounded by high signal intensity foraminal fat. A 45° oblique sagittal image is also useful in displaying intervertebral foraminal anatomy in the cervical spine.

Hyaline cartilage, imaging with intermediate signal intensity, can be seen between the obliquely oriented inferior and superior articular facets (Fig. 8-3). The signal void of the anterior vertebral artery can be seen on parasagittal sections through the dorsal root ganglion and articular pillars. The subarachnoid space anterior and posterior to the cord is of equal dimensions. The ability to differentiate gray and white matter varies, depending on CSF pulsation and truncation artifacts. Truncation artifacts are visualized as bands, parallel to the cervical cord, and are related to FOV, acquisition times, and pixel size. Bright signal intensity from marrow is imaged in both the anterior and posterior arches of C1 and in the body of C2. Signal intensity in the body of C2 is higher than that visualized in the adjacent odontoid process. However, there is a fat pad of high signal intensity directly superior to the odontoid.

T2-Weighted Images

On T2*-weighted gradient echo images the intervertebral discs and CSF demonstrate high signal intensity (Fig. 8-4).[36,37] The cord images with low signal intensity, and high signal intensity subarachnoid CSF is seen anteriorly and posteriorly (Fig. 8-5). The marrow and cortex of the cervical vertebrae are of low signal intensity on gradient echo images, allowing sharp delineation of the spinal canal, impinging osteophytes, and the disc-thecal sac interface. The basivertebral vein follows a horizontal course through the midvertebral body, and generates bright signal intensity. Facet cartilage, which is intermediate in signal intensity on conventional T1- or T2-weighted imaging, images with bright signal intensity on gradient echo images (Fig. 8-6); flowing arterial and venous blood image with high signal intensity. Because the contrast between nerve root and fat is diminished on T2-weighted images (fat is imaged with intermediate and not high signal intensity), the anatomy of the neural foramina is not accurately demonstrated on these images. The low signal intensity dura can be identified on T2* gradient echo images, but it is not satisfactorily seen on corresponding conventional T1- or T2-weighted images.

Axial Images

T1-Weighted Images

On T1-weighted axial images, the disc (of intermediate signal intensity), the CSF (black), and the cord (of higher signal intensity) can be differentiated (Fig. 8-7). Differentiation of the nucleus pulposus and annulus, however, is not possible with short TR/TE sequences. The low signal intensity uncinate processes are identified lateral to the disc margins, and the facet joints are demonstrated in their oblique orientation, with greater medial–lateral than superior–inferior dimensions. The ventral and dorsal nerve roots form a triangle of intermediate signal intensity, with the anterolateral apex of the triangle represented by the dorsal root ganglion. Anterior to the dorsal root ganglion, the low signal intensity vertebral artery can be seen. At the level of the cervical body, but not the intervertebral disc, high signal intensity neural foraminal fat may outline the intermediate signal intensity nerve roots and sheaths. Low signal intensity epidural veins are displayed directly posterior to the vertebral body and surrounding the vertebral artery in a venous plexus. Gray and white matter can be separately identified on T1-weighted axial images.

T2-Weighted Images

On T2* gradient echo images the intervertebral disc is visualized with high signal intensity from the nucleus pulposus (Fig. 8-8).[37] Annular fibers remain low in signal intensity. The anterior epidural venous plexus generates bright signal intensity, as do the vertebral arteries, allowing the low to intermediate signal intensity nerve roots and dorsal root ganglion to be seen. It may be difficult to distinguish the exiting nerve roots, because both the roots and neural foraminal fat are intermediate in signal intensity on these images. The thin line of the dural sac is identified anterior to subarachnoid CSF. The common carotid artery and jugular vein (both of bright signal intensity) are defined anteromedially and posterolaterally, respectively, on axial planar images. Cortical bone and marrow are both low in signal intensity on gradient refocused images.

Figure 8-4

High signal intensity discs *(white arrows)* and CSF *(open black arrow)* are imaged with T2* gradient echo contrast. CSF-cord differentiation is poor on this image. TR = 400 msec, TE = 15 msec; flip angle = 45°.

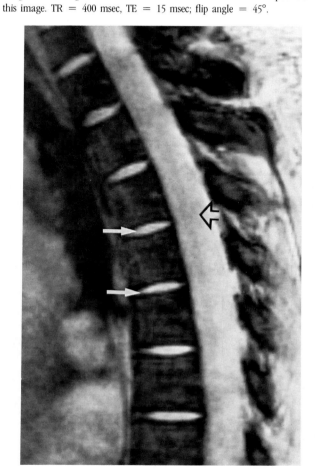

Figure 8-5

Low signal intensity cord *(large black arrows)* is clearly differentiated from bright signal intensity CSF *(small black arrows)* on T2* gradient echo image. Extradural defect is visualized as minimal C5–6 disc bulge *(white arrows)*. TR = 400 msec, TE = 15 msec; flip angle = 30°.

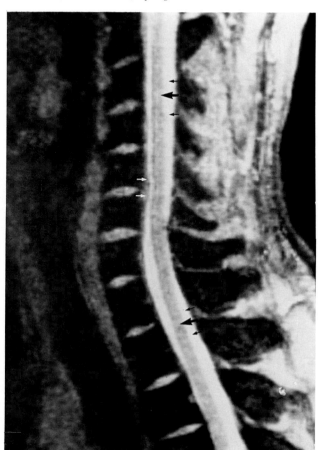

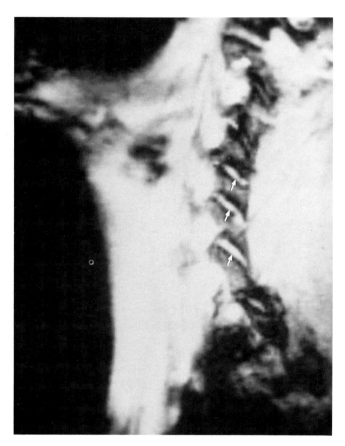

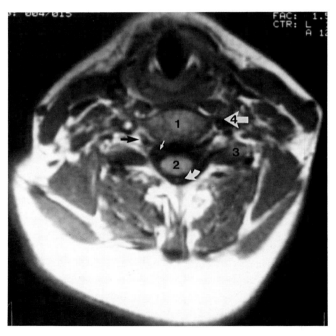

Figure 8-7

T1-weighted axial image through cervical intervertebral disc: intervertebral disc *(1)*, cord *(2)*, articular pillar *(3)*, vertebral artery *(4)*. Root sleeve *(black arrow)*, ventral nerve root *(straight white arrow)*, and CSF *(curved white arrow)* are identified.

Figure 8-6

Apophyseal joint visualized on sagittal gradient echo image. The facet articular cartilage images with high signal intensity *(arrows)* on T2* gradient echo image. TR = 400 msec, TE = 15 msec; flip angle = 15°.

Figure 8-8

Axial T2* gradient echo image at midcervical level: intervertebral disc *(1)*, cord *(2)*, common carotid artery *(3)*, jugular vein *(4)*, vertebral artery *(5)*, dorsal root ganglion *(6)*, superior articular process *(7)*, inferior articular process *(8)*, facet cartilage *(9)*, uncinate process *(10)*. TR = 400 msec, TE = 30 msec; flip angle = 30°.

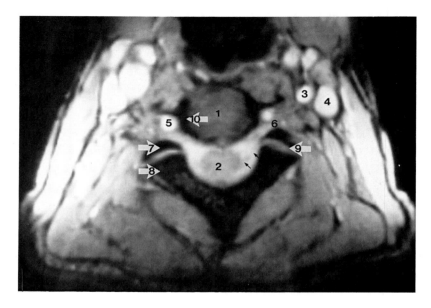

IMAGING PROTOCOLS FOR THORACIC AND LUMBAR SPINES

The thoracic and lumbar spines are imaged using a planar surface coil with its long axis oriented parallel to the spine. This permits acquisition with an FOV approximating the anatomic region of interest. When the area of interest is restricted to one or two vertebral levels, a 5-inch circular spine coil may be used to provide better signal-to-noise.

Sagittal images of the thoracic and lumbar spines are obtained with T1- and T2-weighting.[36–38] Routine T1-weighted images are acquired with a TR of 600 msec, a TE of 20 msec, 5-mm thick sections, a 20- to 24-cm FOV, a 256 × 256 acquisition matrix, and four NEX. This sequence allows adequate bilateral coverage of the canal and neural foramina. Conventional T2-weighted images are acquired with a TR of 2000 msec, a TE of 20, 60 msec, a 256 × 128 acquisition matrix, and four NEX. Although less pronounced than in the cervical spine, low signal intensity pulsatile CSF motion artifact, secondary to spin dephasing, may degrade image quality or

Figure 8-9
T1-weighted sagittal image of thoracic spine: cord *(1)*, CSF *(2)*, epidural fat *(3)*, thoracic disc herniation without cord compression *(4)*, intervertebral disc *(5)*. TR = 600 msec, TE = 20 msec.

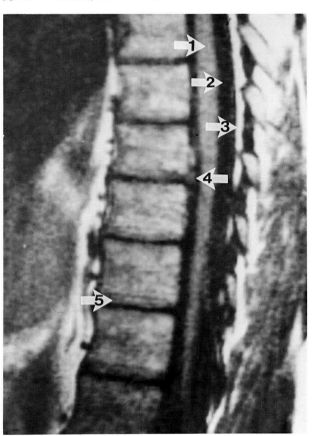

obscure pathology in the thoracic spine. Cardiac gating of studies in the upper thoracic spine minimizes the effects of flow. Aortic pulsation artifacts may also be problematic in thoracic spine studies that use long TR/TE sequences. Compared to conventional spin echo techniques, T2* gradient echo images of the thoracic and lumbar spines minimize artifact from pulsatile CSF and generate increased signal-to-noise and contrast. Gradient echo sequences use a TR of 400 msec, a TE of 15 msec, and a flip angle of 30°. Even though T2* gradient echo contrast may be substituted for conventional T2-weighting, contrast properties are not equivalent. For instance, desiccated discs that image with low signal intensity on T2-weighted images may remain isointense with intact intervertebral discs on T2* gradient refocused images.

In the *axial plane,* T1-weighted images are obtained using a TR of 1000 msec, a TE of 20 msec, 5-mm sections, a 16-cm FOV, a 256 × 256 acquisition matrix, and four NEX. This sequence provides anatomic coverage from L3 to S1. A supplementary spin echo T2-weighted sequence can be obtained by using a TR of 2000 msec, a TE of 20, 60 msec, and a 256 × 128 acquisition matrix. Instead of conventional T2-weighting, a T2* gradient echo sequence can be used to supplement the T1-weighted acquisition.

NORMAL MR ANATOMY OF THE THORACIC AND LUMBAR SPINES

Sagittal Images

T-1 Weighted Images

In the thoracic spine the posterior subarachnoid space is larger than the subarachnoid space anterior to the cord (Fig. 8-9). CSF within the subarachnoid space is visualized with low signal intensity, in contrast to the brighter (intermediate) signal intensity of the cord, and posterior epidural fat images with high signal intensity. Anterior epidural fat is prominent in the L5–S1 region. Yellow or fatty marrow within the vertebral bodies of the thoracic and lumbar spine images with high signal intensity, in contrast to the intermediate signal intensity of intervertebral discs. Nuclear annular differentiation is not precisely defined on T1-weighted images (Fig. 8-10). The cord is of uniform intermediate signal intensity. The conus medullaris is tapered and terminates posteriorly at the level of L1. Sagittal images of the lumbar spine with a 24-cm FOV demonstrate the conus medullaris. The cauda equina is of lower signal intensity than the conus medullaris, secondary to greater surface contact with surrounding CSF. On T1-weighted images anterior and posterior longitudinal ligaments are difficult to distinguish from low signal intensity cortical bone. The exiting nerve roots are visualized with intermediate signal

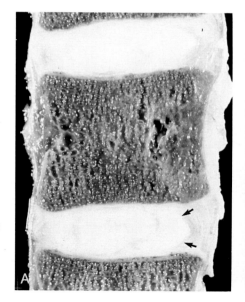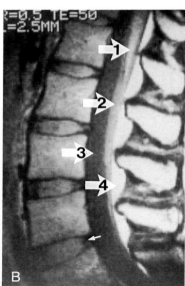

Figure 8-10

Lumbar spine. **(A)** Gross sagittal specimen demonstrating nuclear-annular separation *(arrows).* **(B)** T1-weighted midsagittal image of the lumbar spine identifying: conus medullaris *(1),* cauda equina *(2),* CSF *(3),* epidural fat *(4),* and annular fibers *(small arrow).* TR = 500 msec, TE = 50 msec.

Figure 8-11

Intervertebral foramina. Parasagittal T1-weighted image demonstrating high signal intensity epidural fat *(large black arrow),* intermediate signal intensity dorsal root ganglion *(small black arrow),* and low signal intensity radicular vein *(curved white arrow).* TR = 600 msec, TE = 20 msec.

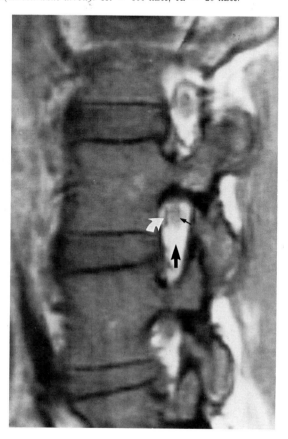

intensity within the tear drop shaped intervertebral foramina and are surrounded by high signal intensity fat (Fig. 8-11). On parasagittal images, the low signal intensity radicular vein and intermediate signal dorsal root are demarcated by abundant high signal intensity fat within the lumbar neural foramina.

T2-Weighted Images

On T2-weighted images the low signal intensity thoracic cord is visualized in contrast to high signal intensity CSF. Thoracic and lumbar intervertebral discs image with bright signal intensity on T2- and T2*-weighted images (Fig. 8-12). Epidural fat is visualized with intermediate signal intensity (Fig. 8-13). Vertebral body marrow is intermediate in signal intensity on T2-weighted images and is low in signal intensity on T2*-weighted images. On T2-weighted images, the conus medullaris demonstrates lower signal intensity than the surrounding bright CSF. The nucleus pulposus and inner annular fibers image with increased signal intensity on T2-weighted images, whereas peripheral annular fibers maintain low signal intensity. A low signal intensity band in the midportion of the intervertebral disc is thought to represent an invagination of annular fibers, although an anatomic correlate has not yet been found. The basivertebral vein is identified as a high signal intensity segment in the midposterior aspect of the vertebral body.

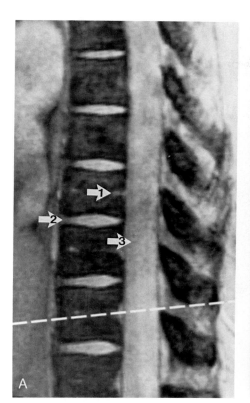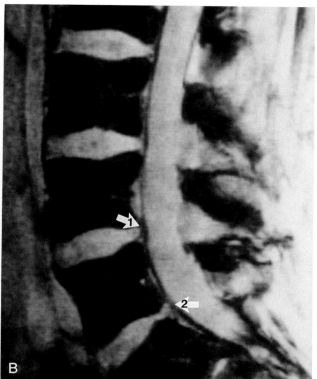

Figure 8-12
Thoracic and lumbar spines. (T2* gradient echo sagittal images; TR = 400 msec, TE = 15 msec; flip angle = 30°) **(A)** Thoracic spine: basivertebral vein *(1)*, high signal intensity intervertebral disc *(2)*, high signal intensity CSF and cord, not differentiated on this image *(3)*. **(B)** Lumbar spine: low signal intensity annulus *(1)*, low signal intensity dural interface *(2)*.

Axial Images

T1-Weighted Images

In cross section, the thoracic cord is imaged with intermediate signal intensity, and surrounding CSF demonstrates low signal intensity. High signal intensity from fatty marrow is visualized in the body, pedicle, lamina, and transverse and spinous processes of the vertebra. The intraforaminal vein (of low signal intensity) can be seen anterior to the dorsal root ganglion (of intermediate signal intensity). The dorsal root ganglion budding and exiting nerve roots are well defined and image with intermediate signal intensity surrounded by bright signal intensity fat (Fig. 8-14). Nerve roots are often identified within the lower signal intensity thecal sac. Posterior epidural fat is identified behind the low signal intensity subarachnoid space. The basivertebral vein, retrovertebral plexus, and anterior epidural veins are displayed as low signal intensity structures. The ligamentum flavum parallels the inner surface of the lamina and demonstrates intermediate signal intensity.

T2-Weighted Images

An axial myelographic effect can be generated with gradient refocused images in a fraction of the time required for conventional spin echo techniques (Fig. 8-15). On T2-weighted images, the thoracic cord and lumbar cauda equina are visualized with low signal intensity, in contrast to the high signal intensity of CSF (Fig. 8-16). Facet cartilage images with high signal intensity on gradient echo images and with intermediate signal intensity on conventional T2-weighted images. High signal intensity nuclear material and inner annular fibers are distinguished from low signal intensity peripheral collagen fibers of the annulus (Fig. 8-17). Anterior signal void within the thecal sac is more frequent with long TR/TE sequences that accentuate CSF pulsation artifacts.

Text continues on p. 332

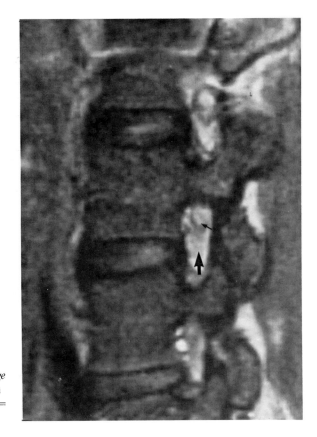

Figure 8-13
Intervertebral foramina. Intermediate signal intensity neural foraminal fat is shown *(large arrow)* with poor contrast compared to intermediate signal intensity dorsal root ganglion *(small arrow)* on conventional T2-weighted parasagittal image. TR = 2000 msec, TE = 60 msec.

Figure 8-14
T1-weighted axial anatomy of lumbar spine at level of superior neural foramina: L5 nerve root sheath *(1)*, thecal sac *(2)*, budding S1 nerve root *(3)*, anterior epidural vein *(4)*.

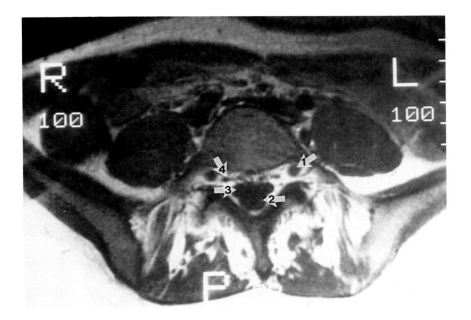

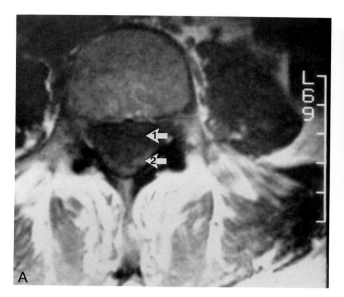 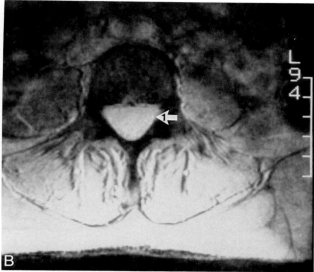

Figure 8-15

Axial myelographic contrast. T1-weighted *(A)* and T2* gradient echo *(B)* axial images at midlumbar body level: thecal sac *(1)*, cauda equina *(2)*. The thecal sac is shown as bright signal intensity on T2* contrast.

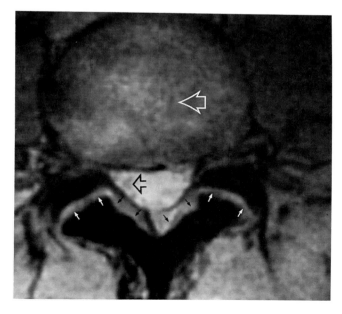

Figure 8-16

T2* gradient echo axial image of lumbar intervertebral disc identifying high signal intensity disc *(open white arrow)*, articular cartilage *(solid white arrows)*, ligamentum flavum *(solid black arrows)* and low signal intensity cauda equina *(open black arrow)*. TR = 400 msec, TE = 15 msec; flip angle = 30°.

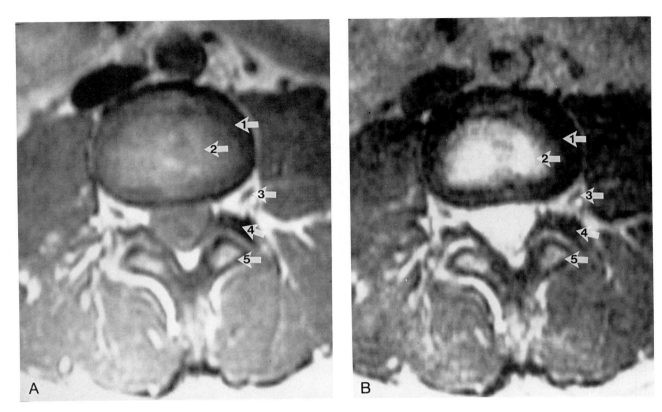

Figure 8-17

Conventional T2-weighted axial sequence at the intervertebral disc. Intermediate *(A)* and T2-weighted *(B)* axial images demonstrating increased signal intensity in the nucleus pulposus on T2-weighted contrast: low signal intensity annular fibers *(1)*, nucleus pulposus *(2)*, exiting nerve root *(3)*, superior articular facet *(4)*, inferior articular facet *(5)*. TR = 2000 msec, TE = 20, 60 msec.

PATHOLOGY OF THE SPINE

In addition to assessing degenerative disc disease in the cervical spine (see below), MR is applicable in the evaluation of infection, trauma, and neoplasia involving osseous structures, soft tissue, and the cord.[6-35] Direct marrow imaging facilitates early detection of marrow replacement disorders such as leukemia, multiple myeloma, and metastasis. Atlantoaxial instability can be functionally imaged using separate acquisitions with the patient positioned in flexion and extension.[39] Signal characteristics of cystic lesions (syringomyelia and hydromyelia) are similar to those of CSF. Intramedullary lipomas image with high signal intensity on T1-weighted images, intermediate to high signal intensity on T2-weighted images, and are dark on STIR sequences (Fig. 8-18). Lipomas can sometimes be confused with subacute hemorrhage, also bright on T1-weighted images, but hemorrhage shows increased signal intensity on long TR/TE (T2-weighted) sequences. Detection of neurofibromas[40] and meningiomas, common intradural extramedullary tumors, may require the use of intravenous gadolinium-DTPA (a paramagnetic contrast agent) to improve their visualization.

Degenerative Disc Disease

Cervical Spine

T1-weighted sagittal images display the subarachnoid disc and cervical cord outlines, directly assessing cord impingement (Fig. 8-19).[6-18,41] Early degenerative disc disease may be identified on a conventional T2-weighted sagittal image and is characterized by loss of signal intensity in a desiccated intervertebral disc. Corresponding gradient echo images are not as sensitive to changes in intradisc signal intensity, and only in more advanced stages of degeneration are regions of low signal intensity from clefting, cavitation, or complete desication demonstrated. T2* gradient echo sequences are useful in producing a myelographic CSF effect, important in assessing spinal canal stenosis and buckling of the ligamentum flavum. With gradient echo techniques, there is nonslice-selective acquisition without degradation or loss of signal intensity from pulsatile flow columns of CSF. Image quality with conventional spin echo techniques degrades with CSF flow artifact, and accuracy in interpreting extradural impressions (disc herniations and osteophytosis) may be compromised. The absence of flow artifact, along with excellent differentiation be-

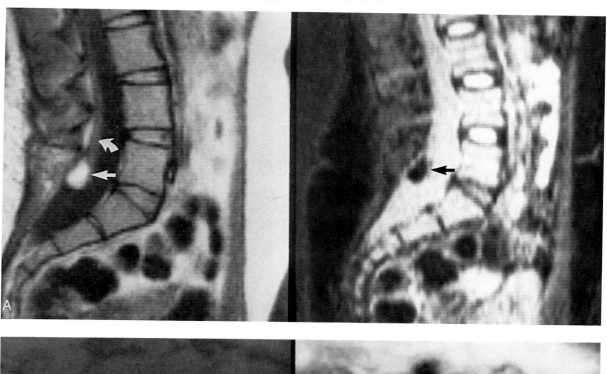

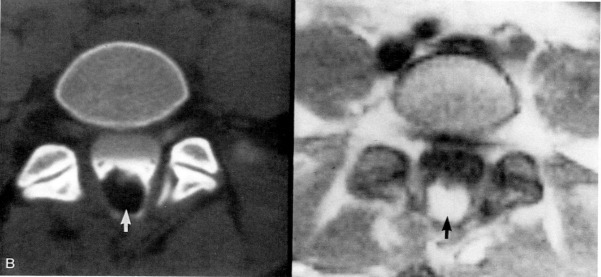

Figure 8-18

Tethered cord with lipoma. **(A)** Intermediate signal intensity tethered cord *(curved arrow)* and associated lipoma *(straight arrow)* are imaged on T1-weighted *(left)* and STIR *(right)* images. Lipoma is imaged with high signal intensity on the T1-weighted image and is dark on the STIR image. **(B)** Corresponding CT scan *(right)* demonstrates low attenuation lipoma *(arrow)* that images with high signal intensity on T1-weighted axial MR image *(left)*.

tween the cord and CSF, eliminates the need for cardiac gating in gradient refocused images.

A decrease in disc height and bulging of the peripheral annular fibers may contribute to spinal stenosis (Fig. 8-20). Associated osteophytes may project from both the anterior and posterior vertebral body margins, and posterior osteophytes may be confused with low signal intensity annular bulges (Fig. 8-21). Enlarged osteophytes that compromise the subarachnoid space contribute to the development of cord myelopathy. Radiculopathy may result from impingement on the dural sac or root sleeve. Neural foraminal stenosis and associated radiculopathy can also be caused by degenerative changes at the facets and uncinate *(uncinate process hypertrophy)*. Severe disc herniations may demonstrate resultant deformity or kinking of the cord. Herniated nuclear material commonly maintains high signal intensity on T2* gradient echo images. Effacement of intervertebral foraminal fat is associated with posterolateral disc herniations, although the uncinate process in the cervical spine, unlike the lumbar spine, affords some protection from posterolateral disc herniations. Lateral disc herniations, however, do occur and can be visualized on peripheral parasagittal (Fig. 8-22) and axial (Fig. 8-23) images.

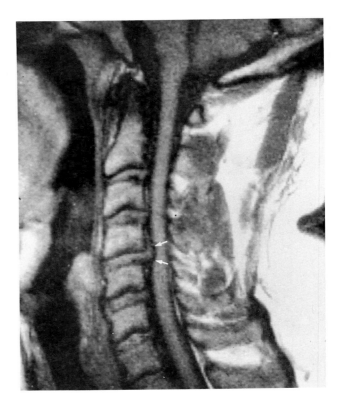

Figure 8-19

C4–5 disc herniation *(arrows)* deforming the spinal cord on midsagittal T1-weighted image. TR = 500 msec, TE = 40 msec.

Figure 8-20

Multiple disc herniations in the cervical spine. C3–4, C4–5, and C5–6 disc herniations *(white arrows)* indenting the spinal cord are identified on T1-weighted sagittal image. Anterior disc bulges *(black arrows)* and loss of disc space height are shown in levels C3–4 and C4–5. TR = 600 msec, TE = 20 msec.

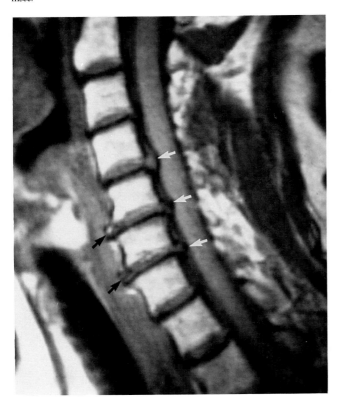

Figure 8-21

Cervical osteophytosis. Degenerative cervical spine with osteophytes *(black arrows)* and desiccated C3–4 disc *(white arrow)*. T2* gradient echo sagittal image; TR = 400 msec, TE = 15 msec.

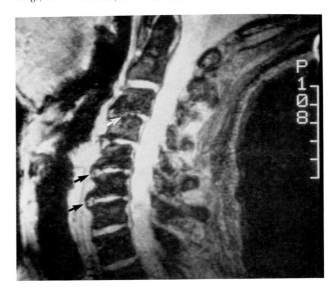

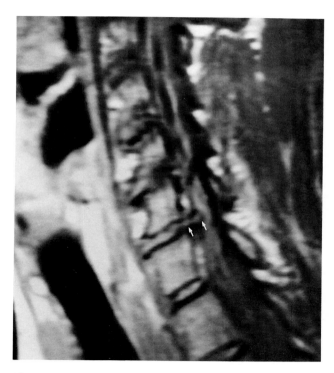

Figure 8-22

Lateral C6–7 disc herniation *(arrows)* visualized on T1-weighted parasagittal image. TR = 600 msec, TE = 20 msec.

Thoracic and Lumbar Spines

The accuracy of MR has been shown to be equivalent to CT and myelography in the assessment of thoracic and lumbar disc herniation.[19–27,42–45] Herniations identified in the sagittal plane should be confirmed on axial images, and thin (3 mm) sections may be necessary to characterize the disc abnormality. Associated Schmorl's nodes and decreased intervertebral signal intensity can be seen on T2-weighted images (Fig. 8-24). Marginal osteophytes contribute to extrinsic (extradural) impression on the thecal sac. Flow artifacts in the lumbar spine should not be mistaken for intrinsic pathology, and may be accentuated around areas of stenosis (Fig. 8-25).

In early lumbar degenerative disc disease there may be a loss of hydropic integrity or intradiscal desiccation, characterized by decreased signal intensity on conventional T2-weighted images (Figs. 8-26 and 8-27). Inhomogeneity and areas of decreased signal intensity on T2* gradient echo images are usually associated with severe degenerative disc disease (Fig. 8-28).[37] Disc-CSF separation may be difficult on T1-weighted images because the posterior disc margin and thecal sac both image with low signal intensity (Fig. 8-29). Most herniated discs are depicted as degenerative or desiccated on conventional T2-weighted images in contrast to T2* gradient refocused images. Lateral disc herniations can efface the

Text continues on p. 339

Figure 8-23

Lateral disc herniation *(curved white arrow)* lateralizing to the left on a T1-weighted axial image. Intervertebral disc *(large black arrow)* and uncinate process *(small black arrow)* are visualized at this level. TR = 1000 msec, TE = 20 msec.

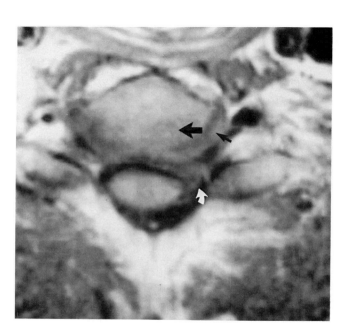

Figure 8-24

Loss of intervertebral thoracic disc height and signal intensity *(arrows)* is shown on T2* gradient refocused image. TR = 400 msec, TE = 15 msec; flip angle = 30°.

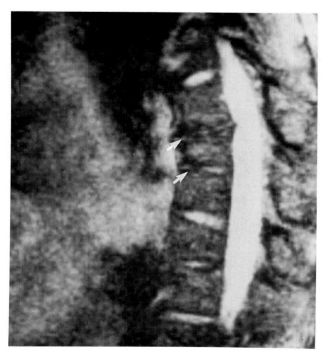

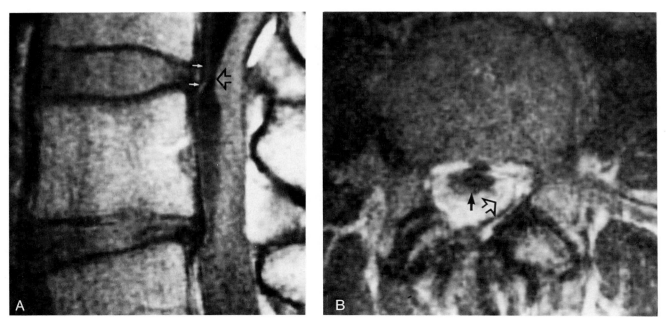

Figure 8-25

Flow artifact in lumbar spine. **(A)** Low signal intensity CSF flow artifact *(open arrow)* is visualized in the anterior aspect of the thecal sac on a T1-weighted sagittal image. Adjacent disc herniation *(white arrows)* creates a tapering deformity within the artifact. TR = 600 msec, TE = 20 msec. **(B)** Corresponding T2-weighted axial image demonstrates the prominent flow void artifact *(solid arrow)* with surrounding bright signal intensity CSF *(open arrow)*. TR = 2000 msec, TE = 60 msec.

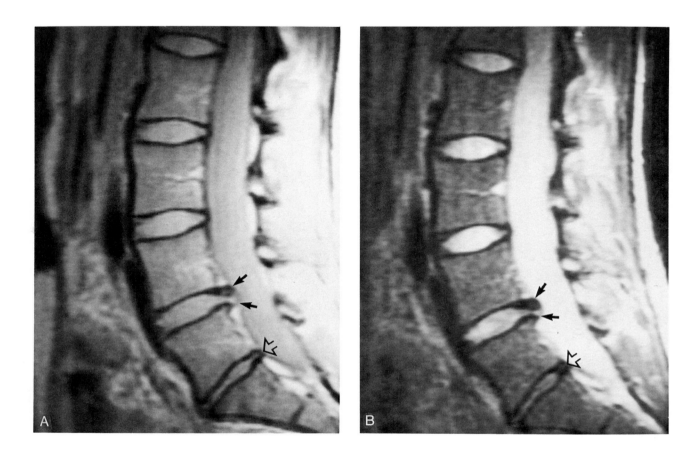

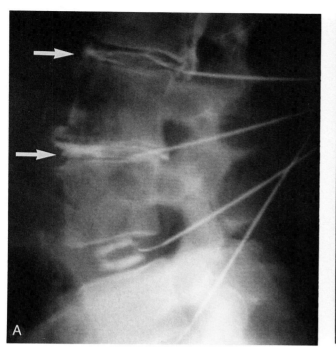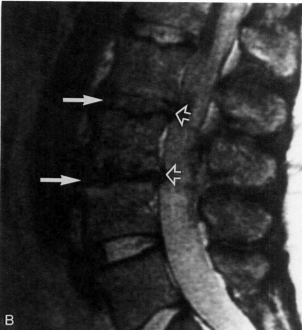

Figure 8-27

Discogram-MR correlation. Desiccated and herniated L2–3 and L3–4 discs are displayed with abnormal contrast distribution *(solid arrows)* in lateral discogram *(A)* and with loss of signal intensity *(solid arrows)* on T2-weighted sagittal image *(B)*. Disc bulges deforming the ventral aspect of the thecal sac are identified on sagittal MR image *(open arrows)*. TR = 2000 msec, TE = 60 msec.

Figure 8-28

Severe intervertebral L4–5 disc desiccation *(arrows)* with loss of signal intensity and disc space height on T2* gradient echo sagittal image. TR = 400 msec, TE = 15 msec; flip angle = 30°.

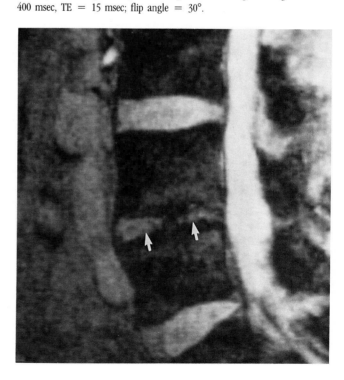

◄ Figure 8-26

Desiccated lumbar disc. Intermediate-weighted *(A)* and T2-weighted *(B)* sagittal images demonstrate isointense and low signal intensity desiccated L5–S1 lumbar disc, respectively *(open arrow)*. Deformity of the anterior thecal sac from L4–5 disc bulge *(solid arrows)* is best appreciated on the T2-weighted image. TR = 2000 msec, TE = 20, 60 msec.

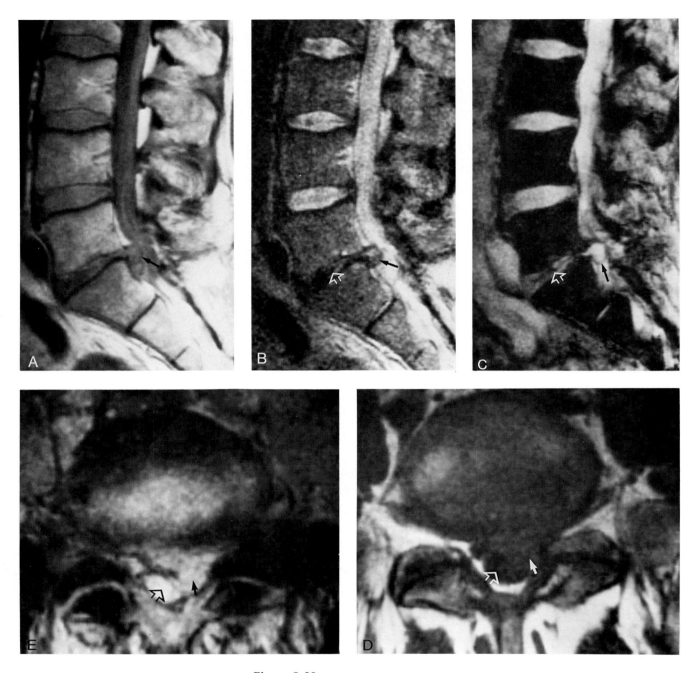

Figure 8-29

Disc herniation on conventional spin echo and gradient echo techniques. T1-weighted *(A)*, T2-weighted *(B)*, and T2* gradient echo *(C)* images demonstrate herniated and extruded L5–S1 nuclear material *(black arrow)*. Intervertebral disc contents *(open arrow)* remain low in signal intensity on conventional T2-weighted sequences *(B)*. On T2* gradient echo contrast, nuclear material generates high signal intensity whereas adjacent desiccated disc is visualized with signal inhomogeneity and low signal intensity clefting *(open arrow in C)*. *(A)* TR = 600 msec, TE = 20 msec; *(B)* TR = 2000 msec, TE = 60 msec; *(C)* TR = 400 msec, TE = 15 msec, flip angle = 30°. Corresponding T1-weighted *(D)* and T2* weighted *(E)* axial images displaying superior contrast definition of herniated nuclear material *(solid arrow)* and deformed thecal sac *(open arrow)* on gradient echo sequence *(E)*. *(D)* TR = 1000 msec, TE = 20 msec; *(E)* TR = 400 msec, TE = 15 msec; flip angle = 30°.

bright signal intensity neural foraminal fat, without compromising the thecal sac (Fig. 8-30). Large posterolateral disc herniations may compromise both the thecal sac and exiting nerve root (Fig. 8-31). The sagittal imaging plane may be more sensitive for defining deformities of the thecal sac at the disc-thecal sac interface. T2-weighted images are effective in increasing contrast discrimination between bright signal intensity CSF and low signal intensity annular fibers at the disc-thecal sac boundary. Acute herniations may be associated with increased signal intensity either on conventional T1- or T2-weighted images (Fig. 8-32). On gradient echo images the posterior annular fibers and longitudinal ligament image with low signal intensity (Fig. 8-33), facilitating differentiation of the disc and CSF. Gradient echo images also display the black line of the dura in the

lumbar spine that may be displaced in posterior disc herniations. Nuclear material extruded from the disc usually images with low signal intensity on conventional T1- and T2-weighted images (Fig. 8-34), and with high signal intensity on gradient echo sequences (Fig. 8-35).

Axial images are important in evaluating neural foramina and nerve root effacement in cases of lateral and posterolateral disc herniations. Axial gradient echo images help distinguish herniated disc material from brighter signal intensity CSF. The path of extruded nuclear material may be outlined on axial T2-weighted images (discogramlike effect; Fig. 8-36). Disc material or fragments superior or inferior to the intervertebral disc level may represent free fragments (Fig. 8-37). Calcified cysts of the facet joint may mimic a calcified free fragment (Fig. 8-38).

Text continues on p. 344

Figure 8-30

Lateral disc herniation. **(A)** T1-weighted parasagittal image showing absent foraminal fat in L3–L4 intervertebral foramina *(solid arrows)*. Intact L2–3 disc level demonstrates normal high signal intensity foraminal fat for comparison *(open arrow)*. TR = 600 msec, TE = 20 msec. **(B)** Corresponding axial CT identifies left lateral disc material encroaching on the intervertebral foramina with resultant stenosis *(open arrow)*.

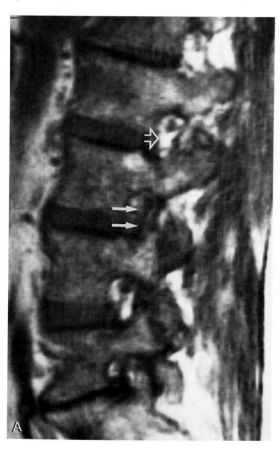
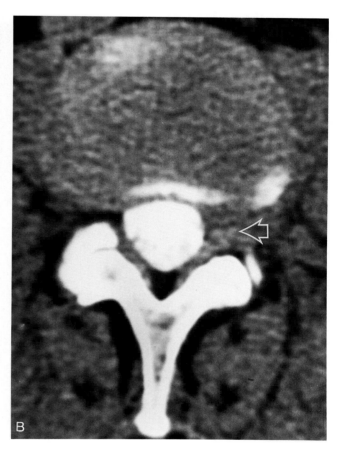

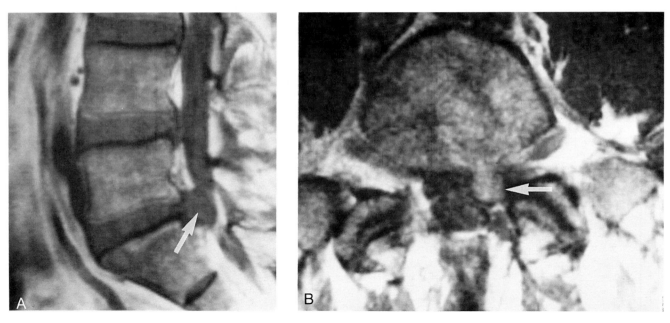

Figure 8-31

L5–S1 disc herniation *(arrow)* with nuclear material impressing the thecal sac and effacing the epidural fat on T1-weighted sagittal *(A)* and axial *(B)* images. Left S1 nerve root involvement is appreciated on axial image. TR = 1000 msec, TE = 20 msec.

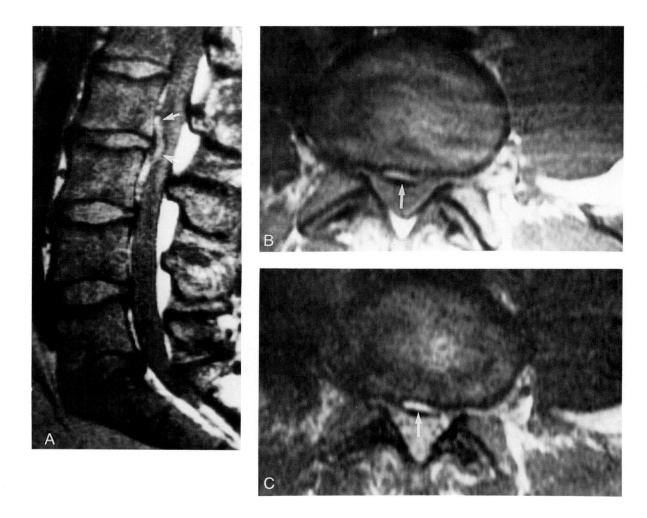

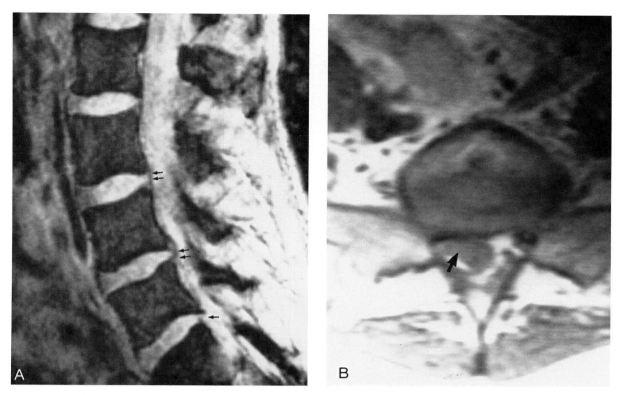

Figure 8-33

Annular disruption. **(A)** Intact *(double arrows)* and disrupted *(single arrow)* annular complex on T2* gradient refocused image. TR = 400 msec, TE = 15 msec; flip angle = 30°. **(B)** Corresponding T1-weighted axial image identifying left posterolateral disc herniation *(arrow)*. TR = 1000 msec, TE = 20 msec.

◄ **Figure 8-32**

Acute disc herniations. **(A)** Conventional T2-weighted sagittal image identifying high signal intensity nuclear extrusion *(arrows)*. TR = 2000 msec, TE = 60 msec. Acute L4–5 central disc herniation *(arrow)* in another patient displaying high signal intensity on T1-weighted **(B)** and T2-weighted **(C)** axial images. **(B)** TR = 1000 msec, TE = 20 msec; **(C)** TR = 2000 msec, TE = 60 msec.

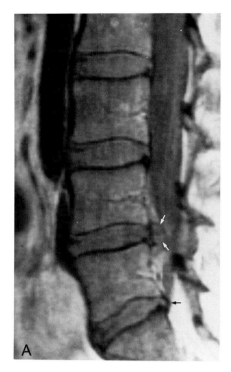
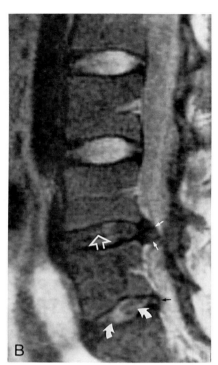

Figure 8-34

Lumbar disc herniation. T1-weighted *(A)* and T2-weighted *(B)* sagittal images displaying mild L5–S1 *(black arrow)* and severe L4–5 disc herniations *(solid white arrows)*. Signal intensity is still present in early L5–S1 disc desiccation *(curved arrows)* while no signal intensity is observed in the L4–5 intervertebral disc *(open arrow)* on T2-weighted sequence. *(A)* TR = 600 msec, TE = 20 msec; *(B)* TR = 2000 msec, TE = 60 msec.

Figure 8-35

Nuclear herniation *(arrows)* is isointense with the intervertebral disc at L5–S1 using T2* gradient echo technique. TR = 400 msec, TE = 15 msec; flip angle = 30°.

Figure 8-36

Discogramlike effect showing the path of extruded nuclear material *(arrows)* on T2* gradient echo axial image. TR = 400 msec, TE = 15 msec; flip angle = 30°.

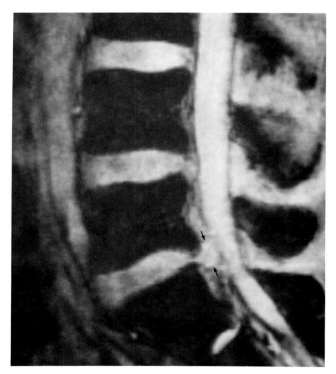

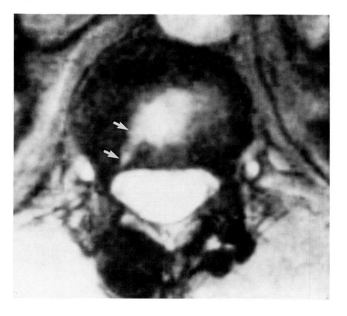

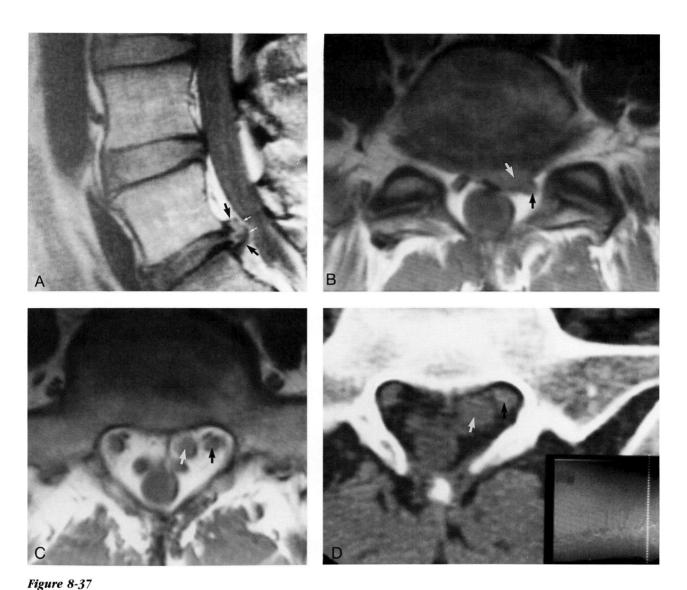

Figure 8-37

Free disc fragment. *(A)* Large L5–S1 left posterolateral disc herniation effacing the epidural fat *(black arrows)* and deforming the anterior aspect of the thecal sac *(white arrows)*. T1-weighted sagittal image; TR = 600 msec, TE = 20 msec. *(B)* Axial image at L5–S1 intervertebral disc level demonstrating herniated disc *(white arrow)* and involved left S1 nerve root *(black arrow)*. T1-weighted axial image; TR = 600 msec, TE = 20 msec. T1-weighted axial MR image *(C)* and axial CT scan *(D)* at a more inferior level identifying free disc fragment *(white arrow)* and adjacent intact left S2 nerve root *(black arrow)*.

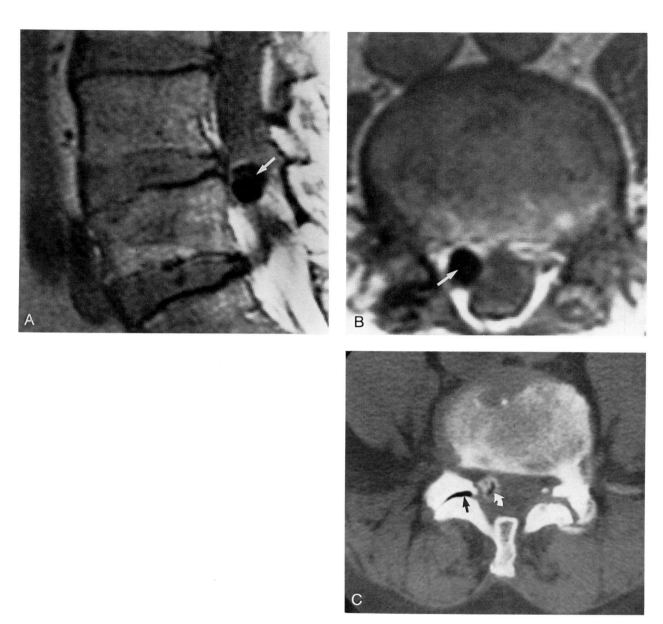

Figure 8-38
Apophyseal joint cyst. Dark signal intensity circular structure *(arrow)* is imaged on T1-weighted sagittal *(A)* and axial *(B)* images. TR = 1000 msec, TE = 20 msec. *(C)* Corresponding axial CT demonstrating air within the left facet joint *(straight arrow)* and contiguous calcified cyst *(curved arrow)*.

Decreased or effacement of epidural fat is seen with lumbar *canal stenosis* (Fig. 8-39).[27] Indentations of the thecal sac are caused by both disc and osteophytic impingement (Fig. 8-40). Facet and ligamentum flavum hypertrophy contribute to neural foraminal and central canal stenosis (Figs. 8-41 and 8-42). Canal dimensions in stenosis are most accurately assessed on T2-weighted images where there is a bright CSF-extradural interface (Fig. 8-43).

Pars defects and grades of spondylolisthesis can be assessed on sagittal and axial images (Figs. 8-44 and 8-45). The sclerosis associated with a pars interarticularis defect is imaged as low signal intensity on T1- and T2-weighted images (Fig. 8-46).

Text continues on p. 349

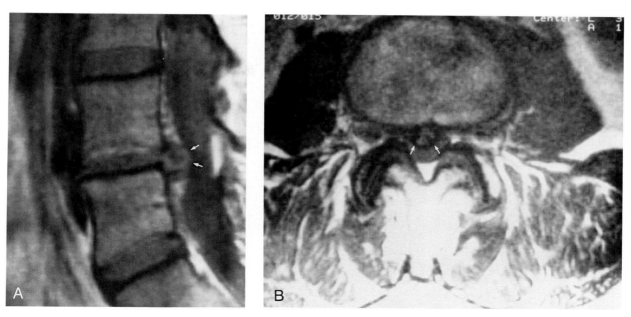

Figure 8-39

Central spinal stenosis secondary to disc herniation. Two examples of central spinal stenosis resulting from severe posterior disc herniation are presented. **(A)** Recurrent disc *(arrows)* after a percutaneous nuclectomy is shown on a T1-weighted sagittal image. **(B)** Spontaneous central herniation *(arrows)* displayed in another patient on a T1-weighted axial image.

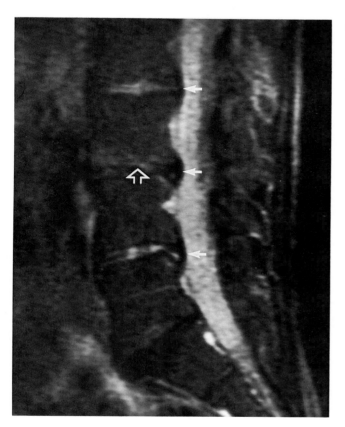

Figure 8-40

Spinal stenosis with osteophytosis. T2-weighted sagittal image demonstrating osteophytic encroachment on the anterior aspect of thecal sac *(solid arrows)*. One of multiple low signal intensity desiccated discs is identified *(open arrow)*. TR = 2000 msec, TE = 60 msec.

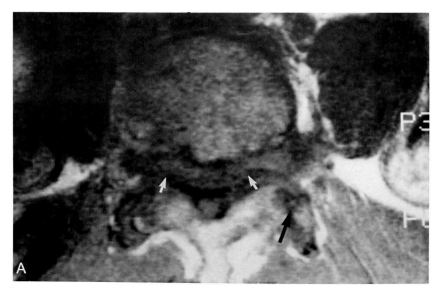

Figure 8-41

Central canal and neural foraminal stenosis. Broad-based disc herniation *(white arrows)* and degenerative facets *(black arrow)* contribute to central and neural foraminal stenosis as visualized on T1-weighted axial MR image *(A)* and on axial CT scan *(B)*. TR = 1000 msec, TE = 20 msec.

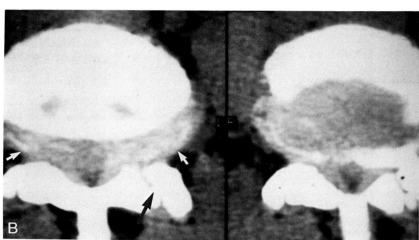

Figure 8-42

Hypertrophied apophyseal joints *(large arrow)* visualized on T1-weighted axial image. Intermediate signal intensity articular cartilage is identified *(small arrows)*. TR = 1000 msec, TE = 20 msec.

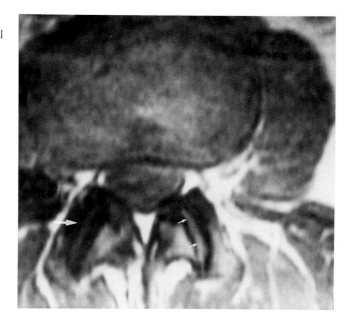

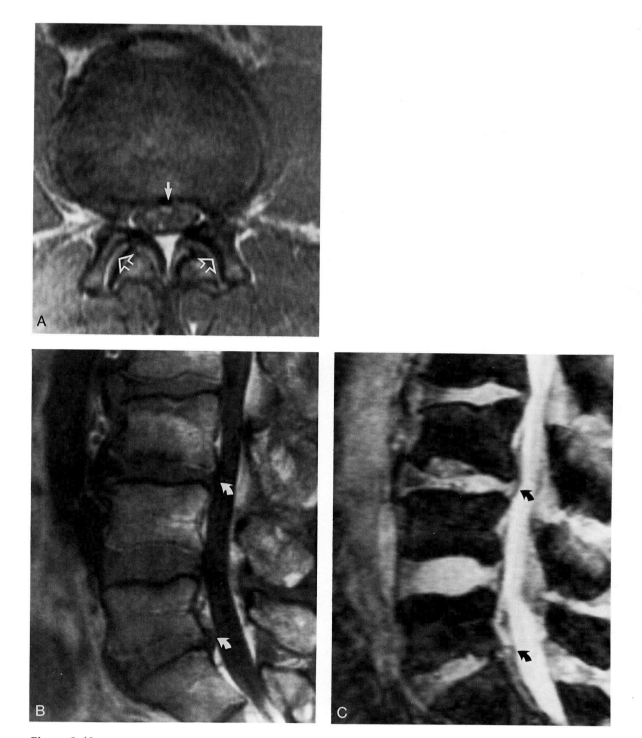

Figure 8-43

Lumbar canal stenosis. Narrowed vertebral canal with multiple level disc bulges *(curved arrows),* vertebral bony encroachment, hypertrophied articular facets *(open arrows),* and small thecal sac *(straight arrow)* visualized on T1-weighted axial *(A),* sagittal *(B)* images, and T2* gradient refocused sagittal image *(C). (A–B)* TR = 1000 msec, TE = 20 msec; *(C)* TR = 400 msec, TE = 15 msec; flip angle = 30°.

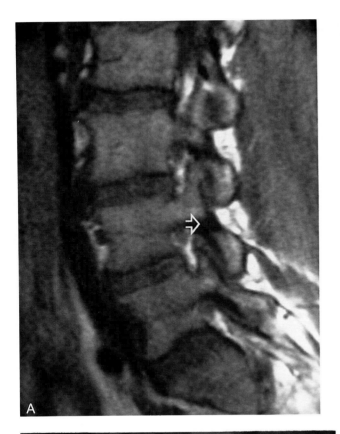

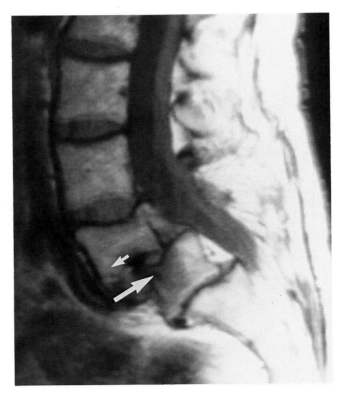

Figure 8-45
Spondylolisthesis, grade 3. Greater than 50% anterior displacement of L5 *(small arrow)* on S1 *(large arrow)*. T1-weighted sagittal image; TR = 600 msec, TE = 20 msec.

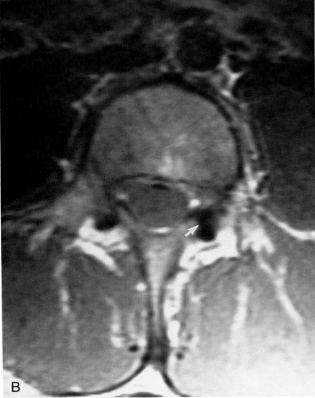

Figure 8-44
Spondylolisthesis, grade 1. Sclerotic pars defect *(arrow)* is imaged as a low signal intensity band on T1-weighted sagittal *(A)* and on axial *(B)* images. TR = 600 msec, TE = 20 msec.

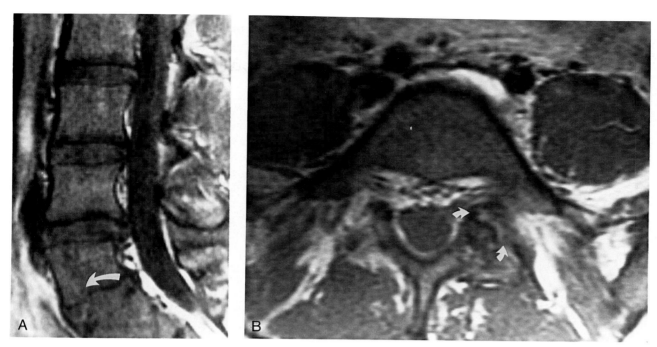

Figure 8-46

Spondylolisthesis, grade 1. **(A)** Anterior displacement of L5 on S1 *(curved arrow)*. T1-weighted sagittal image; TR = 600 msec, TE = 20 msec. **(B)** Pars defect irregularity with associated low signal intensity sclerosis *(curved arrows)* is identified on a T1-weighted axial image. TR = 1000 msec, TE = 20 msec.

Postoperative Spine

CT plays an important role in assessing postoperative bony detail, especially in evaluating pseudoarthrosis in lumbar spine fusions.[46] MR imaging, however, is also useful in characterizing endplate and associated marrow changes.[47] Preliminary work indicates that stable *fusions of the lumbar spine* are associated with fatty marrow conversion at the endplates of the corresponding levels (Fig. 8-47).[48] This yellow or fatty marrow conversion images with increased signal intensity on T1-weighted images and becomes isointense with adjacent marrow on T2-weighted images (Fig. 8-48). On T1-weighted images, fusion instability frequently demonstrates low signal intensity adjacent to the endplates that increases with progressive T2 weighting (Fig. 8-49). Focal fatty marrow conversion also has been documented in cases of degenerated discs (Fig. 8-50).[47] Endplate sclerosis is visualized with low signal intensity on T1- and T2-weighted images.

MR imaging has also been used to assess postoperative changes in *fusion* (Fig. 8-51) and *laminectomy* and in *chymopapain* and *percutaneous nucleotomy.*[48–50] The sensitivity and specificity of MR have been shown to be equal to intravenous contrast CT in distinguishing recurrent disc herniations from scar or fibrosis (Fig. 8-52). Scar tissue demonstrates low to intermediate

Figure 8-47

Stable fusion. Increased signal intensity *(arrows)* in superior endplate of L5 and inferior endplate of L4 in area of yellow marrow conversion associated with stable lumbar fusion. T1-weighted sagittal image; TR = 600 msec, TE = 20 msec.

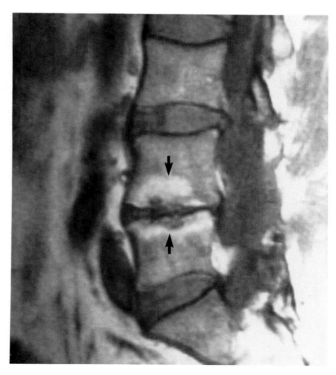

signal intensity on T1-weighted images and intermediate to increased signal intensity without mass effect on T2-weighted images (Fig. 8-53). Gadolinium contrast has been shown to have a role in defining and enhancing epidural fibrosis.[51] Disc herniations (protrusions and extrusions) demonstrate mass effect and do not increase in signal intensity on conventional T2-weighted images (Fig. 8-54). On gradient echo images, herniated disc material may generate higher signal than adjacent fibrosis or scar. When interpreting MR studies of the spine with metallic artifact, the increased sensitivity to magnetic susceptibility with gradient echo imaging must be appreciated (Fig. 8-55).

Clumping and irregular separation of the nerve roots are characteristic of *arachnoiditis*,[52] which often requires T2-weighted axial images to display the distortion of thecal sac and roots. A postoperative fluid collection or *pseudomeningocele* images with signal characteristics analogous to CSF—low signal intensity on T1-weighted images and high signal intensity on T2-weighted images (Fig. 8-56). Focal collections of Pantopaque in the thecal sac have a characteristic appearance on MR and image with high signal intensity on T1-weighted images and with low signal intensity on T2-weighted images (Fig. 8-57).[53] Lipomas also image with increased signal intensity on T1-weighted images and may be confused with residual Pantopaque. Associated spinal dysraphism or nulled fat signal intensity on STIR sequences is characteristic of a lipomatous lesion, and helps distinguish the two.[54]

Text continues on p. 356

Figure 8-48

Stable lumbar fusion. L5–S1 yellow marrow conversion *(arrows)* images with bright signal intensity on T1-weighted image *(A)* and is isointense with adjacent marrow on T2* gradient echo image *(B)*. *(A)* TR = 600 msec, TE = 20 msec; *(B)* TR = 400 msec, TE = 15 msec; flip angle = 30°

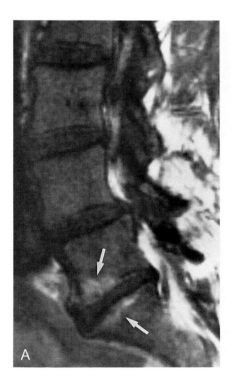
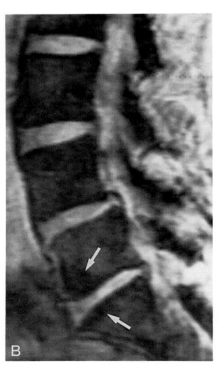

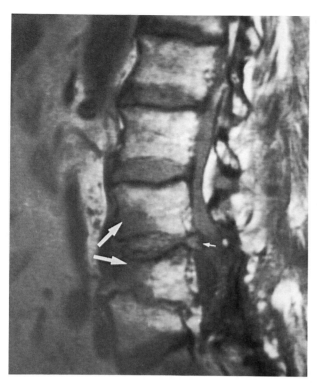

Figure 8-49
Unstable lumbar segmental fusion associated with low signal intensity regions in L3–4 endplates *(large arrows)*. Herniated disc is identified *(small arrow)*. T1-weighted sagittal image; TR = 600 msec, TE = 20 msec.

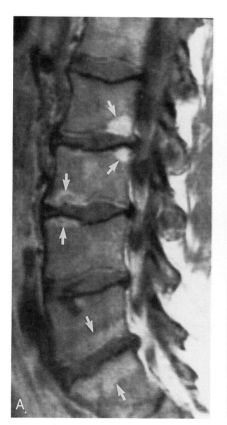

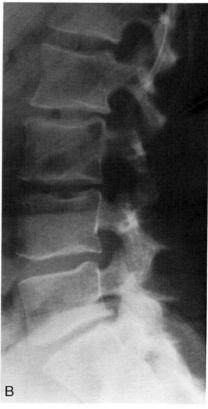

Figure 8-50
Endplate changes in degenerative disease. *(A)* Focal areas of endplate yellow marrow development *(arrows)* in degenerative spine. T1-weighted sagittal image; TR = 600 msec, TE = 20 msec. *(B)* Conventional radiograph for comparison.

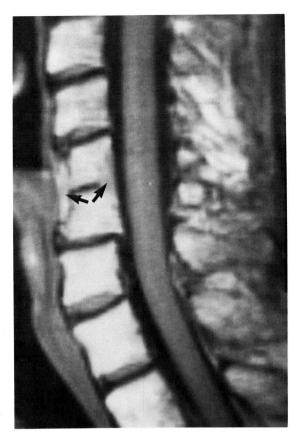

Figure 8-51

Solid osseous fusion (between C5 and C6 cervical vertebrae *(arrows)*. T1-weighted sagittal image; TR = 600 msec, TE = 20 msec.

Figure 8-52

Postcontrast CT scan *(A)* and T1-weighted axial image *(B)* demonstrating bilobed recurrent disc *(arrows)* in a post-lumbar laminectomy patient. Superior soft tissue contrast is obtained with MR image without the need for contrast administration. TR = 1000 msec, TE = 20 msec.

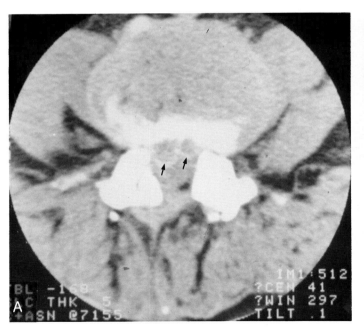

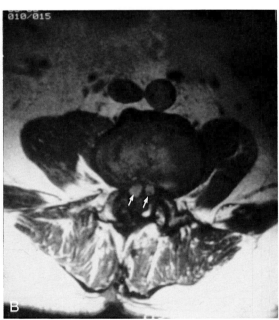

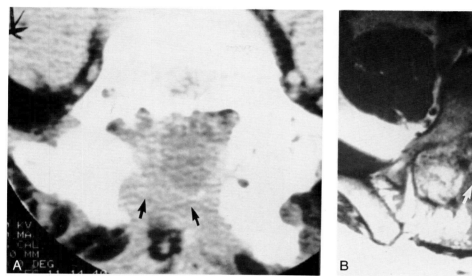
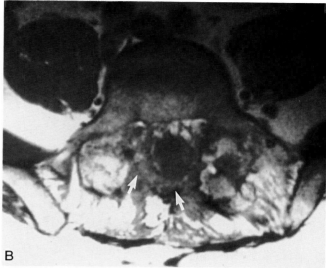

Figure 8-53

Postoperative scar *(arrows)* following lumbar laminectomy is identified on axial CT scan *(A)* and T1-weighted axial image *(B).* Scar images with intermediate signal intensity on MR. TR = 1000 msec, TE = 20 msec.

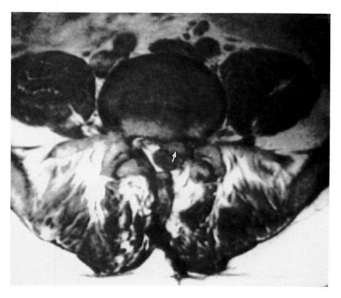

Figure 8-54

Mass effect is demonstrated on anterior aspect of the thecal sac at site of left posterolateral disc herniation *(arrow),* following left laminectomy. T1-weighted axial image; TR = 500 msec, TE = 40 msec.

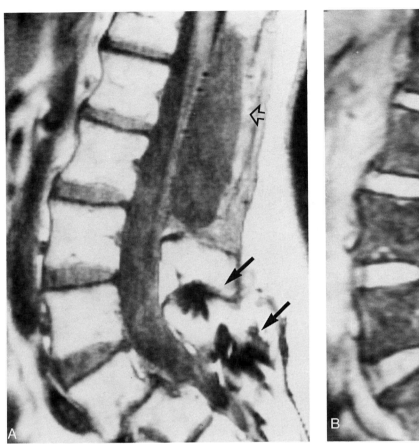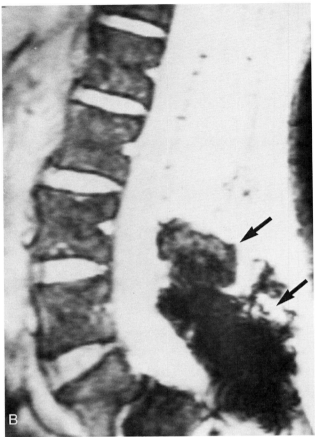

Figure 8-55
Postoperative fusion with signal void in metallic artifact *(solid arrows)* on T1-weighted *(A)* and on T2*
gradient refocused *(B)* images. Low signal intensity artifact is accentuated on gradient echo image.
Postoperative fluid collection is indicated on T1-weighted image *(open arrow)*. *(A)* TR = 600 msec, TE
= 20 msec; *(B)* TR = 400 msec, TE = 15 msec; flip angle = 30°.

Figure 8-57   ▶
High signal intensity Pantopaque *(arrows)* on T1-weighted sagittal *(A)* and axial *(B)* images. *(A)* TR
= 600 msec, TE = 20 msec; *(B)* TR = 1000 msec, TE = 20 msec.

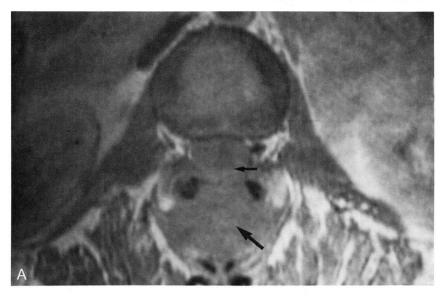

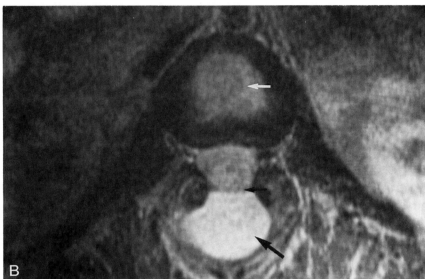

Figure 8-56
Postoperative pseudomeningocele *(large black arrow)* images with low signal intensity on intermediate-weighted image *(A)* and with high signal intensity on T2-weighted image *(B)*. Thecal sac-fluid interface *(small black arrow)* and bright signal intensity nucleus pulposus *(white arrow)* are best displayed on T2-weighted image. TR = 2000 msec, TE = 20, 60 msec.

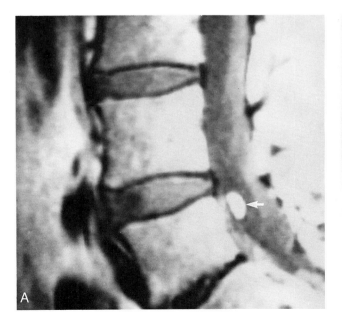

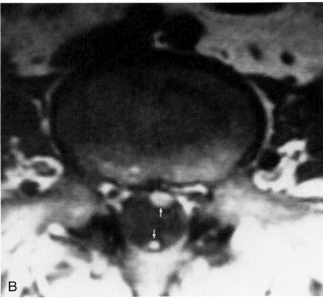

Fractures

MR has been used in the assessment of traumatic and nontraumatic vertebral body fractures.[43,55,56] In *traumatic fractures,* retropulsed fracture fragments are identified relative to the cord, thecal sac, and neural foramina (Figs. 8-58 and 8-59). In the acute and subacute stages, hemorrhage or edema image with low signal intensity on T1-weighted images and with high signal intensity on T2-weighted images. A chronic fracture does not demonstrate increased signal intensity on long TR/TE sequences (Fig. 8-60). *Osteoporotic* or *nontraumatic compression fractures* may be characterized on T1-weighted images by low signal intensity bands parallel to the endplates that increase in signal intensity on T2-weighted images (Figs. 8-61 and 8-62). In some cases compression fractures cannot be differentiated from metastatic disease, although associated convexity or bulging of the posterior vertebral body margin suggests neoplastic disease and a pathologic fracture (Fig. 8-63). On T2-weighted images the branching pattern of the high signal intensity basivertebral plexus may simulate fracture.

Text continues on p. 360

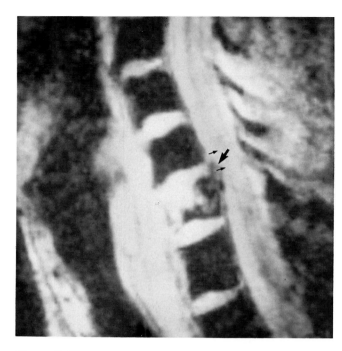

Figure 8-58

Traumatic cervical fracture. Retropulsed cervical fracture *(large arrow)* impinging on the lower cervical cord *(small arrows).* T2* gradient echo image; TR = 400 msec, TE = 15 msec; flip angle = 30°.

Figure 8-59

Posttraumatic L1 vertebral body fracture *(large arrow)* images with low signal intensity hemorrhagic marrow on T1-weighted image *(A)* and with increased signal intensity on T2* gradient echo image *(B).* Retropulsed fracture segment *(small arrow)* is identified impressing on the thecal sac.

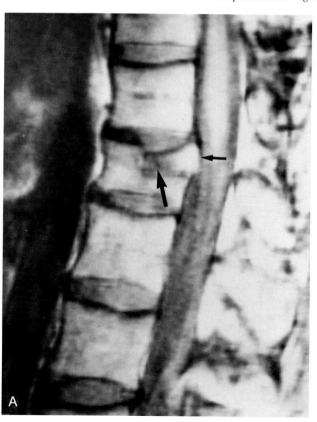

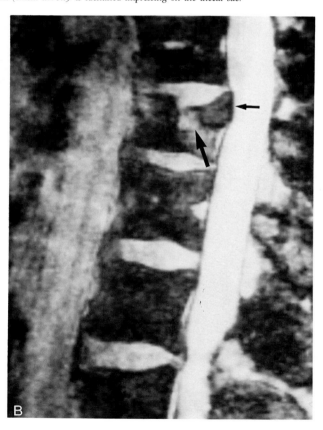

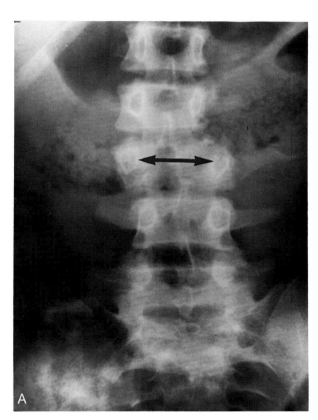

Figure 8-60

Chronic burst fracture. **(A)** AP radiograph of L3 burst fracture demonstrating splayed pedicles *(arrows)*. T1-weighted **(B)** and T2-weighted **(C)** sagittal images identifying the fracture site *(white arrow)* and deformity of the anterior thecal sac *(black arrows)*. No marrow edema is associated with this chronic fracture. **(B)** TR = 1000 msec, TE = 20 msec; **(C)** TR = 2000 msec, TE = 60 msec.

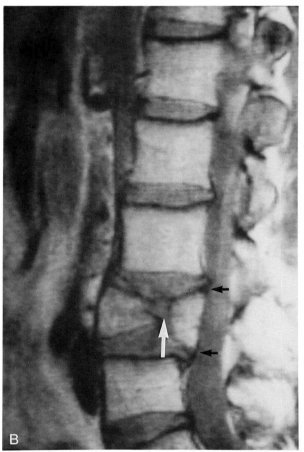

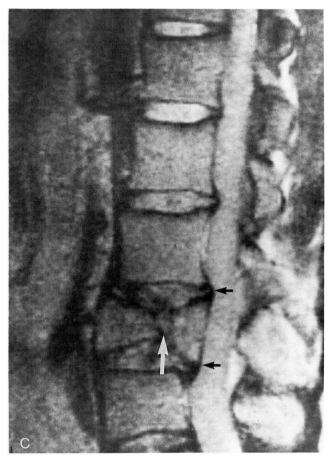

Figure 8-61
Osteoporotic compression fractures. *(A)* Lateral radiograph with multiple vertebral body wedge compression fractures *(arrows)*. Corresponding T1-weighted *(B)* and T2*-weighted *(C)* images identifying compression fractures *(white arrows)* and deformity of the thecal sac *(black arrow)*. *(B)* TR = 600 msec, TE = 20 msec; *(C)* TR = 400 msec, TE = 30 msec; flip angle = 30°.

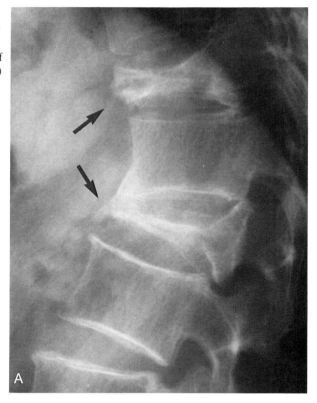

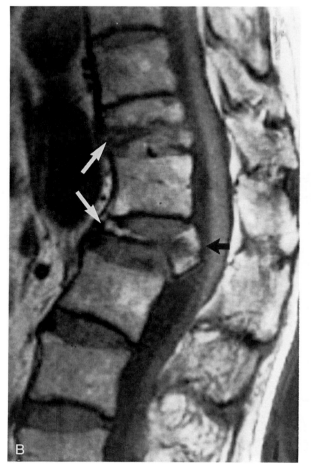

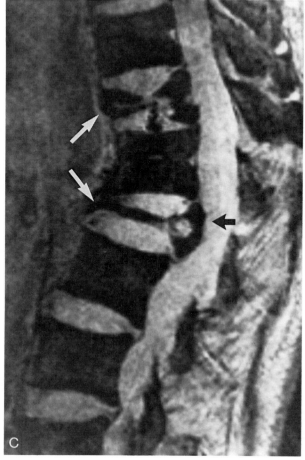

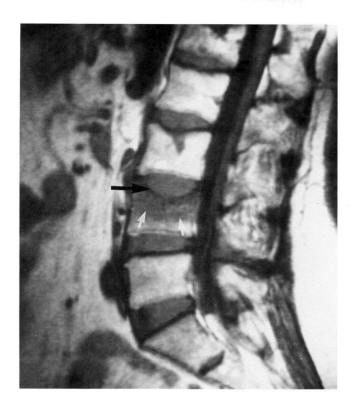

Figure 8-62

Low signal intensity band of marrow edema *(white arrows)* is seen in association with L4 osteoporotic compression fracture *(black arrow)* on T1-weighted sagittal image. TR = 600 msec, TE = 20 msec.

Figure 8-63

Pathologic fracture. Thoracic vertebral body collapse with posterior convexity and soft tissue mass in a patient with non-Hodgkin's lymphoma, as imaged on T1-weighted *(A)* and T2-weighted *(B)* sagittal images. Soft tissue component is visualized with increased signal intensity on T2-weighted image, isointense with CSF *(B). (A)* TR = 600 msec, TE = 20 msec; *(B)* TR = 2000 msec, TE = 60 msec.

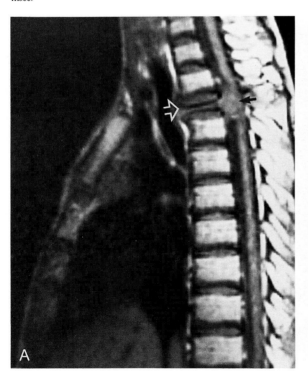

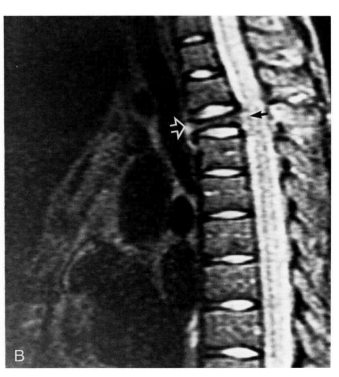

Infection

MR imaging is more sensitive in the detection of vertebral *osteomyelitis* than either conventional radiography or CT.[57] Specificity rates of MR are also superior to corresponding nuclear scintigraphic studies. Infection of vertebral bodies and adjacent intervertebral disc spaces is visualized on T1-weighted images as areas of low signal intensity (Fig. 8-64). On T2-weighted images, high signal intensity is observed crossing the involved bone and disc space, with irregularity of cortical margins (Fig. 8-65). In advanced stages of infection such as tuberculous spondylitis, a soft tissue mass (of low signal intensity on T1- and of high signal intensity on T2-weighted images) is frequently observed (Fig. 8-66).[58] Unlike neoplastic disease, infection is associated with loss of disc space height and the low signal intensity intranuclear cleft normally seen on T2-weighted images.

Figure 8-64

E. coli osteomyelitis. T1-weighted sagittal **(A)** and axial **(B)** images displaying low signal intensity *E. coli* abscess anterior to the L4 through S2 vertebral bodies *(solid white arrows)*, with adjacent cortical and cancellous destruction. Low signal intensity marrow involvement *(open white arrows)* and epidural spread *(straight black arrows)* are indicated. Prior posterior fusion mass is shown on axial image *(curved black arrow)*. TR = 1000 msec, TE = 20 msec.

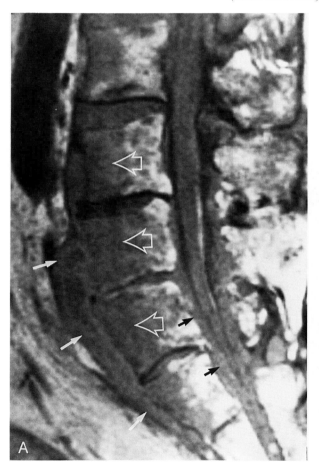

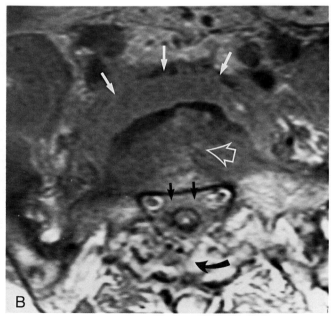

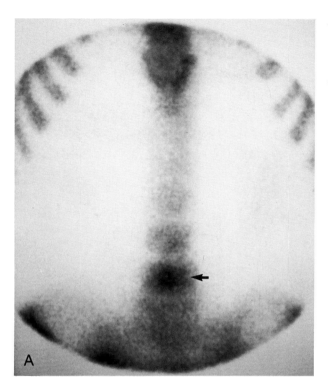

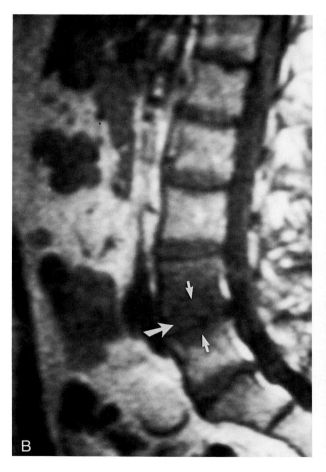

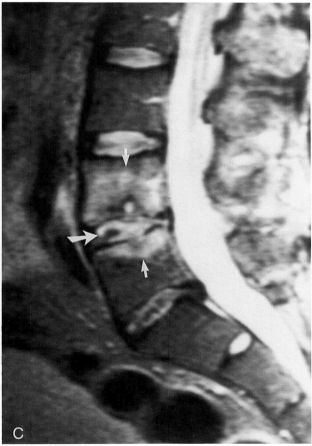

Figure 8-65

Staphylococcal osteomyelitis. **(A)** Nonspecific vertebral body uptake of 99mTc-MDP bone tracer on nuclear scintigraphy *(arrow)*. Low signal intensity marrow involvement *(small arrows)* of L4 and L5 crossing the discovertebral junction *(large arrow)* images with low signal intensity on T1-weighted image **(B)** and with high signal intensity on T2-weighted image **(C)**. **(A)** TR = 600 msec, TE = 20 msec; **(B)** TR = 2000 msec, TE = 60 msec.

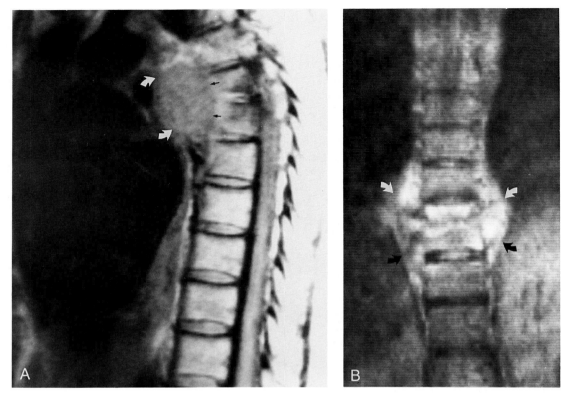

Figure 8-66

Tuberculous spondylitis. Two separate cases of tuberculous infection of the thoracic spine. Paraspinal mass *(curved arrows)* images with intermediate signal intensity on T1-weighted sagittal image *(A)* and with high signal intensity on T2-weighted image *(B)*. Adjacent vertebral body erosion is indicated *(small black arrows in A)*.

Metastatic and Marrow Disease

MR directly images fatty or yellow marrow with high signal intensity and hematopoietic or red marrow with low signal intensity in normal and pathologic states.[59–65] T1, T2, T2* gradient echo, and STIR sequences have complementary roles in visualizing replacement of normal marrow in primary (Fig. 8-67),[66] metastatic, and infiltrative disease processes (Fig. 8-68). MR is also useful in differentiating benign processes that may mimic malignancy on conventional radiography (Fig. 8-69).

Since most *metastatic tumors* are characterized by long T1 and T2 values, there is good contrast discrimination between normal adult marrow and marrow infiltrated by metastatic processes.[67] On STIR images signal from normal yellow marrow is suppressed, and T1 and T2 prolongation effects are additive. Metastatic lesions from carcinoma of the breast (Fig. 8-70), prostate (Fig. 8-71), lung, colon (Fig. 8-72), and testes (Fig. 8-73); from Ewing sarcoma (Fig. 8-74); and from multiple myeloma (Fig. 8-75) have been visualized with increased signal intensity on conventional T2-weighted images, on T2*-weighted images, and on STIR images, even in cases where nuclear scintigraphy was equivocal (Fig. 8-76). Blastic lesions generally image with low signal intensity, regardless of the selected pulse parameters (Fig. 8-77). With STIR images, however, metastatic foci with a blastic reaction have been observed to image with increased signal intensity.[68] Epidural involvement, with posterior cortical disruption, is best appreciated on T2, T2*, STIR, or gadolinium-enhanced studies.[69,70] Gadolinium generates increased signal intensity in neoplastic tissue on short TR/TE sequences (the effect of T1 and T2 shortening), while adjacent CSF remains dark (Fig. 8-78). This precisely defines the boundary between tumor and thecal sac, not possible with conventional T2-weighting or even with STIR images where CSF and tumor both image with bright signal intensity.

MR is also sensitive to the replacement of marrow fat with tumor cell populations that have T1 values significantly longer than normal yellow marrow.[64,68] Marrow infiltrates from *leukemia* (Fig. 8-79) and *lymphoma* (Fig. 8-80) have been successfully identified on STIR sequences as areas of bright signal intensity within a black or gray background of nulled fat signal from uninvolved marrow. Since lymphomatous involvement of marrow may present with a patchy or nodular involvement of the spine and pelvis, MR localization prior to biopsy reduced false negatives from sampling error.

Fatty replacement of affected marrow in patients undergoing *radiation* and *chemotherapy* can be imaged on T1, T2, and STIR sequences (Fig. 8-81).[71] Normal red or hematopoietic elements in the spine image with gray contrast on stir sequences while areas of fatty or yellow marrow replacement will image with dark nulled signal.

Text continues on p. 374

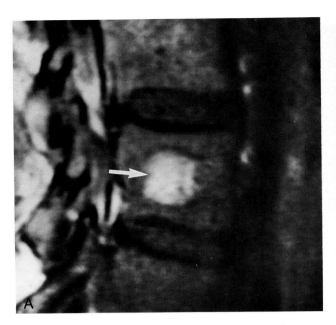

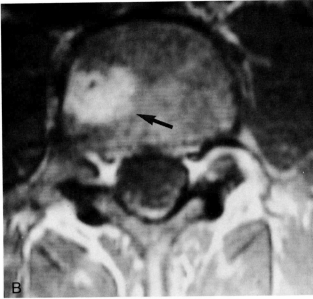

Figure 8-67
High signal intensity hemangioma of L4 vertebral body *(arrow)* on T1-weighted sagittal *(A)* and on axial *(B)* images. *(A)* TR = 600 msec, TE = 20 msec; *(B)* TR = 1000 msec, TE = 60 msec.

Figure 8-68
Iron deposition in hemochromatosis is visualized as diffuse low signal intensity on T1-weighted axial image. This simulates the appearance of a gradient refocused or STIR sequence. TR = 1000 msec, TE = 20 msec.

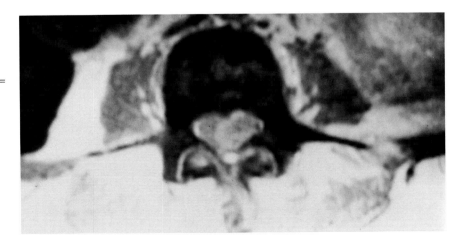

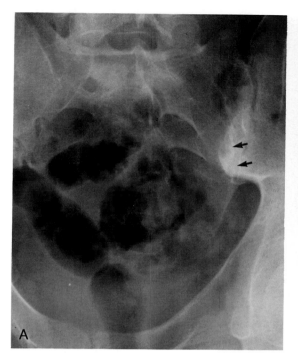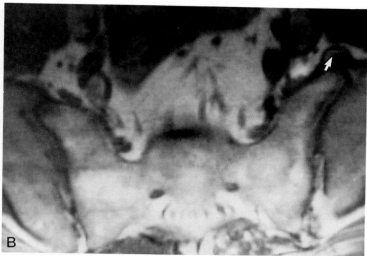

Figure 8-69

Osteophyte. *(A)* AP radiograph with sclerosis overlying the left sacroiliac joint *(arrows)*. Axial T1-weighted MR image *(B)* and CT scan *(C)* identify degenerative bridging osteophyte *(arrow)* and not sclerotic metastasis. TR = 1000 msec, TE = 20 msec.

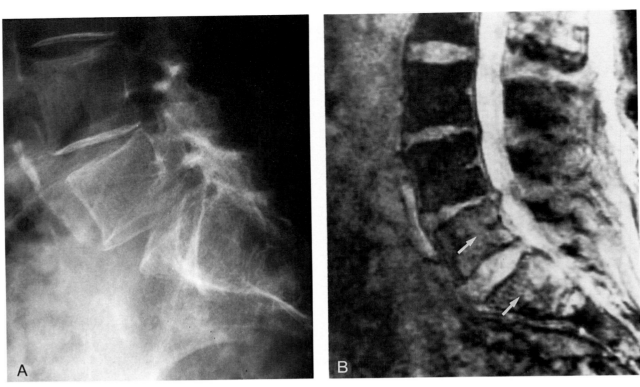

Figure 8-70

Metastatic breast carcinoma. **(A)** Negative lateral radiograph. **(B)** T2* gradient refocused sagittal image demonstrating high signal intensity metastatic infiltration of marrow in L5 and S1 vertebral bodies *(arrows)*. TR = 400 msec, TE = 15 msec; flip angle = 30°.

Figure 8-71

Metastatic prostate carcinoma *(straight arrow)* to the spine is visualized with low signal intensity on T1-weighted sagittal image **(A)** and with high signal intensity on STIR sequence **(B)**. In addition, posterior element involvement *(curved arrow)* is uniquely demonstrated on the STIR image **(B)**.

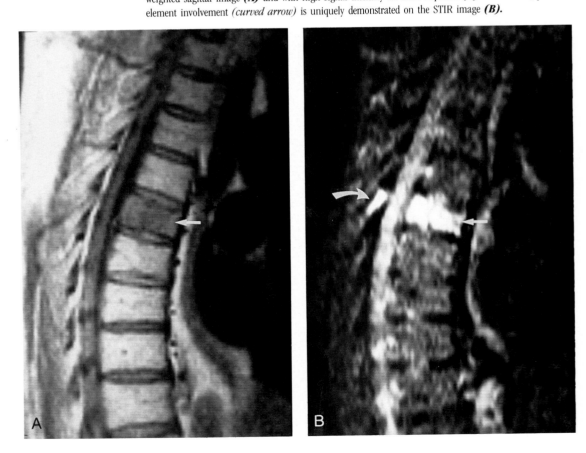

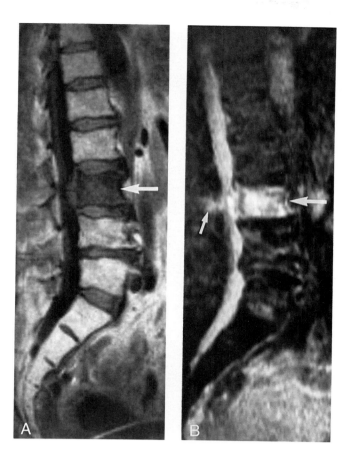

Figure 8-72

Metastatic colon carcinoma of L4 *(large arrow)* images with low signal intensity on T1-weighted sagittal image *(A)* and with high signal intensity on STIR sequence *(B)*. The STIR image displays spinous process involvement as well *(small arrow)*.

Figure 8-73

Metastatic carcinoma of the testis involving the lumbar spine *(straight arrows)* and paraortic lymph nodes *(curved arrows)* images with low signal intensity on T1-weighted image *(A)* and with high signal intensity on STIR sequence *(B)*.

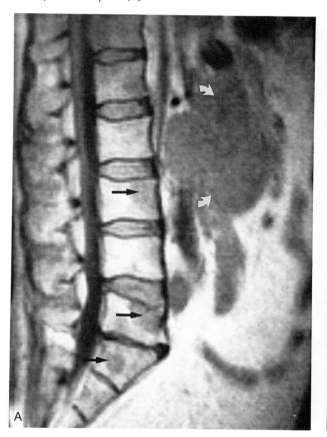
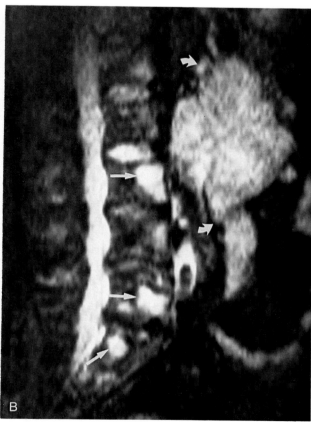

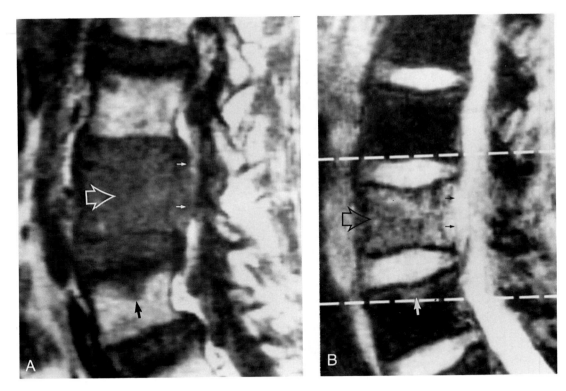

Figure 8-74

Ewing sarcoma metastatic to L3 *(open arrow)* with epidural involvement *(small solid arrows)* is seen as low signal intensity on T1-weighted image *(A)* and as high signal intensity on T2* gradient echo image *(B)*. Schmorl's node of L5 endplate *(large solid arrow)* should not be mistaken for tumor. *(A)* TR = 600 msec, TE = 20 msec; *(B)* TR = 400 msec, TE = 25 msec; flip angle = 30°.

Figure 8-75   ▶

Multiple myeloma. *(A)* Multiple foci of myelomatous involvement in the lumbar spine visualized as low signal intensity on T1-weighted sagittal image. Collapse of L5 *(straight arrow)* and convexity to the posterior margin of L2 *(curved arrows)* are characteristic of metastatic disease. Corresponding T1-weighted *(B)* and STIR *(C)* coronal images in the same patient demonstrating deposits of multiple myeloma *(arrows)* which generate increased signal intensity on STIR contrast. *(D)* On a T1-weighted image in a separate patient, diffuse pattern of multiple myeloma *(arrows)* images with low signal intensity replacement of normally bright signal intensity marrow.

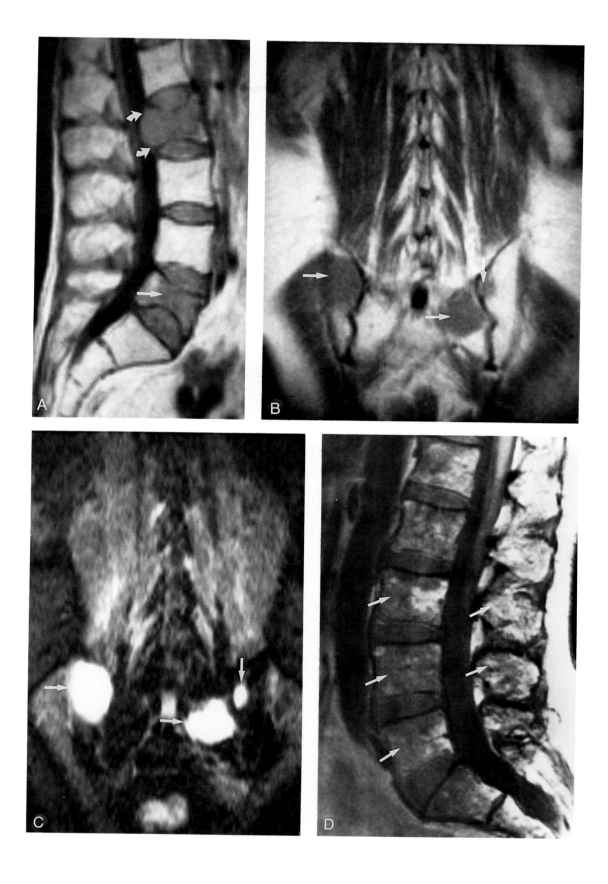

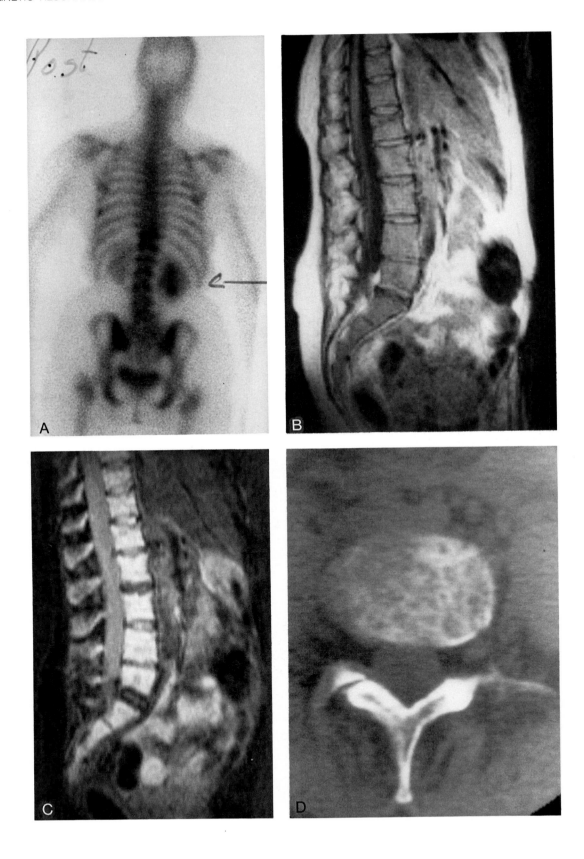

◄ *Figure 8-76*

Metastatic breast carcinoma. *(A)* Unremarkable bone scan in a patient with aggressive metastatic breast carcinoma. T1-weighted *(B)* and STIR *(C)* images showing low and high signal intensity, respectively, in diffuse marrow involvement of the entire thoracic and lumbar spines. *(D)* Corresponding axial CT scan confirms lytic destruction of cancellous cortical bone.

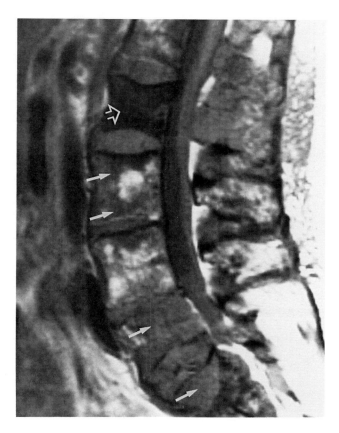

Figure 8-77

Lytic and blastic metastases. T1-weighted sagittal image identifying low signal intensity metastatic breast carcinoma *(solid arrows)* and isolated blastic vertebrae *(open arrow)* imaging with diffuse dark signal intensity. TR = 600 msec, TE = 20 msec.

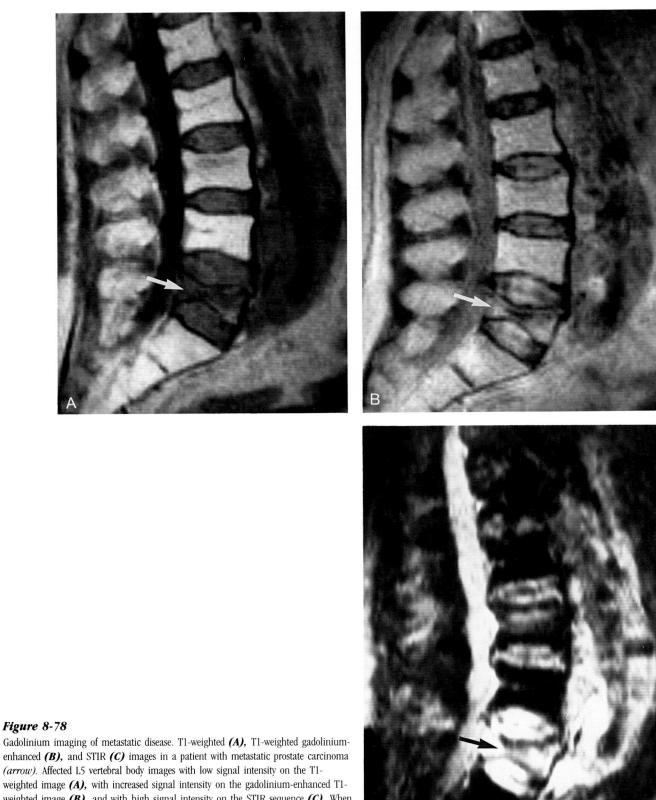

Figure 8-78

Gadolinium imaging of metastatic disease. T1-weighted *(A)*, T1-weighted gadolinium-enhanced *(B)*, and STIR *(C)* images in a patient with metastatic prostate carcinoma *(arrow)*. Affected L5 vertebral body images with low signal intensity on the T1-weighted image *(A)*, with increased signal intensity on the gadolinium-enhanced T1-weighted image *(B)*, and with high signal intensity on the STIR sequence *(C)*. When using T1-weighted sequences, gadolinium offers the advantage of imaging tumor with high signal intensity while CSF remains low in signal.

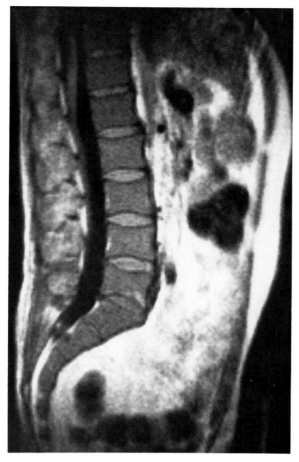

Figure 8-79
Acute lymphocytic leukemia. Diffuse low signal intensity leukemic infiltration of marrow on T1-weighted sagittal image. TR = 600 msec, TE = 20 msec.

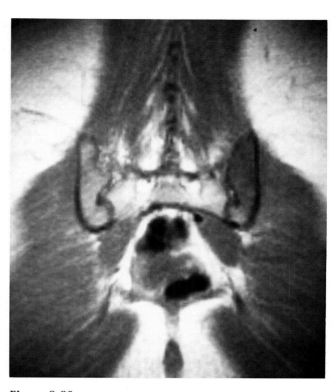

Figure 8-80
Characteristic asymmetric involvement of lymphoma (arrow) shown as low signal intensity infiltration in left posterior iliac bone on T1-weighted coronal image. TR = 600 msec, TE = 20 msec.

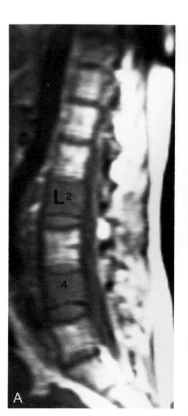

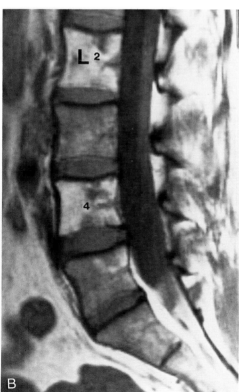

Figure 8-81
Marrow response to chemotherapy. T1-weighted images of the lumbar spine prechemotherapy *(A)* and post chemotherapy *(B)* for metastatic colonic carcinoma. Metastatic disease images with low signal intensity on L2 and L4 prior to chemotherapy, and shows evidence of high signal intensity fatty replacement after chemotherapy *(B).* Adjacent uninvolved vertebral bodies also show a flip-flop in signal intensity as red marrow is activated.

PERSPECTIVE ON MR IMAGING OF THE SPINE

MR affords a unique perspective for noninvasive imaging of the spine in degenerative disc disease affecting both osseous and disc structures. The ability to directly image the nucleus pulposus, CSF, and cord facilitates discrimination of the disc-thecal sac interface without the use of CT or myelography. In studies comparing MR with conventional diagnostic imaging modalities, further potential for MR imaging in characterization of trauma, infection, and neoplasia has been documented. Direct marrow imaging has expanded the application of MR in identifying and monitoring patients with leukemia, lymphoma, and metastatic disease involving the spine. The postoperative spine presents a unique clinical and radiologic challenge to which MR imaging can contribute valuable information regarding postoperative scarring, recurrent disc disease, and fusion stability.

REFERENCES

1. Dixon AK, Bannon RP: Computed tomography of the postoperative lumbar spine: The need for, and optimal dose of, intravenous contrast medium. Br J Radiol, 60:215, 1987

2. Braun IF, et al: Contrast enhancement in CT differentiation between recurrent disk herniation and postoperative scar: Prospective study. AJNR, 6:607, 1985

3. Zinreich SJ, et al: CT myelography for outpatients: An inpatient/outpatient pilot study to assess methodology. Radiology, 157:387, 1985

4. Helms CA, et al: CT of the lumbar spine: Normal variants and pitfalls. RadioGraphics, 7:447, 1987

5. Weiss T, et al: CT of the postoperative lumbar spine: Value of intravenous contrast. Neuroradiol, 28:241, 1986

6. Mills DG: Imaging of the cervical spine. Proceedings of the MR Clinical Symposium, vol 3, no 5. Milwaukee, GE Medical Systems 1987

7. Berger PE, et al: High resolution surface coil magnetic resonance imaging of the spine: Normal and pathologic anatomy. RadioGraphics, 6:573, 1986

8. Smoker WRK, et al: MRI versus conventional radiologic examinations in the evaluation of the craniovertebral and cervicomedullary junction. RadioGraphics, 6:953, 1986

9. Maravilla KR, et al: Magnetic resonance demonstration of multiple sclerosis plaques in the cervical cord. AJNR, 5:685, 1984

10. Kulkarni MV, et al: Acute spinal cord injury: MR imaging at 1.5T. Radiology, 164:837, 1987

11. Modic MT, et al: Cervical radiculopathy: Value of oblique MR imaging. Radiology, 163:227, 1987

12. Rubin JB, Enzmann DR: Optimizing conventional MR imaging of the spine. Radiology, 163:777, 1987

13. Enzmann DR, et al: Cervical spine MR imaging: Generating high-signal CSF in sagittal and axial images. Radiology, 163:233, 1987

14. Modic MT, et al: Magnetic resonance imaging of the cervical spine: Technical and clinical observations. AJNR, 5:15, 1984

15. Flannigan BD, et al: MR imaging of the cervical spine: Neurovascular anatomy. AJR, 148:785, 1987

16. Burnett KR, et al: MRI evaluation of the cervical spine at high field strength. Applied Radiol, Nov/Dec 1985

17. Yu S, et al: Facet joint menisci of the cervical spine: Correlative MR imaging and cryomicrotomy study. Radiology, 164:79, 1987

18. Teresi LM, et al: Asymptomatic degenerative disk disease and spondylosis of the cervical spine: MR imaging. Radiology, 164:83, 1987

19. Ross JS, et al: Thoracic disk herniation: MR imaging. Radiology, 165:511, 1987

20. Modic MT, et al: Magnetic resonance imaging of intervertebral disk disease: Clinical and pulse sequence considerations. Radiology, 152:103, 1984

21. Grenier N, et al: Degenerative lumbar disk disease: Pitfalls and usefulness of MR imaging in detection of vacuum phenomenon. Radiology, 164:861, 1987

22. Ramsey RG: MRI's reputation grows in herniated disk evaluation. Diagnostic Imaging, June:120, 1987

23. Pech, Haughton VM: Lumbar intervertebral disk: Correlative MR and anatomic study. Radiology, 156:699, 1985

24. Chafetz NI, et al: Recognition of lumbar disk herniation with NMR. AJR, 141:1153, 1983

25. Schellinger D, et al: Facet joint disorders and their role in the production of back pain and sciatica. RadioGraphics, 7:923, 1987

26. Grenier N, et al: Normal and degenerative posterior spinal structures: MR imaging. Radiology, 165:517, 1987

27. Ross JS, et al: Lumbar spine: Postoperative assessment with surface-coil MR imaging. Radiology, 164:851, 1987

28. Nokes SR, et al: Childhood scoliosis: MR imaging. Radiology, 164:791, 1987

29. Heithoff KB: Spontaneous lumbar epidural hematoma. Proceedings of the MR Clinical Symposium, vol 3, no 3. Milwaukee, GE Medical Systems, 1987

30. Glenn WV, et al: Magnetic resonance imaging of the lumbar spine: Nerve root canals, disc abnormalities, anatomic correlations, and case examples. Milwaukee, GE Medical Systems, 1986

31. Haughton VM: MR imaging of the spine. Radiology, 166:297, 1988

32. Porter BA: MR may become routine for imaging bone marrow. Diagnostic Imaging, February 1987

33. Porter BA, et al: Magnetic resonance imaging of bone marrow disorders. Radiol Clin North America, 24:269.

34. Kaplan PA, et al: Bone marrow patterns in aplastic anemia: Observations with 1.5T MR imaging. Radiology, 164:441, 1987

35. McKinstry CS, et al: Bone marrow in leukemia and aplastic anemia: MR imaging before, during, and after treatment. Radiology, 162:701, 1987

36. Stoller DW, Genant HK: MRI helps characterize disorders of the spine. Diagnostic Imaging, 9:128, September 1987

37. Enzmann DR, Rubin JB: Cervical spine: MR imaging with a partial flip angle, gradient-refocused pulse sequence, Part I: General considerations and disk disease. Radiology, 166:467, 1988

38. Stoller DW, Genant HK: Fast imaging of the spine. In Genant HK (ed): Spine Update pp 47–54. San Francisco, Radiology Research and Education Foundation, 1987

39. Reynolds H, et al: Cervical rheumatoid arthritis: Value of

flexion and extension views in imaging. Radiology, 164:215, 1987

40. Burk DL, et al: Spinal and paraspinal neurofibromatosis: Surface coil MR imaging at 1.5T. Radiology, 162:797, 1987

41. Flannigan BD, et al: MR imaging of the cervical spine: Neurovascular anatomy. AJRN, 8:27.

42. Reicher MA, et al: MR imaging of the lumbar spine: Anatomic correlations and the effects of technical variations. AJR, 147:891, 1986

43. Modic MT, et al: Magnetic resonance imaging of the spine. Radiol Clin N Am, 24:229, 1986

44. Edelman RR, et al: High-resolution MRI: Imaging anatomy of the lumbosacral spine. Magn Res Imag, 4:515, 1986

45. Berger PE, et al: High resolution surface coil magnetic resonance imaging of the spine: Normal and pathologic anatomy. RadioGraphics, 6:573, 1986

46. Stoller DW, et al: Applications of computed tomography in the musculoskeletal system. Current Orthopaedics, 1:219, 1987

47. Modic MT, et al: Degenerative disk disease. Assessment of changes in vertebral body marrow with MR imaging. Radiology, 166:193, 1988

48. Lang P, et al: Magnetic resonance imaging in the assessment of functional lumbar spinal stability (abstr) p 149. Sixth Annual Meeting and Exhibition of the Society of Magnetic Resonance in Medicine, New York City, August 17–21, 1987

49. Huckman MS, et al: Chemonucleation and changes observed on lumbar MR scan: Preliminary report. AJRN, 8:1, 1987

50. Onik G, et al: Percutaneous lumbar diskectomy using a new aspiration probe. AJRN, 6:290, 1985

51. Ross JS, et al: MR enhancement of epidural fibrosis by Gd-DPTA: Biodistribution and mechanism. Radiology, 165P:142, 1987

52. Ross JS, et al: MR imaging of lumbar arachnoiditis. AJR, 149:1025, 1987

53. Hackney DB, et al: MR characteristics of iophendylate (Pantopaque). JCTA, 10:401, 1986

54. Altman NR, Altman DH: MR imaging of spinal dysraphism. AJNR, 8:533, 1987

55. Sartoris DJ, et al: Vertebral-body collapse in focal and diffuse disease: Patterns of pathologic processes. Radiology, 160:479, 1986

56. Kaplan PA, et al: Osteoporosis with vertebral compression fractures, retropulsed fragments, and neurologic compromise. Radiology, 165:533, 1987

57. Modic MT, et al: Vertebral osteomyelitis: Assessment using MR. Radiology, 157:157, 1985

58. deRoss A, et al: MRI of tuberculous spondylitis. AJR, 146:79, 1986

59. Sugimura K, et al: Bone marrow diseases of the spine: Differentiation with T1 and T2 relaxation times in MR imaging. Radiology, 165:541, 1987

60. Daffner RH, et al: MRI in the detection of malignant infiltration of bone marrow. AJR, 146:353, 1986

61. Kricun ME: Red-yellow marrow conversion: Its effect on the location of some solitary bone lesions. Skeletal Radiol, 14:10, 1985

62. Hajek PC, et al: Focal fat deposition in axial bone marrow: MR characteristics. Radiology, 162:245, 1987

63. Weaver GR, Sandler MP: Increased sensitivity of magnetic resonance imaging compared to radionuclide bone scintigraphy in the detection of lymphoma of the spine. Clin Nucl Med, 12:333, 1987

64. Olson D, et al: Magnetic resonance imaging of the bone marrow in patients with leukemia, aplastic anemia and lymphoma. Investigative Radiology, June 1986

65. Beltran J, et al: Tumors of the osseous spine: Staging with MR imaging versus CT. Radiology, 162:565, 1987

66. Ross JS, et al: Vertebral hemangiomas: MR imaging. Radiology, 165:165, 1987

67. Sarpel S, et al: Early diagnosis of spinal-epidural metastasis by magnetic resonance imaging. Radiology, 164:887, 1987

68. Porter BA, et al: Low-field STIR imaging of marrow malignancies. Radiology, 165P:275, 1987

69. Emory TH, et al: Comparison of Gd-DPTA MR imaging and radionuclide bone scans (WIP). Radiology, 165P:342, 1987

70. Berry I, et al: Gd-DPTA enhancement of cerebral and spinal tumors on MR imaging. Radiology, 165P:38, 1987

71. Ramsey RG, Zacharias CE: MR imaging of the spine after radiation therapy: Easily recognizable effects. JNR, 6:247, 1985

David W. Stoller
Clyde A. Helms
Gregory W. Doyle

Chapter 9   # THE TEMPOROMANDIBULAR JOINT

OUTLINE

Imaging Protocols for the TMJ
Normal MR Anatomy of the TMJ in the Sagittal Plane
Pathology of the TMJ
    Internal Derangement

Trauma
Arthritis
Neoplasms
Perspectives on MR Imaging of the TMJ

Primary interest in the temporomandibular joint (TMJ) is in evaluation of internal disc derangements. Abnormalities in both position and morphology of the TMJ meniscus (disc) have been implicated in myofacial pain syndromes and in biomechanical joint dysfunction. Young and middle-age women are thought to represent a significant proportion of patients with TMJ abnormalities, mostly caused by "bruxism" or grinding of the teeth. However, internal disc derangements may also result from direct trauma, indirect trauma (prolonged dental procedures), or they may occur spontaneously.

Clinical diagnosis and documentation of TMJ disorders are difficult, and patients may present with symptoms of dysfunction without objective joint disease. The articular disc cannot be visualized with conventional radiography or tomography, since these modalities rely on the assessment of osseous structures. With arthrography, the lower compartment of the TMJ is filled with contrast material in order to assess the position of the disc or presence of perforation indirectly.[1-5] This is an invasive procedure, with associated morbidity and limitations in

accuracy (i.e., inability to inject contrast material into the lower joint compartment or injection into both compartments that mimic disc perforation). Computed tomography (CT) requires the use of ionizing radiation and only allows visualization of the TMJ disc through the use of reformatted sagittal images obtained from a series of transaxial joint scans.[6-10]

Magnetic resonance (MR) imaging is rapidly replacing arthrography and CT as the examination of choice in evaluating the TMJ.[11-19] MR is noninvasive and provides direct sagittal images that not only display the TMJ meniscus, but also differentiate cortex, marrow, hyaline cartilage, muscle, fluid, fibrous tissue, and adhesions. This inherent soft tissue discrimination facilitates thin section acquisitions with specialized surface coils. The development of faster imaging techniques has facilitated routine bilateral examinations, with functional or dynamic positioning of the joint.[20,21] MR can also be used to study other disease processes affecting the TMJ including trauma, arthritis, neoplasia, and postsurgical assessments.[22-25]

IMAGING PROTOCOLS FOR THE TMJ

Direct sagittal images through the TMJ are acquired with the use of a small (3″) diameter surface coil placed over the region of interest (Fig. 9-1). High signal-to-noise is achieved by using thin (3 mm) sections at a 12-cm field of view (FOV), with a 256 × 256 acquisition matrix, and two excitations (NEX). Axial and coronal images, if obtained, are used as localizers for the sagittal plane scans. A series of sagittal images can provide information about medial and lateral disc position without a separate coronal acquisition. Routine imaging is obtained using a T1-weighted protocol with a recovery time (TR) of 600 msec and echo time (TE) of 20 msec. The addition of a T2-weighted sequence can highlight joint effusions (bright signal intensity), but will double imaging time and is not routinely used. Recently introduced partial flip angle, fast scan techniques permit acquisition of gradient echo effective T2*-weighted images of the TMJ in a fraction of the time needed for conventional spin echo techniques.[21] Using multiplanar gradient echo software (MPGR; General Electric), we have gained preliminary experience with T2*-gradient refocused images using a TR of 400 msec, TE of 30 msec and a theta of 30°.

Simultaneous, bilateral imaging of the TMJ is possible with newer coil designs in production that will eliminate the need for separate unilateral studies.[26,27] While many dentists find studies of only the affected or symptomatic side acceptable, others prefer to evaluate both sides routinely because of the known incidence of bilateral involvement in internal disc derangements.

There has been some controversy concerning the position of the mouth (closed, partially open, or open) for MR evaluation of TMJ disc displacements. Advocates of the partially open mouth position feel that in this position the morphology of the TMJ meniscus is not as distorted as it is in the closed mouth position. In the closed mouth position, the articular disc may become compressed between the articular eminence of the temporal bone and the condyle. In studies comparing closed and partially open mouth positions, it was found that up to one third of patients inadvertently reduce the meniscus with partial mouth opening.[28,29] We do not routinely evaluate the TMJ in a full open mouth position to verify meniscal reduction, since this is frequently evident on clinical examination. In some cases of chronic meniscal derangements, however, full open and closed mouth studies are ordered to document meniscus position and degree of reduction. If time permits only one acquisition, then closed mouth imaging will eliminate the possibility of a recaptured disc during forward translation of the condyle.

NORMAL MR ANATOMY OF THE TMJ IN THE SAGITTAL PLANE

The bony support of the TMJ, the articular eminence of the temporal bone, and the condyle of the mandible image with the high signal intensity of marrow fat (Fig. 9-2). The TMJ disc, or meniscus, is not true fibrocartilage. Rather, it is a condensation of fibrous tissue, positioned on the superior surface of the condyle.

The meniscus is composed of three parts: an anterior band, a thin intermediate zone, and a thicker posterior band (Fig. 9-3).[11–19] Although all three parts of the normal biconcave disc visualize with low signal intensity, a central portion of intermediate signal intensity in the posterior band is a normal finding (Fig. 9-4). The anterior band, positioned in front of the condyle, is anchored to the superior belly of the lateral pterygoid muscle. The oblique orientation of the lateral pterygoid tends to direct most meniscal displacements in an anteromedial direction. The thin intermediate zone is identified between the low signal intensity cortical surfaces of the articular eminence and condylar head. The inter-

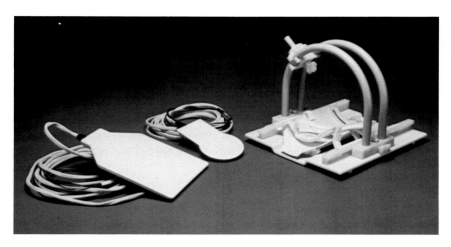

Figure 9-1
Flat TMJ surface coil *(left)* and corresponding holder *(right)*.

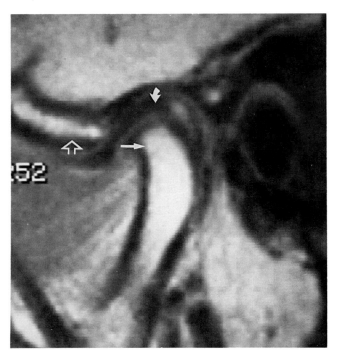

Figure 9-2
High signal intensity yellow marrow in articular eminence *(open arrow)* and mandibular condyle *(straight arrow)*. Posterior band located in expected position superior to condylar head *(curved arrow)*. T1-weighted sagittal image at .35 Tesla; TR = 1000 msec, TE = 40 msec.

mediate zone, also referred to as the weight-bearing zone, maintains a consistent relationship to the condyle and temporal eminence during translation. The thick posterior band is attached to a vascularized bilaminar zone in the retrodiscal tissue complex anchored to the temporal bone (Fig. 9-5). Within the bilaminar zone, a parallel band of low signal intensity may be distinguished coursing through its midsubstance. The transition between the posterior band and the bilaminar-retrodiscal complex may be marked by a vertical line of intermediate signal intensity. In the closed mouth position the posterior band occupies a 12-o'clock position in relation to the condylar head. In the open mouth position, with forward translation and posterior disc rotation, the posterior band may be visualized just dorsal to the 12-o'clock position. The articular disc defines and separates the upper and lower joint compartments.

PATHOLOGY OF THE TMJ

Internal Derangement

Internal derangements of the TMJ usually involve an anteromedial *displacement of the meniscus* in relation to the condyle and temporal fossa (Figs. 9-6 and 9-7).[11–]

[19,30–32] Trauma, degeneration, ligamentous laxity, and retrodiscal rents can be contributing factors. Such an anteriorly positioned disc blocks normal forward translation of the condyle, and the patient may present clinically with limited jaw opening and deviation of the mandible toward the affected side. An opening click is usually associated with relocation of the thick posterior band as it moves posteriorly in the open mouth position, recaptured by the condylar head (Fig. 9-8). Less frequently, a reciprocal click may occur during closure, as the posterior band redislocates, anterior to the condyle. A patient with the jaw locked in the closed mouth position *(closed lock)* has a displaced meniscus in both closed and open mouth positions, preventing anterior condylar motion (Fig. 9-9).

A grading system for characterizing disc displacements by both morphology and MR signal characteristics has been developed (Fig. 9-10).[29] This system is based on an evaluation of the shape of the disc and on a region of intermediate signal intensity which is best visualized within the posterior band in the partially open mouth position. The normal meniscus has a drumstick contour with a bull's-eye or target region of intermediate signal intensity in the posterior band. A similar region of intermediate signal intensity, but with meniscal dislocation, represents a grade 1 meniscus (Fig. 9-11). A normal drumstick morphology, but absence of intermediate signal intensity, is classified as a grade 2 displacement (Fig. 9-12). A grade 2 meniscus images with uniform low signal intensity. Abnormal disc morphology (loss of the drumstick shape) and no internal signal intensity is seen in grade 3 displacements (Fig. 9-13). A grade 3 meniscus has the highest association with degenerative joint disease, and may not be repairable at surgery. Preliminary clinical evidence indicates that increased grades of internal disc derangements correlate not only with degenerative joint disease, but with severity of pain, chronicity, and restriction of joint motion. Thus MR imaging provides the potential to identify a displaced meniscus and to evaluate the severity of the derangement and the possible response to therapy.

Conservative splint therapy is used to position the mandible and condyle more anteriorly, to recapture the displaced meniscus and to relax the lateral pterygoid muscle that may be in spasm. MR studies can be performed both pre- and post-splint application to assess the location of the TMJ meniscus and to measure condylar translation (Fig. 9-14). We have also had limited experience imaging patients undergoing an experimental arthroscopic procedure in which saline is injected into the lower joint recess to force reduction of a displaced disc (Fig. 9-15).

Disc perforations are more difficult to identify on MR images than with arthrography.[25] With arthrography, a small disc perforation may be demonstrated by communication of contrast material between the superior and inferior joint recesses; however, false-positive rates

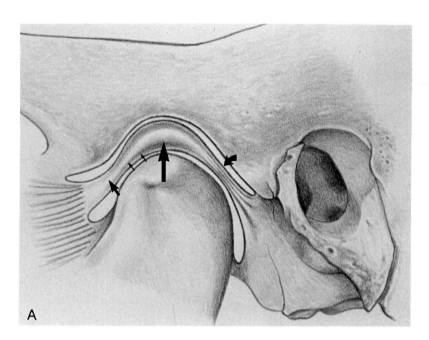

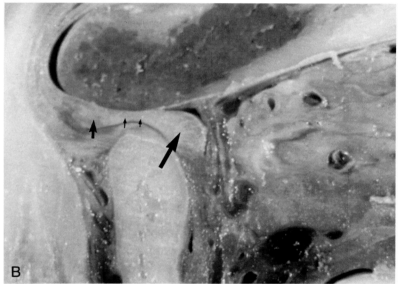

Figure 9-3
Normal anatomy. *(A)* Illustration demonstrating normal relationships of the TMJ meniscus to the joint landmarks in the closed mouth position. The posterior band *(large arrow)* is in a 12-o'clock position (superior to the condylar head). The intermediate zone *(small double arrow)* is between the articular eminence and the condylar head, and the anterior band *(medium arrow)* is anterior to the condyle and attached to the lateral pterygoid muscle. The bilaminar attachment is identified posteriorly *(curved arrow).* *(B)* Gross anatomic section in open mouth position displaying the thick posterior band *(large arrow),* thin intermediate zone *(small double arrows),* and anterior band *(medium arrow).*

as high as 20% have been reported. The majority of these perforations, however, are associated with a dislocated meniscus that would be detected on MR.

Scarring or *adhesions* within the TMJ image with intermediate signal intensity on T1- and T2-weighted images. In contrast, *joint fluid* images with high signal intensity on T2-weighted images.

Engorged veins in the vascular pterygoid attachments can mimic upper and lower joint compartment fluid and may result in a false-positive diagnosis of effusion (Fig. 9-16).

Postsurgical plication (Fig. 9-17) and *proplast prosthetic replacements* of the TMJ meniscus should have the same anatomic relationships to the condylar

and articular eminences as the native disc, and they are evaluated with the same criteria.[33,34]

Trauma

In complex fractures about the mandible and TMJ, CT is useful in demonstrating osseous fragments and their degree of displacement.[25,35] In selected cases, MR may provide additional information regarding soft tissue injury and the integrity of the articular disc (Fig. 9-18). Internal derangement of the TMJ can occur without fracture as forces are transmitted through the condyle. A direct mandibular blow may stretch the meniscus, causing lat-

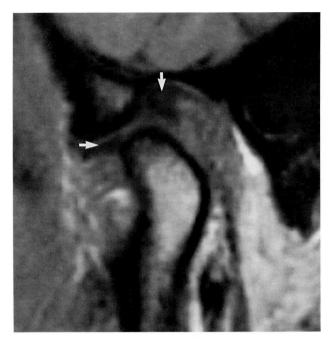

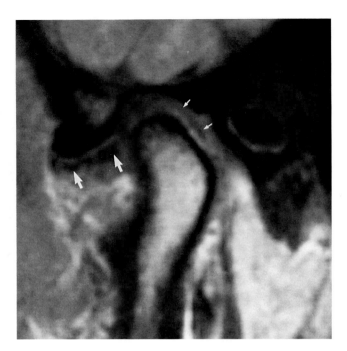

Figure 9-4

Intact TMJ meniscus with central region of intermediate signal intensity in the posterior band *(vertical arrow)*. Anterior band is visualized with uniform dark signal *(horizontal arrow)*. TR = 600 msec, TE = 20 msec.

Figure 9-6

Complete anterior displacement of the TMJ meniscus *(two large arrows)*. Anterior band, intermediate zone, and posterior band are all anterior to the condylar head. Retrodiscal bilaminar zone *(small double arrows)* is indicated. T1-weighted image; TR = 600 msec, TE = 20 msec.

Figure 9-5

Normal meniscus anatomy showing anterior band *(curved arrow)*, intermediate zone *(medium straight arrow)*, posterior band *(large straight arrow)*, and low signal intensity band within the bilaminar zone *(small double arrows)*. T1-weighted image; TR = 600 msec, TE = 20 msec.

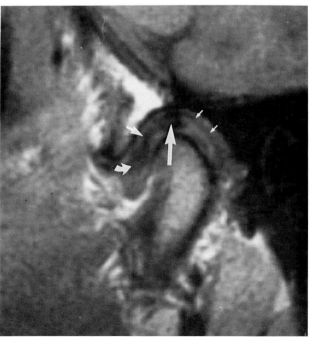

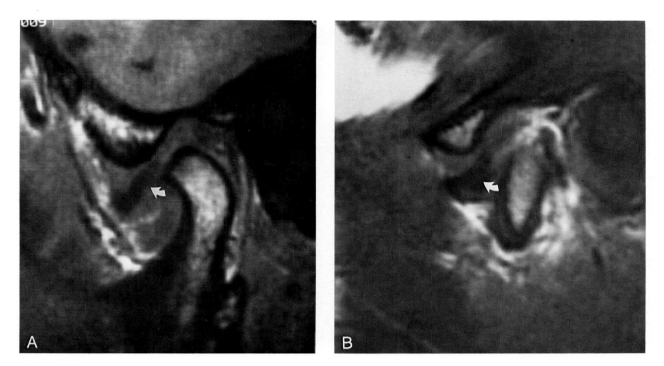

Figure 9-7
Less common anterolateral disc displacement. Meniscus *(curved arrow)* demonstrated anterior *(A)* and medial *(B)* to condylar head.

eral pterygoid spasm and anterior disc displacement. TMJ trauma in children may, in addition result in disruption of the condylar growth center of the jaw.

Arthritis

In the adult, osteoarthritis may occur as a sequela to TMJ trauma and internal disc derangements.[25] The TMJ may be affected in episodes of gout, rheumatoid arthritis, lupus, or the seronegative arthropathies such as psoriatic arthritis[36] and ankylosing spondylitis. In the presence of synovitis and articular destruction, the disc is vulnerable to perforation and displacement. TMJ pain may be present even in the absence of significant appendicular joint involvement.

In osteoarthritis, cortical and articular cartilage thinning, with flattening and deformity of the condylar head, is visualized on MR images. Osteophytes (usually anterior), joint space narrowing, and erosions of both the temporal eminence and condyle are frequently seen in degenerative joint disease (Fig. 9-19). Extensive subchondral or bony sclerosis visualizes on T1- and T2-weighted images as diffuse low signal intensity in the condylar head, neck, and articular eminence (Fig. 9-20). This low signal intensity may also represent the development of avascular necrosis.[34] Joint effusions, articular erosions, and synovial proliferation are all identifiable on T1- and T2-weighted images. On T2-weighted images, hyperplastic synovium and pannus do not generate the high signal intensity seen with associated fluid.

Rarely is the TMJ involved with cartilaginous metaplasia in synovial chondromatosis.[24] MR examination is characterized by small calcifications and associated soft tissue mass.

Neoplasms

Tumors of the TMJ are rare, especially in malignant processes.[25] In primary chondrosarcoma of the TMJ, MR has been found to be superior to CT in delineating tumor extension into the middle cranial fossa, whereas CT is more effective in identifying areas of cortical destruction (Fig. 9-21). On T2-weighted images, chondrosarcoma visualizes with uniform high signal intensity.

Text continues on p. 387

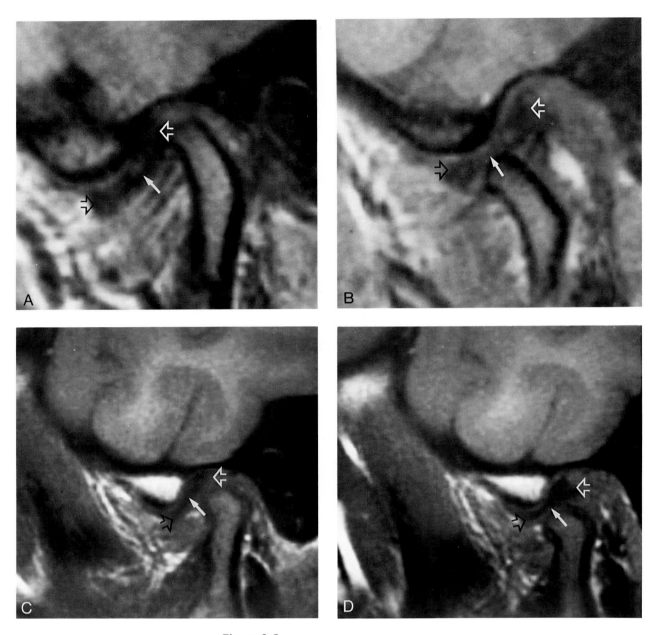

Figure 9-8
Two examples of an anteriorly displaced TMJ meniscus as imaged in the closed mouth position **(A** and
C), with recapture of the disc in the open mouth position **(B** and **D)**. Anterior band *(open black
arrow)*, intermediate zone *(closed arrow)*, and posterior band *(open white arrow)* are displayed. In the
closed mouth position the posterior band is anterior to the condylar head, and in the open mouth
position with reduction, the posterior band is seen directly superior to the condylar head.

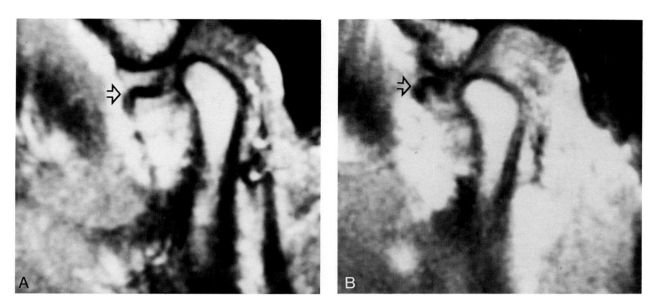

Figure 9-9

Displaced meniscus. Nonreducible anteriorly displaced meniscus *(arrow)* is visualized in both the closed **(A)** and open **(B)** mouth positions. Limited condylar translation and deformity of the meniscus is demonstrated in the open mouth image.

Figure 9-11

Grade 1 displacement with intact morphology and internal signal intensity *(white arrows)*. Condylar head with overlying retrodiscal tissue is identified *(black arrow)*.

Figure 9-10

Grades of TMJ disc displacements include a displaced meniscus with (grade 1) and without (grade 2) internal signal intensity in the posterior band, and displacement with abnormal disc morphology and no internal disc signal intensity (grade 3).

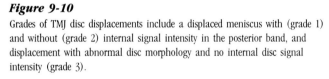

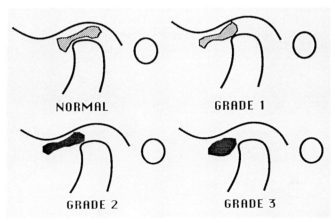

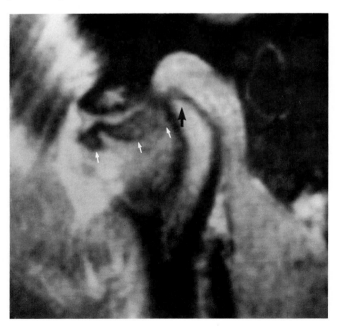

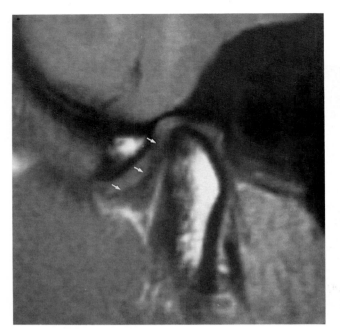

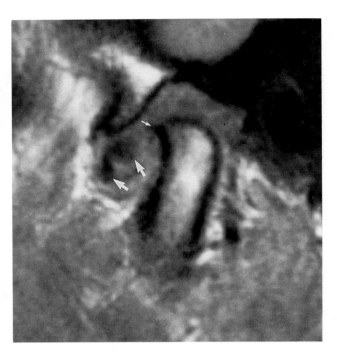

Figure 9-12
Grade 2 displacement with loss of internal disc signal intensity and intact morphology *(arrows)*. T1-weighted image; TR = 600 msec, TE = 20 msec.

Figure 9-13
Grade 3 meniscal derangement with complete loss of normal morphology and internal signal characteristics. The meniscus is identified redundantly compressed anterior to the condylar head *(large arrows)*. Associated degenerative change is identified as low signal intensity anterior osteophyte *(small arrow)*. T1-weighted image; TR = 600 msec, TE = 20 msec.

Figure 9-14
TMJ meniscus imaged in a patient with removal *(A)* and insertion *(B)* of an internal splint. The posterior band *(arrow)* is visualized anterior to the condylar head without internal splint (mildly anteriorly displaced). With insertion of the internal splint it is positioned directly superior to the condylar head.

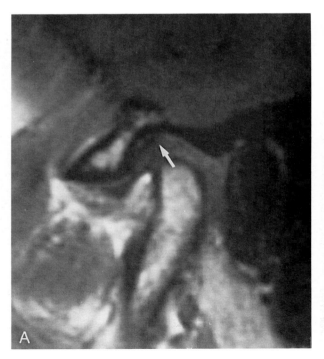

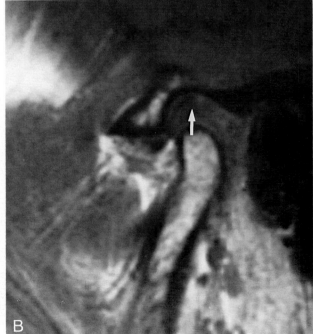

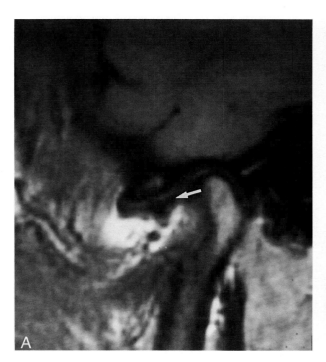
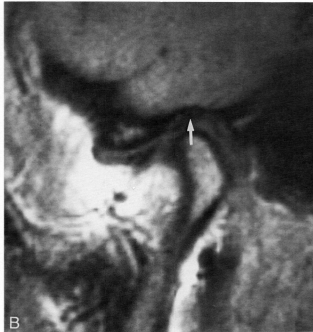

Figure 9-15
TMJ meniscus *(arrow)* before *(A)* and after *(B)* arthroscopic saline reduction.

Figure 9-16
High signal intensity in enlarged veins *(black arrowheads)* in lateral pterygoid attachment *(black arrow)* to the TMJ meniscus. Intact posterior band is visualized superior to the condylar head between the 11 o'clock and 12 o'clock positions *(white arrow)*. T2* gradient echo image; TR = 400 msec, TE = 30 msec; flip angle = 30°.

Figure 9-17
Postsurgical primary plication of the TMJ meniscus in normal position *(small arrows)*. Focus of low signal intensity subchondral sclerosis is visualized *(open arrow)*.

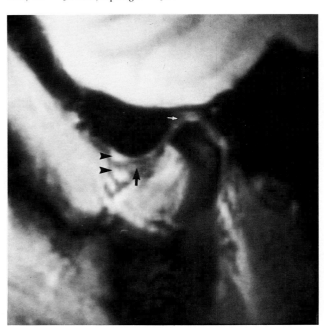
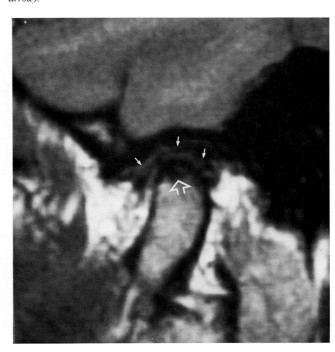

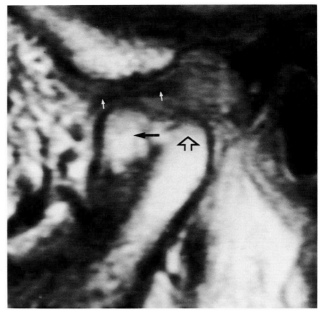

Figure 9-18
Pseudo-double condyle in posttraumatic fracture of the mandibular condyle with displacement of the articular head *(solid black arrow)* anterior to the condylar neck *(open arrow).* Associated TMJ meniscus is identified *(white arrows).*

Figure 9-19
Large anterior osteophyte *(small arrows)* images with low signal intensity (cortical bone signal). Associated anterior meniscal displacement is also demonstrated *(curved arrow).*

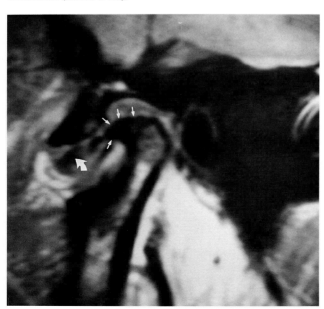

Figure 9-20
Degenerative sclerosis *(open arrows)* images with low signal intensity in mandibular condyle. Anteriorly displaced meniscus *(black arrow)* and articular head deformity *(curved arrow)* are shown.

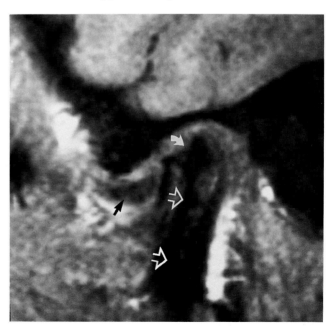

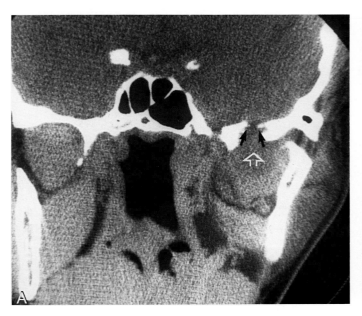
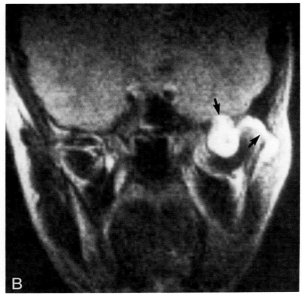

Figure 9-21

Chondrosarcoma of the TMJ. **(A)** Lesion demonstrates vague low attenuation mass *(open arrow)* and cortical destruction *(solid arrows)* extending to the middle cranial fossa on direct coronal CT. **(B)** Corresponding T2-weighted coronal image identifies the exact location and boundaries of the bright signal intensity tumor *(arrows)*.

PERSPECTIVES ON MR IMAGING OF THE TMJ

Whereas accurate clinical and diagnostic evaluation of the TMJ are difficult with conventional imaging modalities, MR affords excellent soft-tissue discrimination and direct imaging of the TMJ disc without the reformations and contrast agents necessary with CT. It is noninvasive and is equally or more accurate than dynamic contrast arthrography in identifying disc position. Besides, the ability to appreciate internal disc morphology is an added advantage that MR examination of the TMJ affords.

Documentation of internal disc derangements is now being required by third-party payers before long-term treatment or surgical intervention is approved. With the timely introduction of fast scan MR techniques, dynamic and functional imaging of the TMJ meniscus may provide valuable information to supplement routine static images in the assessment of joint performance. MR has also demonstrated potential in the evaluation and assessment of arthritic, neoplastic, and traumatic pathology about the TMJ, but further investigation is needed in these areas.

REFERENCES

1. Jacobs JM, Manaster BJ: Digital subtraction arthrography of the temporomandibular joint. AJR, 148:344, 1987

2. Kaplan PA, et al: Inferior joint space arthrography of normal temporomandibular joints: Reassessment of diagnostic criteria. Radiology, 159:585, 1986

3. Kaplan PA, et al: Temporomandibular joint arthrography following surgical treatment of internal derangements. Radiology, 163:217, 1987

4. Kaplan PA, et al: Temporomandibular joint arthrography of normal subjects: Prevalence of pain with ionic versus nonionic contrast agents. Radiology, 156:825, 1985

5. Katzberg RW, et al: Temporomandibular joint arthrography: Comparison of morbidity with ionic and low osmolality contrast media. Radiology, 155:245, 1985

6. Christiansen EL, et al: Correlative thin section temporomandibular joint anatomy and computed tomography. RadioGraphics, 6:703, 1986

7. Christiansen EL, et al: CT number characteristics of malpositioned TMJ menisci: Diagnosis with CT number highlighting (blinkmode). Invest Radiol, 22:315, 1987

8. Larheim TA, Kolbenstvedt A: High resolution computed tomography of the osseous temporomandibular joint. Radiology, 157:573, 1985

9. Swartz JD, et al: High-resolution computed tomography, Part 5: Evaluation of the temporomandibular joint. Radiology, 159:823, 1986

10. Manco LG, et al: Internal derangements of the temporomandibular joint evaluated with direct sagittal CT: Prospective study. Radiology, 157:407, 1985

11. Kneeland JB, et al: High-resolution MR imaging using loop-gap resonators (work in progress). Radiology, 158:247, 1986

12. Middleton WD, et al: High resolution surface coil magnetic resonance imaging of the joints: Anatomic correlation. RadioGraphics, 7:645, 1987

13. Helms CA, et al: Magnetic resonance imaging of internal derangement of the temporomandibular joint. Radiol Clin North Am, 24:189, 1986

14. Harms SE, Wilk RM: Magnetic resonance imaging of the temporomandibular joint. RadioGraphics, 7:521, 1987

15. Katzberg RW, et al: Normal and abnormal temporomandibular joint: MR imaging with surface coil. Radiology, 158:183, 1986

16. Wetesson PL, et al: Temporomandibular joint: Comparison of MR images with cryosectional anatomy. Radiology, 164:59, 1987

17. Roberts D, et al: Temporomandibular joint: Magnetic resonance imaging. Radiology, 154:829, 1985

18. Harms SE, et al: Temporomandibular joint: Magnetic resonance imaging using surface coils. Radiology, 157:133, 1985

19. Laurell KA, et al: Magnetic resonance imaging of the temporomandibular joint, Part I: Literature review. J Prosthet Dent, 58:83, 1987

20. Burnett KR, et al: Dynamic display of the temporomandibular joint meniscus by using "fast-scan" MR imaging. AJR, 149:959, 1987

21. Stoller DW, et al: Fast MR improves imaging of the musculoskeletal system. Diagnostic Imaging, February:98, 1988

22. Manco LG, DeLuke DM: CT diagnosis of synovial chondromatosis of the temporomandibular joint. AJR, 148:574, 1987

23. Kneeland JB, et al: Failed temporomandibular joint prostheses: MR imaging. Radiology, 165:179, 1987

24. Nokes ST, et al: Temporomandibular joint chondromatosis with intracranial extension: MR and CT contributions. AJR, 148:1173, 1987

25. Murphy WA: The temporomandibular joint. In Resnick D, Niwayama, G (eds): Diagnosis of Bone and Joint Disorders, 2nd ed, vol 3, chapter 53. Philadelphia, WB Saunders, 1988

26. Hardy CJ, et al: Simultaneous MR image acquisition with electronically decoupled surface receiver coils. Radiology, 165(P):91, 1987

27. Harms SE, et al: Specialized receiver coils for bilateral MR imaging examinations of the temporomandibular joint. Radiology, 165(P):159, 1987

28. Drace J, Enzmann DR: MR imaging of the temporomandibular joint (TMJ): Closed-, partially open-, and open-mouth views of the abnormal TMJ. Radiology, 165(P):149, 1987

29. Helms CA, et al: Staging of internal derangements of the temporomandibular joint with MR imaging, and optimal mouth position for diagnosis. Radiology, 165(P):149, 1987

30. Katzberg RW, et al: Magnetic resonance imaging of the temporomandibular joint meniscus. Oral Surg Oral Med Oral Pathol, 59:332, 1985

31. Schellhas KP, et al: Temporomandibular joint: Diagnosis of internal derangements using magnetic resonance imaging. Minn Med, 69:516, 1986

32. Cirbus MT, et al: Magnetic resonance imaging in confirming internal derangement of the temporomandibular joint. J Prosthet Dent, 57:488, 1987

33. Kneeland JB, et al: MR imaging of a fractured temporomandibular disk prosthesis. JCAT, 11:199, 1987

34. Schellhas KP, et al: Temporomandibular joint: MR imaging of internal derangements and postoperative changes. AJR, 150:381, 1988

35. Katzberg RW, et al: Dislocation of jaws. Radiology, 154:556, 1985

36. Kononen M: Radiographic changes in the condyle of the temporomandibular joint in psoriatic arthritis. Acta Radiol, 28:185, 1987

Index

Index

NOTE: Page numbers followed by an *(f)* indicate that the item is found on that page in an illustration. Page numbers followed by a *(t)* indicate that the item is found on that page in a table.

ISBN 0-397-50958-8

90000